Teaching the Mindful Self-Compassion Program

Also from Christopher Germer and Kristin Neff

FOR PROFESSIONALS

Mindfulness and Psychotherapy, Second Edition
Edited by Christopher Germer, Ronald D. Siegel,
and Paul R. Fulton

*Wisdom and Compassion in Psychotherapy:
Deepening Mindfulness in Clinical Practice*
Edited by Christopher Germer and Ronald D. Siegel

FOR GENERAL READERS

*The Mindful Path to Self-Compassion: Freeing Yourself
from Destructive Thoughts and Emotions*
Christopher Germer

*The Mindful Self-Compassion Workbook: A Proven Way
to Accept Yourself, Build Inner Strength, and Thrive*
Kristin Neff and Christopher Germer

Teaching the Mindful Self-Compassion Program

A GUIDE FOR PROFESSIONALS

Christopher Germer
Kristin Neff

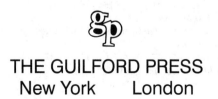

THE GUILFORD PRESS
New York   London

See page 452 for terms of use for audio files.

Printed in the United States of America

This book is printed on acid-free paper.

Last digit is print number: 9 8 7 6 5 4 3 2

The authors have checked with sources believed to be reliable in their efforts to
provide information that is complete and generally in accord with the standards
of practice that are accepted at the time of publication. However, in view of the
possibility of human error or changes in behavioral, mental health, or medical
sciences, neither the authors, nor the editors and publisher, nor any other party
who has been involved in the preparation or publication of this work warrants
that the information contained herein is in every respect accurate or complete,
and they are not responsible for any errors or omissions or the results obtained
from the use of such information. Readers are encouraged to confirm the
information contained in this book with other sources.

Library of Congress Cataloging-in-Publication Data

Names: Germer, Christopher K., author. | Neff, Kristin, author.
Title: Teaching the mindful self-compassion program : a guide for professionals /
    Christopher Germer, Kristin Neff.
Description: New York : Guilford Press, [2019] | Includes bibliographical
    references and index.
Identifiers: LCCN 2018041446 | ISBN 9781462538898 (pbk.) |
    ISBN 9781462539048 (hardcover)
Subjects: LCSH: Self-acceptance. | Compassion. | Mindfulness (Psychology) |
    Meditation—Therapeutic use.
Classification: LCC BF575.S37 G47 2019 | DDC 158.1/3071—dc23
LC record available at *https://lccn.loc.gov/2018041446*

About the Authors

Christopher Germer, PhD, has a private practice in mindfulness- and compassion-based psychotherapy in Arlington, Massachusetts, and is a part-time Lecturer on Psychiatry at Harvard Medical School/Cambridge Health Alliance. He is a founding faculty member of the Institute for Meditation and Psychotherapy and of the Center for Mindfulness and Compassion. Dr. Germer's books include *The Mindful Self-Compassion Workbook* and *The Mindful Path to Self-Compassion* (for the general public) and *Wisdom and Compassion in Psychotherapy* and *Mindfulness and Psychotherapy, Second Edition* (for professionals). He lectures and leads workshops internationally. His website is *www.chrisgermer.com*.

Kristin Neff, PhD, is Associate Professor of Human Development and Culture at the University of Texas at Austin and a pioneer in the field of self-compassion research. Her books include *The Mindful Self-Compassion Workbook* and *Self-Compassion*. She is also author of an audio program, *Self-Compassion: Step by Step,* and has published numerous academic articles. Dr. Neff lectures and offers workshops worldwide. Together with Christopher Germer, she hosts an 8-hour online course, "The Power of Self-Compassion." Her website is *www.self-compassion.org*.

Authors' Note

This book describes the theory, research, pedagogy, and curriculum of the Mindful Self-Compassion (MSC) program. It is designed to help readers understand the principles and practices of MSC and apply them in the context of their professional activities. Before teaching self-compassion to others in any form, however, readers are strongly encouraged to have a personal practice of mindfulness and self-compassion, and to participate as students in an MSC course to understand the subtleties of learning self-compassion. Anyone who wishes to go on to teach the 8-week MSC program described in this book must successfully complete formal MSC teacher training. For more on the teacher training pathway, go to *https://centerformsc.org.*

Preface: The Authors' Journey

The Mindful Self-Compassion (MSC) program has been a work in progress since 2008, when we met at the first scientists' meditation retreat at the Insight Meditation Society in Barre, Massachusetts, co-sponsored by the Mind and Life Institute. Kristin is a developmental psychologist who operationally defined *self-compassion* in the early 2000s (Neff, 2003b); she also developed the Self-Compassion Scale (Neff, 2003a), which is used in most research in the field. Chris is a clinical psychologist who has been integrating mindfulness into psychotherapy since the mid-1980s. On the drive back to the airport from the retreat, I (Chris) suggested to Kristin that she create a program to teach self-compassion. She responded, "What, *me*? I've never taught a workshop in my life. You've been leading workshops and teaching mindfulness for years. *You* should do it." And at that moment it clicked—we would do it together!

I (Kristin) first came across the idea of self-compassion in 1997, during my last year of graduate school in the Human Development program at the University of California, Berkeley. I was struggling to complete my PhD and was experiencing a lot of the stress that usually accompanies the dissertation process. My first marriage had also recently fallen apart, and even though I was in a new relationship, I was still feeling shame and self-doubt. I had been interested in Eastern spirituality from the time I was a small child, having been raised by an open-minded mother just outside Los Angeles, but I had never taken meditation seriously or studied Buddhist philosophy. Nonetheless, I soon found myself starting to read American Buddhist classics such as Sharon Salzberg's (1995) *Lovingkindness* and Jack Kornfield's (1993) *A Path with Heart*, and my life took a new turn, never to be the same again.

Although I knew that Buddhists talked a lot about the importance of compassion, I never considered that having compassion for *oneself* might be as important as having compassion for others. Yet the first night I went to a local meditation group, the woman leading the group spoke about how essential it was to have compassion for oneself *as well as* others—that we need to treat ourselves with the same kindness and understanding as those we deeply care about. My initial reaction was "What? You mean we're *allowed* to be nice to ourselves? Isn't that selfish?" Soon, however, I came to the conclusion that you have to care about yourself in order to really be connected with other people. If you are continually judging and criticizing yourself while trying to be kind to others, you are drawing artificial boundaries and distinctions that only lead to feelings of separation and isolation. This is the opposite of oneness, interconnection, and universal love—the ultimate goals of most spiritual paths, regardless of the traditions from which they stem. So I tried it, and my newfound practice of self-compassion allowed me to cope with my life struggles with greater strength and grace.

After receiving my PhD, I did 2 years of postdoctoral training with a leading self-esteem researcher at the University of Denver, Susan Harter. I wanted to know more about how people develop their self-concept and sense of self-worth. I soon learned that the field of psychology was falling out of love with self-esteem as the ultimate marker of positive mental health. Although thousands of articles had been written on the importance of self-esteem, researchers were starting to point out all the traps that people can fall into when they try to get and keep a high level of self-esteem: narcissism, constant comparisons with others, ego-defensive anger, prejudice, and so on. I realized that self-compassion was the perfect alternative to the relentless pursuit of self-esteem. Why? Because self-compassion offered the same protection against self-hatred as self-esteem, but without the need to see oneself as perfect or as better than others.

In 1999 I received an Assistant Professorship in the Educational Psychology Department at the University of Texas at Austin, and soon made the decision to conduct research on self-compassion. At that point, no one had published an academic article defining self-compassion, let alone done any research on it. So I decided to enter uncharted territory and began what has now become my life's work.

The power of self-compassion didn't fully dawn on me, however, until some years later. My son, Rowan, was diagnosed with autism in 2007, and I believe that the practice of self-compassion is what kept me sane during Rowan's early years. Because of the intense sensory issues experienced by autistic children, they are prone to violent tantrums. The only thing a parent of such a child can do at such times is try to keep the child safe and wait until the storm passes. When my son screamed and flailed away in the grocery store for no discernible reason, and strangers inevitably gave me reproachful looks, there was nothing left for me to do but practice self-compassion. In the midst of my confusion, shame, and helplessness, all I could do was soothe and comfort myself, giving myself the emotional support I so desperately needed. Self-compassion gradually helped me get through self-pity and anger; it also allowed me to remain reasonably calm and loving toward Rowan, despite the intense stress and despair that would inevitably arise. Of course, I would still become frustrated or overwhelmed at times, but I noticed that whenever I became agitated with Rowan, he would inevitably become more agitated himself. On the other hand, whenever I had the presence of mind to give myself compassion for what I was going through, he would calm down. Furthermore, when I was kind toward myself, I discovered that I had more emotional resources to be patient and compassionate toward Rowan. I quickly learned that practicing self-compassion was one of the most effective ways I could help my son, as well as myself, in times of stress or struggle.

It is not uncommon in the field of psychology that new knowledge emerges when psychologists find solutions to their own personal problems. This is also how Chris became involved in self-compassion.

I (Chris) had been practicing meditation since the late 1970s, when I took a year to travel the length and breadth of India, visiting saints, sages, indigenous healers, and meditation masters. I also learned mindfulness meditation at a hermitage in Sri Lanka. Afterward, I went to graduate school, received a PhD in clinical psychology, and joined a study group on mindfulness and psychotherapy in Cambridge, Massachusetts. This study group morphed into the Institute for Meditation and Psychotherapy, and we eventually wrote a popular professional text, *Mindfulness and Psychotherapy* (now in its second edition; Germer, Siegel, & Fulton, 2013), which began to articulate this new model of therapy.

The initial publication of the book, together with the public's burgeoning interest in mindfulness and psychotherapy, meant that I would be asked to do more public speaking—a long-standing source of fear and panic. Despite maintaining a regular practice of meditation and periodically being in therapy during my adult life, I continued to be dogged by debilitating public speaking anxiety. In the run-up to just about any speech, my heart started pounding, my hands began to sweat, and I found it harder and harder to think clearly. I tried everything I could think of to counter this anxiety—exposure, meditation, mindfulness- and acceptance-based strategies, diaphragmatic breathing, strenuous exercise, beta blockers, you name it—but nothing worked. Once, while I was trying to make some opening comments at a lecture in Santa Fe, my anxiety got so bad that a well-meaning audience member called out from the back of the lecture hall, "Take a breath!" I was supposed to be talking about the benefits of mindfulness and could hardly get a word out.

Not long afterward, I was scheduled to speak at a Harvard Medical School conference. I'd been safely tucked in the shadows as a clinical instructor on the faculty of the medical school for many years, but this gathering meant that I'd have to stand up in front of a crowd of colleagues and expose my shameful secret yet again. With 4 months to go before the conference, I went on a silent meditation retreat where there was no escape from my fears. Whenever my mind wandered to the upcoming conference, I could feel my body surge with anxiety at the prospect of making a fool of myself. No amount of trying to hold the fear in spacious awareness— mindfulness—alleviated the distress.

Eventually, I had an interview with a very experienced meditation teacher who was among those running the retreat. I sheepishly reported my failure to meditate, but was still too ashamed to fully disclose the content of my distress. She flashed a sweet, knowing smile and then offered a suggestion so simple that it was almost mortifying for me to think I'd not yet done it on my own. I don't remember the exact words, but they were something like these: "Just love yourself. Just repeat loving-kindness phrases like 'May I be safe. May I be happy. May I be healthy. May I live with ease.' " That was it.

Willing to try anything at that point, I returned to my cushion in the meditation hall and immediately began repeating the phrases. In spite of all the years I'd been meditating and reflecting on my inner life as a psychologist, I'd never spoken to myself in that tender, comforting way. Right off the bat, I started to feel soothed. I even wondered if maybe I was cheating— aren't retreats supposed to be *hard*?—until I realized that something had loosened up inside and I could feel my breath again. During the breaks in the retreat, the world became alive in a new way. I could actually see the people around me and savor the beautiful surroundings of the retreat center. It was as if someone had opened the door to a different way of being.

When I got home, I adopted loving-kindness as my primary meditation practice. Whenever anxiety arose about the upcoming conference, I just said the loving-kindness phrases to myself, day after day, week after week. I didn't do this particularly to calm down, but simply because I needed some comfort. (I had learned long ago that *trying* to calm down only made me more anxious.) Eventually, however, the day of the conference arrived. When I was called to the podium to speak, the usual fear rose up in the usual way. But this time there was something new—a little faint background whisper saying, "May you be safe. May you be happy. . . ." And when I looked out over the crowd, I thought, "Oh, may *everyone* be safe. May *everyone* be happy. . . ." In that moment, for the first time, excitement and joy rose up and took the place of fear.

What happened in that seminal moment? Perhaps the reason why I couldn't accept my anxiety and let it flow through me earlier was that something deeper was the real issue. Perhaps my public speaking anxiety wasn't an *anxiety* disorder after all, but a *shame* disorder—and shame was just too overwhelming to bear. Whenever I imagined myself at the podium, trembling and unable to speak, I was fundamentally unwilling to accept the experience of anxiety because of the intolerable possibility of being perceived as incompetent or fraudulent by my esteemed colleagues: "Of course I'm a fraud if I'm talking about mindfulness but I'm too frightened to speak!" But as I continued to practice loving-kindness meditation, it felt as if a good friend was available to support me even in these dark moments, and would *continue* to support me even if everyone in the audience thought I was a fool. I had begun learning *self-compassion.*

I realized that sometimes all of us need to hold *ourselves* in loving awareness before we can hold our *experience* with the same attitude. That's where compassion comes into mindfulness practice. When we're in the midst of intense and disturbing emotions, we need extra support to be able to see clearly and take positive action in our lives. As a therapist, moreover, I intuitively knew the importance of compassion. When a new client arrives, we therapists instinctively offer compassion as a foundation for exploring the person's life, especially the shameful parts. However, it's entirely another matter to offer kindness to *ourselves* when we need it the most. Somehow this insight and capacity elude even highly introspective people like mindfulness meditation practitioners and mental health professionals.

After my epiphany, I began exploring the potential of self-compassion training for my clients, especially those suffering from disorders with a shame component ("I'm defective," "I'm bad"), such as social anxiety, complex trauma, addiction, and depression. I wrote *The Mindful Path to Self-Compassion* (Germer, 2009) in an effort to share what I had learned, especially in terms of how self-compassion helped the clients I saw in psychotherapy. Soon afterward, Kristin published *Self-Compassion* (Neff, 2011b), which reviewed the theory and research on self-compassion, provided many techniques for enhancing self-compassion, and described the impact of self-compassion in her personal life.

We held our first MSC program in 2010 in the Fritz Perls house at the Esalen Institute in Big Sur, California. We remember with amusement that 12 people attended our launch program, and 3 participants dropped out by the second day. Perhaps our participants could sense our uncertainty, or maybe we had made it too emotionally challenging? But we persisted. After a rough start, we have devoted a tremendous amount of time and energy to developing the 8-week MSC curriculum and making it safe, enjoyable, and effective for a wide range of people in different cultures. We conducted a randomized controlled trial of MSC in 2012 (Germer & Neff, 2013; Neff & Germer, 2013); we founded a nonprofit organization called the Center for Mindful Self-Compassion the same year, to meet the demand for disseminating the protocol; and in 2014 we initiated an MSC teacher training program under the expert guidance of Steve Hickman and Michelle Becker at the Center for Mindfulness, University of California, San Diego.

Currently, over 50,000 people have taken the MSC program, taught by over 1,000 teachers around the world. Since MSC teachers receive online consultation while teaching their first MSC class, we have been able to refine the MSC curriculum further, based on their feedback. The book you hold in your hands can best be described as a project of the entire MSC teaching community, and we hope that it will remain a living document, evolving as we continue to practice and learn together.

Who Is This Book For?

We have written this book on MSC for professionals who are interested in practicing and teaching self-compassion for psychological well-being. Most readers will probably want to bring self-compassion into their *ongoing* work activities, such as psychotherapy, coaching, medicine, business, and education. Others are already trained MSC teachers, or want to become MSC teachers, and wish to explore the theoretical, empirical, and pedagogical underpinnings of MSC more fully. Some readers will primarily have a scholarly interest in self-compassion (e.g., professors, researchers), and still others are interested in self-compassion only for personal reasons. This book has been written to support all these efforts.

If your goal is to teach the 8-week MSC program itself, please understand that you still have to complete the formal MSC teacher training before you teach. For information on how to become an MSC teacher, see the information under the "Teach" tab at *https://centerformsc.org*. Formal teacher training is necessary because *how* MSC is taught matters as much as *what* is taught, and the information in this book about the pedagogy of MSC needs to be augmented by working with qualified teacher trainers within a teaching community. Personal practice is also necessary to transmit the essence of mindfulness and self-compassion to others. Therefore, we hope that this book will deepen your understanding of self-compassion; inspire you to practice self-compassion for yourself; and, if it feels right, connect with other professionals who are interested in self-compassion and share the gift with others.

Acknowledgments

So many talented people have been part of the development of MSC that they could never be properly acknowledged. This book is the fruit of a rapidly expanding community of mindfulness and self-compassion practitioners, teachers, clinicians, and researchers who are committed to bringing more compassion into the world, starting with compassion for ourselves.

First, we would like to express appreciation to our teachers who have kept the light of compassion burning brightly for a long time, including the Dalai Lama, Thich Nhat Hanh, Jon Kabat-Zinn, Sharon Salzberg, Jack Kornfield, Tara Brach, Pema Chödrön, and Thupten Jinpa. We are also grateful to the poets who manage to find just the right words for what we're trying to say and do—Rumi, Hafez, Mary Oliver, Naomi Nye, David Whyte, John O'Donohue, Miller Williams, and Mark Nepo, to name a few.

The efforts of our community depend largely on brilliant researchers in the field of compassion and mindfulness who continually inspire the secular contemplative community, such as Richie Davidson, Tania Singer, Paul Gilbert, Shauna Shapiro, Barbara Fredrickson, Mark Leary, Juliana Breines, Emma Seppälä, Zindel Segal, Jud Brewer, Mark Williams, Sara Lazar, and Rebecca Crane; on outstanding teachers of contemplative science, such as Rick Hanson, Dan Siegel, Dan Goleman, and Kelly McGonigal; and on groundbreaking psychotherapists, such as Steve Hayes, Marsha Linehan, Mark Epstein, Dick Schwartz, and Ron Siegel.

Loyal friends and colleagues were with us from the start, providing encouragement and support as we struggled to discover the best way to teach self-compassion. Our earliest 8-week MSC courses were taught with Susan Pollak in Massachusetts and Pittman McGehee in Texas. Two years later, in 2012, we discovered Michelle Becker, who became the first person to teach MSC on her own (at the Center for Mindfulness, University of California, San Diego). Her colleague Steve Hickman was inspired by Michelle's passion for the subject, and Steve eventually became the Executive Director and Director of Professional Training of the Center for Mindful Self-Compassion. Christine Brähler joined the team from Germany and has been instrumental in cultivating our global vision. Michelle, Steve, and Christine have also contributed significantly to the MSC curriculum, as well as to the content and style of this book. Another key figure from those early days is Kristy Arbon, who anticipated the demand for self-compassion training and helped us create an organization to meet the demand. Jim Douglass continues to monitor our progress and keep us growing in a sustainable manner.

The MSC program is always evolving through interactions with and among our talented teacher trainers, including Hilde Steinhauser and Arve Thurman in Germany; Regula Saner in Switzerland; Mila de Koning and Rob Brandsma in the Netherlands; Hailan Guo and Joy Huang in China; Soegwang Snim in Korea; Judith Soulsby, Vanessa Hope, and Ali Lambie in the United Kingdom; Marta Alonso Maynar and Luis de la Fuenta in Spain; Tina Gibson in Australia; Dawn MacDonald and Micheline St. Hilaire in Canada; and Beth Mulligan in the United States. Additionally, many MSC teachers such as Martin Thomson-Jones, Bal de Buitlear, Sydney Spears, and Liz Fitzgerald have taken special effort to help us improve the curriculum. The most enriching experience of all—as MSC teachers know so well—is being touched by the authenticity of our MSC students, who teach us more about the program and ourselves than we could possibly have imagined.

Closer to home, Kristin would like to thank two of her graduate students in educational psychology at the University of Texas at Austin, Marissa Knox and Phoebe Long, as well as the Rev. Krista Gregory at Dell Children's Hospital (all three are MSC teachers), for helping to explore how MSC may be adapted for health care and educational contexts. She would also like to thank her many research collaborators for providing a wealth of empirical evidence for the benefits of self-compassion. Chris is especially grateful to his friends at the Institute for Meditation and Psychotherapy, Cambridge, Massachusetts, for over 30 years of support, and more recently to Zev Schumann-Olivier and colleagues at the Center for Mindfulness and Compassion, Cambridge Health Alliance.

Which brings us to writing this book. Special appreciation goes to our clear-headed and patient Senior Editor at The Guilford Press, Jim Nageotte, for taking a chance with this project and for enduring umpteen missed deadlines as we gradually learned how to teach self-compassion and describe the process for others. We are also grateful to our developmental editor, Barbara Watkins, who has unrivaled knowledge about books like this and helped us fashion the content into a readable form; to our remarkable and forgiving copyeditor, Marie Sprayberry; and to our production editor, Laura Specht Patchkofsky.

Finally, we will be forever indebted to our nearest and dearest—in particular, to Kristin's son, Rowan, and Chris's wife, Claire—for their love and understanding over the past 5 years. May all beings benefit from their generous natures.

Contents

Purchasers of this book can download audio files
of the meditations at *www.guilford.com/germer4-materials*
for personal use or use with clients (see page 452 for details).

PART I

Self-Compassion

THEORY, RESEARCH, AND TRAINING

I learned a long time ago the wisest thing I can do
is be on my own side.
—MAYA ANGELOU (quoted in Anderson, 2012)

Most people assume that they have some understanding of self-compassion. After all, compassion for others is a central tenet of most world religions, enshrined in the Golden Rule: "Do unto others as you would have them do unto you" (based on Matthew 7:12; see also Armstrong, 2010). Self-compassion simply implies the reverse—learning to treat *ourselves* as we might naturally treat others when they suffer, fail, or feel inadequate. This is easier said than done, however. What happens when we close our eyes, pay careful attention, and give ourselves kindness and compassion? Ordinarily we awaken to the *un*lovely parts of ourselves, and also to old wounds that have been hiding in the recesses of our hearts and minds. It requires special training to bring light to those dark places and to linger there long enough to transform what we find.

The next four chapters constitute an effort to put self-compassion training into context. It's good to have a map before we walk the territory. In Chapter 1, readers will learn how mindfulness and self-compassion relate to one another, including some practical differences between the Mindful Self-Compassion (MSC) program and other empirically supported mindfulness-based training programs.

Chapter 2 defines the construct of self-compassion, compares self-compassion and compassion for others, deepens the discussion of the relationship of mindfulness and self-compassion, addresses the yin and yang of self-compassion, and points out differences between self-esteem and self-compassion. Chapter 2 also identifies common misgivings about self-compassion. Chapter 3 offers a broad review of the research literature on self-compassion, which suggests that most misgivings about self-compassion are unfounded. Discussion of the research is grouped into categories such as emotional well-being, health, coping, body image, relationships, caregiving, clinical populations, neurophysiology, and more. Finally, Chapter 4 focuses on the science of *training* self-compassion; it describes research on the MSC program as well as other compassion training programs, supporting the benefits of compassion-based interventions.

We, the co-developers of the MSC program, are both self-compassion practitioners and social scientists. We believe that the benefits of being more self-compassionate are as old as human nature, and that learning self-compassion does not require a particular set of beliefs. Our understanding is built on personal experience and supported by scientific research. The special benefit of understanding the strong research base for self-compassion is the confidence and inspiration it may bring to personal practice. The research offers clues to understanding for what and for whom self-compassion works best; provides insights into the mechanisms of action underlying self-compassion; and points toward new training initiatives. Ultimately, however, it is the *experience* of self-compassion—the direct perception of what happens when we treat ourselves in a warm and supportive manner—that allows us to walk the path with confidence and ease.

Chapter 1

An Introduction
to Mindful Self-Compassion

May there be kindness in your gaze when you look within.
—JOHN O'DONOHUE (2008, p. 44)

Life is difficult for all of us. If we carefully examine our moment-to-moment experience, we discover that we're under some degree of stress from the instant we wake up ("Uh-oh, I'm late!") until the time we fall asleep ("I really should have . . ."). Usually we don't know it. Right now, for example, is there any discomfort in your body? Are you worrying about something? Are you hungry? And shouldn't you really be clearing out your email inbox rather than starting to read a new book? Ironically, recognizing and embracing our challenges, large and small, can substantially enrich our lives. That's mindfulness. And embracing *ourselves* in the midst of our difficulties with care and concern can enrich our lives even more. That's self-compassion. Together, they constitute the resource of *mindful self-compassion*.

Mindfulness and Compassion

The past two decades have seen an explosion of research into the benefits of *mindfulness,* roughly defined as "the awareness that emerges through paying attention, on purpose, in the present moment, and non-judgmentally to the unfolding of experience moment by moment" (Kabat-Zinn, 2003, p. 145). Mindfulness promotes mental and physical well-being in myriad ways, and thus provides a foundation for living our lives wisely and compassionately. The opposite of mindfulness is being on autopilot, daydreaming about past and future events, hardly aware of what's happening in us or around us. A wandering mind, though hardwired in our brains, can lead us

3

into dark corners of regret and worry from which it may take days, weeks, or even longer to break free.

Our modern definitions of mindfulness tend to emphasize attention and awareness over the *qualities* of mindful awareness, such as acceptance, loving-kindness, and compassion. This is unfortunate, and our language surely contributes to this lopsided view of mindfulness. For example, the word *mindfulness* is a translation of the ancient Pali word *sati*, which refers to awareness, and it is associated with the Pali word *citta*, which literally means "heart–mind." We do not have a word for mind or awareness in the English language that captures both the mental and emotional aspects of mindful awareness.

To complicate matters further, when someone says, "I practice mindfulness meditation," they are probably referring to one or more of the following three types of meditation: (1) focused attention, (2) open monitoring, or (3) loving-kindness and compassion (Salzberg, 2011b). *Focused attention* (or concentration) is the practice of returning attention again and again to one object, such as the breath. Concentration helps calm the mind. *Open monitoring* (or *choiceless awareness*) is paying attention to what is most salient and alive in our field of awareness, one moment after the next. Open monitoring helps the practitioner to develop spacious awareness and understand the nature of the mind. *Loving-kindness and compassion* meditation cultivates the qualities of warmth and goodwill toward oneself and others, which are essential for tolerating and transforming difficult states of mind.

Most of the research on mindfulness has been aimed at the practices of focused attention and open monitoring. However, research on loving-kindness and compassion meditation has increased in recent years (Hofmann, Grossman, & Hinton, 2011). Neurological evidence suggests that all three types of meditation produce overlapping, yet distinct, brain patterns (Brewer et al., 2011; Desbordes et al., 2012; Lee et al., 2012; Leung et al., 2013; Lutz, Slagter, Dunne, & Davidson, 2008). For the purposes of this book, a simple way of describing mindful awareness that does not leave out the heart qualities is *loving awareness* or *compassionate awareness*.

When mindfulness is in full bloom—when we feel calm and alert amidst the full range of our thoughts, feelings, and sensations—our awareness is permeated with an attitude of loving-kindness and compassion. Full mindfulness feels like love itself. Unfortunately, our mindfulness is rarely complete, commingled as it is with anxiety, longing, or confusion. This is particularly the case when things become difficult in our lives—when we suffer, fail, or feel inadequate. Not only does our awareness become tinged by our moods, but our sense of self is often taken hostage, and we become engulfed in self-criticism and self-doubt. We can go from "I *feel* bad" to "I don't *like* this feeling" to "I don't *want* this feeling" to "I *shouldn't* have this feeling" to "Something is *wrong* with me" to "I'm *bad*!" In the blink of an eye, we move from "I *feel* bad" to "I *am* bad." That's when self-compassion comes in. Sometimes we need to comfort and soothe ourselves—the *experiencer*—before we can relate to our *experience* in a more mindful way.

Self-compassion may be considered the heart of mindfulness when we meet personal suffering. Mindfulness invites us to open to suffering with spacious awareness. Self-compassion adds, "Be kind to yourself in the midst of suffering." Mindfulness asks, "What am I *experiencing*?" and self-compassion adds, "What do I *need*?" Together, mindfulness and self-compassion constitute a state of warmhearted, accepting presence during difficult moments in our lives. They are like best friends.

Research shows that self-compassion is positively associated with psychological well-being, including less psychopathology (such as anxiety, depression, and stress) and more positive states of mind (such as happiness, optimism, and life satisfaction) (Barnard & Curry, 2011; MacBeth & Gumley, 2012; Neff, Long, et al., 2018; Zessin, Dickhauser, & Garbade, 2015). Self-compassion is also associated with increased motivation, healthy behaviors and immune functioning, positive body image, and resilient coping (Allen & Leary, 2010; Braun, Park, & Gorin, 2016; Breines & Chen, 2012; Friis, Johnson, Cutfield, & Consedine, 2016; Terry & Leary, 2011), as well as more caring and compassionate relationship behavior (Neff & Beretvas, 2013; Yarnell & Neff, 2012). In other words, self-compassion has many benefits and is worth cultivating (see Chapter 3).

Mindful Self-Compassion

The Mindful Self-Compassion (MSC) program was the first training program created for the general public that was specifically designed to enhance a person's self-compassion. Mindfulness-based training programs such as mindfulness-based stress reduction (MBSR; Kabat-Zinn, 1990) and mindfulness-based cognitive therapy (MBCT; Segal, Williams, & Teasdale, 2013) also increase self-compassion (see Chapter 4), but they do so implicitly, as a welcome byproduct. We wondered, "What would happen if self-compassion skills were *explicitly* taught as the primary focus of the training?"

MSC is loosely modeled on the MBSR program, especially in its focus on experiential learning and inquiry-based teaching, as well as in its structure (eight weekly sessions of 2+ hours each, plus a retreat). Some key practices in MBSR have been adapted for MSC by highlighting the *quality* of awareness—warmth, kindness—in those practices. Most MSC practices have been specifically designed to cultivate compassion and self-compassion.

MSC can be accurately described as *mindfulness-based self-compassion training*. It is a hybrid of mindfulness and compassion, with an emphasis on self-compassion. Mindfulness is the foundation of self-compassion since we need to be mindfully aware that we're suffering *while* we're suffering (no small feat!) in order to have a compassionate response. Although mindfulness is already part of self-compassion, we named this program Mindful Self-Compassion to highlight the key role of mindfulness in self-compassion training. For more on the integration of mindfulness into MSC, see Chapter 11 (Session 2).

MSC was designed for the general public. It is therapeutic, but it isn't psychotherapy. The focus of MSC is on building the *resources* of mindfulness and self-compassion. In contrast, therapy tends to focus on healing old wounds. Since MSC is a structured classroom training program that takes place over a limited period, we do not have the capacity to focus on the details of each person's life as we might in individual or group therapy. Nonetheless, many MSC participants report that MSC has a profound impact on their psychological well-being, especially by healing old wounds. The therapeutic aspect of MSC may be considered a byproduct of developing the resources of mindfulness and self-compassion. (See Part IV for more on the relationship of self-compassion to psychotherapy.)

The MSC Curriculum

The complete MSC curriculum is presented in Part III of this book. MSC is designed to move participants from a conceptual understanding of mindfulness and self-compassion to a felt sense of those concepts, and to provide tools for evoking mindfulness and self-compassion in daily life and making this evocation a habit. The sessions have been carefully sequenced to build upon one another. Each session includes brief didactic topics, followed by exercises that give participants a visceral sense of the subject, and then by inquiry-based exploration of the participants' direct experience.

The needs of MSC participants tend to vary greatly. Participants are encouraged to be experimental in choosing and adapting the practices to their own needs, and to become their own best teachers. MSC teachers strive to create a safe atmosphere wherein each individual's experience of the practices is honored and appreciated.

Teachers are strongly encouraged to find their own teaching voices—to make the program their own. However, the message is "Find your own voice, not your own curriculum." This is especially important in the initial stages of teaching MSC because the structural integrity of the program only reveals itself after it has been taught a few times. There is some flexibility in the curriculum for minor adjustments, such as what to emphasize when presenting concepts to various participants, but teachers should not create new core practices or adjust the content of the program by more than 15% if they still want to call it MSC. And, again, no one should attempt to teach MSC without formal teacher training.

Teaching MSC

The most powerful teaching tool of an MSC teacher is embodiment of mindful compassion. As the saying goes, "People will want what you know if they know that you care." If you take a moment to reflect upon the teachers who've had the greatest impact in your life, they're likely to be the ones who had compassion for the challenges you faced during the learning process and knew how to help you through them. Therefore, the most effective way to *teach* self-compassion is to *be* compassionate.

MSC teachers are expected to maintain a personal practice of mindfulness and self-compassion of about 30 minutes per day, especially while teaching a course (and particularly the practices taught each week). Personal practice keeps the challenge of learning mindfulness and self-compassion fresh in a teacher's mind. It also gives a teacher's words authenticity and power. Teaching MSC is a heart-to-heart transmission, imparted through emotional resonance between teachers and students. Students in the presence of a teacher who embodies mindfulness and self-compassion will experience a host of qualities—respect, humility, self-awareness, tenderness—that will support the students' personal practice.

MSC includes a particular style of interacting with students known as *inquiry,* which will be familiar to readers who have already been trained to teach mindfulness. Inquiry is a *self-to-other* interaction that mirrors for the student a mindful or compassionate *self-to-self* relationship. Inquiry usually follows a practice or class exercise and begins with the questions "What did you notice?" and "What did you feel?" Teachers help to illuminate students' direct experience through gentle, nonjudgmental questioning. When an experience is difficult to bear, a student is guided to discover how mindfulness and compassion could be brought to that particular experience. For example, the teacher may ask, "Can you bring some kindness to that experience?", "What do you think you *need* right now?", or "What might you say to a friend who felt just as you do?" MSC has its own flavor of inquiry, which is key to teaching the program, so half of the practice sessions in the MSC teacher training program are dedicated to practicing the art of inquiry. Examples of inquiry follow almost every meditation, informal practice, and exercise described in Part III of this book.

Other MSC teaching modalities are delivering didactic topics, guiding meditations, leading class exercises, and reading poems. All these aspects of teaching have one common denominator—*teaching from within.* For example, didactic topics should be delivered in a teacher's own, authentic voice, and teachers should listen to and follow their own instructions while guiding meditations. Teachers can more readily adjust the tone of class exercises when they feel their own words come from within. Poems also have power to transmit subtle states of mind when teachers allow the words to resonate in their own being.

MSC and Mindfulness Training

MSC is designed to cultivate mindfulness *and* self-compassion because we cannot be genuinely compassionate without mindfulness, and, conversely, we need compassion to be fully mindful. Mindfulness has four main roles in MSC: (1) to help students recognize when they are suffering; (2) to anchor awareness in the present moment when students are emotionally activated; (3) to cultivate awareness of emotions in the body to regulate emotion; and (4) to develop equanimity, which makes space for compassionate action. The question may arise: "How is MSC similar or different from established mindfulness training programs?"

The most widely disseminated mindfulness training today is MBSR, originally developed by Jon Kabat-Zinn (1990) to bring relief to patients in a university hospital who were suffering from chronic pain and other difficult-to-treat conditions. Three core practices in MBSR are breath meditation, the body scan, and mindful movement. MBSR instructors teach loving-kindness and compassion implicitly, by embodying those qualities in how they interact with their students and by encouraging a friendly attitude toward all experience. Loving-kindness meditation is also taught during the daylong retreat, but the primary purpose of MBSR is to develop equanimity in the midst of stressful life events through nonjudgmental, moment-to-moment awareness.

MBCT is a cognitive-behavioral therapy adaptation of MBSR for the treatment of recurrent depression, developed by Zindel Segal and colleagues (2013). Both MBSR and MBCT have been shown to enhance self-compassion in practitioners (see Chapter 4). Loving-kindness meditation is not included in the MBCT protocol, due to concern about emotionally activating this vulnerable population; MBCT focuses more on cultivating decentered, mindful awareness of depressive thinking.

Three core practices found in MBSR and MBCT have been adapted for the MSC program, with explicit emphasis on warmth and kindness. For example, the Affectionate Breathing meditation in MSC is a type of breath meditation, but invites participants to savor the gentle rhythm of the breath, especially the experience of being internally rocked and caressed by the breath. This meditation is less about building concentration than about feeling held and nourished by the breath, which inevitably strengthens concentration. The Compassionate Body Scan in MSC is similar to the MBSR body scan, but focuses on appreciating how hard each part of the body works for us, wishing each part well, and allowing the heart to soften with compassion when emotional or physical discomfort arises. MSC also has a movement practice—Compassionate Movement—in which awareness is brought to stress points in the body, and participants are encouraged to allow their bodies to move in a spontaneous manner to alleviate the stress.

While the practice of loving-kindness meditation in MBSR typically only occurs during the retreat day, it has been elevated to a core meditation in MSC. (MSC has an additional practice that helps participants discover their own loving-kindness and self-compassion phrases.) Conversely, whereas the body scan is a core meditation in MBSR, it is typically only taught during the retreat day in MSC. These differences between MBSR and MSC reflect the relative emphases of the two programs: spacious, present-moment awareness in MBSR, and warmth and goodwill toward oneself in MSC. MBSR and MSC teach skills that complement one another.

From our experience, seasoned MBSR and MBCT teachers can learn to teach MSC quite easily when they understand the principles and practices of MSC. Valuable skills that MBSR and MBCT teachers have usually acquired are an established personal meditation practice; sensing the difference between "fixing" and "being with" distress; understanding the centrality of kindness in both teaching and practice; and knowing how to engage a group in a spacious, nonjudgmental manner.

We have found that our best compassion teachers are often steeped in mindfulness, just as some of the finest mindfulness teachers are full of compassion. *Self*-compassion training brings a new lens to mindfulness training, however. When a practitioner is struggling, a mindfulness teacher might ask, "Can you make some room for that experience?" or "Can you hold that experience in tender awareness?" A self-compassion teacher might add, "Can you bring some kindness to *yourself* in this moment?" or "What do you think you *need* right now?" Mindfulness focuses on moment-to-moment experience, whereas compassion focuses on the suffering person, or "self."

Mindfulness teachers may have questions or concerns about MSC that reflect differences between these two approaches. Some of these questions are now discussed.

Isn't warming up awareness with loving-kindness and compassion a subtle way of resisting moment-to-moment experience? This is indeed an inherent danger in self-compassion practice. Beginning students try to throw compassion at suffering to make it go away, introducing a subtle element of striving and resistance to present-moment experience. Over time, however, students discover that self-compassion involves allowing the heart to melt in the heat of suffering by abandoning striving and resistance. While warming up awareness may be more intentional with self-compassion, it isn't more effortful. Mindfulness and self-compassion are both skills that enable practitioners to release their instinctive resistance to discomfort.

Why do we need compassion training at all? Aren't compassion and self-compassion already in mindfulness training? When mindfulness is fully present, it is suffused with kindness and compassion. However, it is very difficult to meet intense and disturbing emotions, such as shame, and remain fully mindful. When we experience shame, for example, our field of awareness tends to narrow in fear, and our attention turns away in disgust. Shame also makes us dissociate from our bodies and hollows out the observing self. That's when we need to reconstitute the observing self with explicit compassion. When we feel safer within the embrace of compassion, we can be mindful again.

If we comfort ourselves when we suffer, won't we bypass important life lessons such as impermanence, suffering, and selflessness? It's true that self-compassion can be used to sugar-coat difficult experience and hamper learning. Any practice can be misused. That's why we first need to *open* to suffering with mindful awareness before comforting ourselves with compassion. How much suffering we allow into our lives before engaging compassion depends, in part, on what we are trying to achieve as practitioners—wisdom or compassion. A wisdom practitioner may wish to linger longer with suffering in order to discover insights such as the impermanence of suffering, whereas a compassion practitioner may prefer to cultivate a tender, spontaneous heart that moves quickly and spontaneously toward alleviation of suffering.

Self-compassion activates old relational wounds. Isn't it dangerous to do that in an 8-week program? The foundation of self-compassion training is a sense of safety (see Chapter 8). MSC students are advised, and shown throughout the program how, to attend to their emotional safety. This may mean *not* engaging in a practice when a student feels too vulnerable, or practicing self-compassion *behaviorally* by drinking a cup of tea or taking a walk. We are all continually opening or closing to our experience throughout the day, and when students need to close, we encourage them to do that. Pushing ourselves to open when we should be closing may lead to emotional harm and isn't self-compassionate. Therefore, learning to practice formal meditation for extended periods, which can be emotionally overwhelming for some participants, is less important in MSC than knowing when we're suffering (mindfulness) and responding with kindness (self-compassion).

Where to Start?

Many people wonder whether they should start learning mindfulness first, or begin with self-compassion training. This is an important empirical question that should be addressed in coming years. Until then, here are a few preliminary guidelines.

Accurate Information

Prospective participants are usually quite knowledgeable about their own needs, and when they receive accurate information, they can usually decide for themselves which training is best for them. An orientation session can help to facilitate this process.

Self-Criticism

Mindfulness practitioners who are self-critical may find it difficult to practice mindfulness consistently until they engage their inner critics. Therefore, self-critical people might benefit from starting with self-compassion practice before taking mindfulness training. Conversely, people who are low in self-criticism may have less need for self-compassion and may benefit more from getting a solid grounding in mindfulness before adding self-compassion to the mix.

Commitment

Inevitably, the best practice for each person is the one they are most committed to. Therefore, after students have tried different mindfulness and self-compassion exercises, it is their responsibility to become their own best teachers. That means knowing which practices are most enjoyable, meaningful, and effective for them, and practicing them regularly.

Self-Compassion and Compassion for Others

Some people feel uncomfortable that the focus of MSC is *self*-compassion rather than compassion for others. Here are some common questions about this.

Doesn't the focus on "self" in self-compassion generate more suffering than it alleviates? We completely agree that a rigid, separate "self" is the source of most unnecessary emotional suffering in our lives, particularly the struggle to protect and promote our egos against ceaseless threats, real and imagined. Paradoxically, however, when we suffer and turn toward ourselves with compassion, our sense of separateness begins to dissolve. An example is what happens when we're struggling, and then we place our hands on the heart to comfort and support ourselves. That act of kindness usually allows us to disengage from self-oriented, ruminative thinking and see the world with new eyes.

Isn't there a better word than "self-compassion"? Our language tends to make ideas more solid than they are. An equivalent expression for self-compassion is "inner compassion." We call it "self-compassion" because it makes sense to beginning practitioners who might be battling with themselves. When a practitioner discovers through meditative inquiry that there is no fixed "self," then "inner compassion" becomes a more fitting expression.

Isn't self-compassion training emotionally activating? Everyone has difficult memories that are likely to resurface during self-compassion training. MSC was designed to meet old wounds in a healthy new way—with mindfulness and compassion. Emotional activation is an essential and unavoidable part of the transformation process. A key reason why mindfulness is taught alongside self-compassion is to stabilize awareness in the midst of strong emotions. Group support is another important part of self-compassion training—holding suffering in a culture of kindness.

Shouldn't MSC focus on training both self-compassion and compassion for others? MSC was never meant to be a complete compassion training program. In our opinion, for compassion to be complete, it should be both inner and outer. Unfortunately, there is a pervasive bias around the world toward valuing compassion for others over compassion for oneself. Hence, our special focus on self-compassion is intended to correct the imbalance. Our agenda is really quite humble—to *include* ourselves in the circle of compassion. MSC also teaches compassion for others, but links it to self-compassion, since that is our main focus. Research shows that MSC training develops compassion for others (Neff & Germer, 2013), but also that enhancing compassion for others helps us grow in self-compassion (Breines & Chen, 2013).

Shall We Begin?

You will now be guided through the MSC program. The remainder of Part I provides the theoretical and research foundations of self-compassion and self-compassion training (Chapters 2–4). Part II describes the pedagogy of self-compassion training. Chapter 5 reviews the structure and curriculum of MSC; Chapter 6 summarizes how to teach didactic topics and to guide meditations and class exercises; Chapter 7 focuses on embodying self-compassion and becoming a compassionate teacher; Chapter 8 offers insights and suggestions for managing group process; and Chapter 9 begins the journey into inquiry-based learning and teaching.

Part III provides an in-depth look at each of the eight sessions of the MSC program (one chapter per session), plus a separate chapter on the half-day retreat. Each chapter begins with an outline of the session (or retreat), followed by a description of a didactic topic; complete instructions for each meditation, informal practice, and class exercise; and samples of inquiry following the experiential activities. (The book's Appendices contain additional resources for study, practice, and teaching.)

Part IV focuses specifically on the integration of self-compassion into psychotherapy. It outlines similarities and differences between MSC and therapy, and addresses special issues like trauma and shame in more detail.

In this text, we alternate between masculine and feminine pronouns when referring to a single individual. We have made this choice to promote ease of reading as our language and culture continue to evolve, and not out of disrespect toward readers who identify with other personal pronouns. We sincerely hope that everyone will feel included. We also use lowercase letters for the full terms for structured training programs such as MBSR or MBCT, in keeping with modern language trends, but readers should use capital letters for the full name of the 8-week program described in this book (Mindful Self-Compassion) and the acronym (MSC®) in other written contexts, such as articles or online content. Finally, we often apply present participles (verbs ending in *-ing*) in meditation instructions; these can seem odd when read in a book, but, when delivered orally, they help to capture a sense of continuity and connection.

We are grateful that you are embarking on the inner journey of self-compassion, and we hope that the material contained in this book will support you in your personal and professional endeavors. If, after reading this book, you wish to teach the 8-week MSC program itself, please review the teacher training pathway at *https://centerformsc.org* for further information. It is essential to take formal MSC teacher training to be prepared to teach the program, no matter the prior skill level or experience of the teacher. Additionally, since MSC can be emotionally activating, in-person training and guidance on teaching the program—especially when difficulties arise—are necessary to ensure the safety of participants.

POINTS TO REMEMBER

* When mindfulness is fully present, it is suffused with the heart qualities of loving-kindness and compassion. Heart qualities are essential for mindful awareness, especially in the midst of difficult emotions, and they can be cultivated through practice.

* MSC is mindfulness-based self-compassion training.

* MSC is a resource-building program designed for the general public. The emphasis of the program is on developing a mindful and compassionate relationship to emotional pain—and to ourselves—rather than healing old wounds. However, old wounds tend to surface and transform in the course of self-compassion training.

* The curriculum contains a variety of formal meditations, informal practices, and exercises, and provides rationales for all these practices. With these skills and understanding, participants are encouraged to become their own teachers.

* MSC has borrowed from MBSR the 8-week training structure and the inquiry-based teaching approach. Three practices have also been adapted from MBSR—breath meditation, the body scan, and mindful movement.

* MSC is the first structured program specifically designed to cultivate self-compassion.

* Formal MSC teacher training is required to safely and effectively teach the program described in this book.

Chapter 2

What Is Self-Compassion?

> What if I should discover that . . . I myself stand in need of the alms
> of my own kindness—that I myself am the enemy who must be loved?
> —C. G. JUNG (1958/2014, p. 520)

Self-compassion isn't really different from compassion for others. The feelings are the same; the experience is the same. The difference is that people usually cut themselves out of the circle of their compassion—they much more readily give compassion to others than themselves (Knox, Neff, & Davidson, 2016). For this reason, examining what compassion is more generally can help us to understand what it means to have compassion for oneself in particular.

Compassion is defined by the Merriam-Webster online dictionary as "sympathetic consciousness of others' distress together with a desire to alleviate it." Goetz, Keltner, and Simon-Thomas (2010) define it as "the feeling that arises when witnessing another's suffering and that motivates a subsequent desire to help" (p. 351). Also central to the definition of compassion is a sense of interconnection with the person who is suffering (Cassell, 2002); the Latin roots of *compassion* literally mean "to suffer" (*passion*) "with" (*com*). Blum (1980) writes that "compassion involves a sense of shared humanity, of regarding the other as a fellow human being" (p. 511). When we feel compassion, therefore, we are willing to be present with the suffering of others and feel a sense of human interconnection. We also experience caring concern in response to their suffering and a desire to help.

For example, let's suppose that you see a homeless man begging for money on your way to work. Rather than rushing past him, or passing judgment that he's a worthless drunk, you may actually stop to consider how difficult this person's life may be. What's his story? Is he getting the mental health services he needs? The moment you see the man as an actual human being who is suffering, your heart connects with him. Instead of

15

ignoring him, you find that you're moved by his pain, and feel the urge to help in some way. And importantly, if what you feel is compassion rather than mere pity, you say to yourself, "He's a human being just like me. If I'd been born into different circumstances, or maybe had just been unlucky, I might also be struggling to survive. We're all vulnerable."

Of course, that may be the moment when you harden your heart completely; your own fear of ending up on the streets may cause you to distance yourself and perhaps to dehumanize the man. But this hardening of the heart, which often involves feeling superior to the homeless person, probably just ends up making you feel isolated and shut down. But let's say you really do experience compassion for the man. How does it feel? Actually, it feels pretty good. It's wonderful when your heart opens—you immediately feel more connected, alive, present.

But what if he was just begging for money to buy alcohol? Should you still give him compassion? Yes. You certainly don't have to offer money if you feel that's irresponsible, but he is still worthy of compassion; all of us are. Compassion is not only relevant to those who are blameless victims, but also to those whose suffering stems from personal failures, weaknesses, or bad decisions—the kinds we all make every day. The very fact that we are conscious human beings experiencing life on the planet means that we are intrinsically valuable and deserving of care. According to the Dalai Lama (1984/2012a), "Human beings by nature want happiness and do not want suffering. With that feeling everyone tries to achieve happiness and tries to get rid of suffering, and everyone has the basic right to do this. . . . Basically, from the viewpoint of real human value we are all the same" (p. 180).

We don't have to earn the right to compassion; it is our birthright. We are human, and our ability to think and feel, combined with our desire to be happy rather than to suffer, warrants compassion for its own sake.

The Elements of Self-Compassion

Self-compassion has the same qualities as compassion for others, but turned inward. It involves the clear seeing of our own suffering, a caring response to our suffering that includes the desire to help, and recognition that suffering is part of the shared human condition (Neff, 2003b). The components of self-compassion are conceptually distinct and tap into different ways that individuals emotionally respond to suffering (with kindness, rather than judgment), cognitively understand their predicament (as part of the human experience, or as isolating), and pay attention to pain (in a mindful, rather than overly identified, manner) (Neff, 2016b). Note that we use the term *suffering* loosely to refer to any moment of pain or discomfort, whether large or small. Self-compassion is relevant when we are considering personal inadequacies, mistakes, and failures, as well as when we are confronting painful life situations outside our control (Germer, 2009).

Self-Kindness versus Self-Judgment

Most of us try to be kind and considerate toward our friends and loved ones when they make a mistake, feel inadequate, or suffer some misfortune. We may offer words of support and understanding to let them know we care—perhaps even a physical gesture of affection such as a hug. We may ask them, "What do you need right now?" and consider what we can do to help. Curiously, we often treat ourselves very differently. We say harsh and cruel things to ourselves that we would never say to a friend. In fact, we're often tougher on ourselves than we are with people we don't like very much. The kindness inherent to self-compassion, however, puts an end to the constant self-judgment and disparaging internal commentary that most of us have come to see as normal. Our internal dialogues become benevolent and encouraging rather than punishing or belittling, reflecting a friendlier and more supportive attitude toward ourselves. We begin to *understand* our weaknesses and failures instead of condemning them. We acknowledge our shortcomings while accepting ourselves unconditionally as flawed, imperfect human beings. Most importantly, we recognize the extent to which we harm ourselves through relentless self-criticism, and choose another way.

Self-kindness involves more than merely ending self-criticism, however. It involves *actively opening up our hearts* to ourselves, responding to our suffering as we would to a dear friend in need. Beyond accepting ourselves without judgment, we may also soothe, comfort, and care for ourselves in the midst of emotional turmoil. We are motivated to try to help ourselves, to ease our own pain if we can. Normally, even when we experience unavoidable problems like having an unforeseeable accident, we focus more on fixing the problem than on caring for ourselves. We treat ourselves with cold stoicism rather than warmth or tender concern, and move straight into problem-solving mode. With self-kindness, however, we learn to nurture ourselves when life is difficult, offering support and encouragement. We allow ourselves to be emotionally moved by our own pain, stopping to say, "This is really difficult right now. How can I care for myself in this moment?" If we are being threatened in some way, we actively try to protect ourselves from harm.

We can't be perfect, and our lives will always involve struggle. When we deny or resist our imperfections, we exacerbate our suffering in the form of stress, frustration, and self-criticism. However, when we respond to ourselves with benevolence and goodwill, we generate positive emotions of love and care that help us cope.

Common Humanity versus Isolation

Self-compassion is embedded within a sense of interconnection rather than separation. One of the biggest problems with harsh self-judgment is that it tends to make us feel isolated and cut off from others. When we fail or feel inadequate in some way, we irrationally feel, "Everyone else is just fine. I'm the only one who is such a hopeless loser." This isn't a logical process, but an emotional reaction that narrows our understanding and distorts reality. Even when things go wrong in our lives that we don't blame ourselves for (and, sadly, we blame ourselves for most things), we tend to feel that somehow other people are having an easier time of it, and that our own situation is abnormal. We act almost as if we had signed a written contract before birth promising that we'd be perfect and that our lives would always go the way we wanted: "Excuse me. There must be some error. I signed up for the 'Everything will go perfectly until the day I die' plan. Can I get my money back?" It's absurd, and yet most of us believe something has gone terribly amiss when we fail or when life takes an unwanted turn. As Tara Brach (2003, p. 6) writes, "Feeling unworthy goes hand in hand with feeling separate from others, separate from life. If we are defective, how can we possibly belong?" This creates a frightening sense of disconnection and loneliness that greatly exacerbates our suffering.

With self-compassion, however, we recognize that life challenges and personal failures are part of being human; these are experiences we all share. In fact, our flaws and weaknesses are what make us card-carrying members of the human race. The element of common humanity also helps us to distinguish self-compassion from mere self-acceptance or self-love. While self-acceptance and self-love are important, they are incomplete by themselves. They leave out an essential factor—other people. Compassion is, by definition, relational. It implies a basic mutuality in the experience of suffering, and springs from the acknowledgment that the human experience is imperfect. Why else would we say, "It's only human," to console someone who has made a mistake? Self-compassion honors the fact that all human beings are fallible, that taking wrong turns is an inevitable part of living. (As the saying goes, a clear conscience is usually the sign of a bad memory.) When we're in touch with our common humanity, we remember that everyone has feelings of inadequacy and disappointment. The pain I feel in difficult times is the same pain that you feel in difficult times. The triggers, the circumstances, and the degree of pain may all be different, but the process is the same. With self-compassion, every moment of suffering is an opportunity to feel closer and more connected to others. It reminds us that we are not alone.

Mindfulness versus Over-identification

In order to have compassion for ourselves, we need to be willing to turn toward our own pain, to acknowledge it with mindfulness. Mindfulness is a type of balanced awareness that neither resists, avoids, nor exaggerates our moment-to-moment experience. Jon Kabat-Zinn (1994, p. 4) writes that mindfulness involves "paying attention in a particular way: on purpose, in the present moment, and nonjudgmentally." In this receptive mind-state, we become aware of our negative thoughts and feelings and are able to just be with them as they are, without fighting or denying them. We recognize when we're suffering, without immediately trying to fix our feelings and make them go away.

We might think that we don't need to become mindfully aware of our suffering. Suffering is obvious, isn't it? Not really. We certainly feel the pain of falling short of our ideals, but our minds tend to focus on the failure itself, rather than the pain caused by failure. This is a crucial difference. When our attention becomes completely absorbed by our perceived inadequacies, we can't step outside ourselves. We become overly identified with our negative thoughts or feelings, and are swept away by our aversive reactions. This type of rumination narrows our focus and exaggerates implications for self-worth (Nolen-Hoeksema, 1991): "Not only did I fail, I AM A FAILURE. Not only am I disappointed, MY LIFE IS DISAPPOINTING." Over-identification means that we reify our moment-to-moment experience, perceiving transitory events as definitive and permanent.

With mindfulness, however, everything changes. Rather than confusing our negative self-concepts with our actual selves, we can recognize that our thoughts and feelings are just that—thoughts and feelings. This helps us to drop our absorption in the storyline of our inadequate, worthless selves. Like a clear, still pool without ripples, mindfulness mirrors what's occurring without distortion, so that we can take a more objective perspective on ourselves and our lives. Mindfulness also provides the mental spaciousness and equanimity we need to see and do things differently. When we are mindful, we can wisely determine the best course of action to help ourselves when in need, even if that means simply holding our experience in gentle, loving awareness. It takes courage to turn toward our pain and acknowledge it, but this act of courage is essential if our hearts are to open in response to suffering. We can't heal what we can't feel. For this reason, mindfulness is the pillar on which self-compassion rests. Sharon Salzberg (2011a) writes:

> Mindfulness, which frees us from the grip of aversive feeling, gives us flexibility of attention, buoyancy and spaciousness of attention. This allows us the suppleness to look at our experience from different angles, to see beyond rigid characterizations, like "I'm so stupid and always will be," and "You're so bad, and that's all you'll be forever." It opens up the door for loving-kindness and compassion to enter. (p. 181)

While the components of self-compassion are conceptually distinct and do not co-vary in a lockstep manner, they do mutually influence one another. For instance, the accepting stance of mindfulness helps to lessen self-judgment and provide the insights we need to recognize our common humanity. Similarly, self-kindness lessens the impact of negative emotional experiences, making it easier to be mindful of them. Realizing that suffering and personal failures are shared with others lessens the degree of self-blame, while also helping to quell the process of over-identification. In this way, self-compassion can be seen as a dynamic system that represents a synergistic state of interaction between its various elements (Neff, 2016b).

How Does Self-Compassion Relate to Mindfulness?

Because so much has been written about the benefits of mindfulness for well-being (Davis & Hayes, 2011; Keng, Smoski, Robins, Ekblad, & Brantley, 2012), and because mindfulness is a core component of self-compassion, it is worth considering how the constructs of mindfulness and self-compassion are similar and how they differ. In an influential paper by Bishop and colleagues (2004), a team of scholars defined *mindfulness* as a metacognitive skill of focusing attention on present-moment experience while also maintaining a curious, nonjudgmental attitude toward that experience. Both components help explain why mindfulness is so powerful. Paying attention to the present moment keeps us from being lost in rumination about the past or anxiety about the future. Acceptance of our experience helps us avoid the frustration and stress that stem from fighting and resisting what we don't like. Put another way, it means that we don't bang our heads against the wall of reality, making an already difficult situation that much worse.

It should be noted that the type of mindfulness that is part of self-compassion is narrower in scope than mindfulness more generally. The mindfulness component of self-compassion refers specifically to awareness of *negative* thoughts and feelings. Mindfulness in general, however, refers to the ability to pay attention to any experience—positive, negative, or neutral—with equanimity. While it's possible to be mindful of eating a raisin (an exercise commonly used to teach mindfulness; see Kabat-Zinn, 1990), it wouldn't make sense to give oneself compassion for eating a raisin—unless perhaps you had a traumatic raisin-eating experience in childhood!

Self-compassion as a total construct is also broader in scope than mindfulness as defined by Bishop and colleagues (2004) because it includes the elements of self-kindness and common humanity: actively soothing and comforting oneself when painful experiences arise, and remembering that such experiences are part of being human. These are not qualities that are inherently part of mindfulness more narrowly defined. Feelings of self-kindness and common humanity may accompany mindfulness of painful experiences, of course, so that self-compassion often co-arises with mindfulness itself. The two do not always co-arise *fully,* however. It is possible to be mindfully aware of painful thoughts and feelings to some extent without actively soothing and comforting oneself, or remembering that these feelings are part of the shared human experience. Our mindfulness is not always in full bloom. Sometimes it takes an extra intentional effort to be compassionate toward our own suffering, especially when our painful thoughts and emotions involve self-judgments and feelings of inadequacy.

Another distinction between mindfulness and self-compassion lies in their respective targets. Whereas mindfulness is a way of relating to experience, self-compassion is a way of relating to the *experiencer* who is suffering (Germer, 2009; Germer & Barnhofer, 2017). Mindfulness nonjudgmentally accepts the thoughts, emotions, and sensations that arise in present-moment awareness. Compassion entails the desire for sentient beings to be happy and free from suffering (Salzberg, 1995). If you are mindful of a stabbing sensation in your knee, for instance, it means that you are aware of the hot pulsating sensation without judgment or resistance, providing mental space for the sensation to be experienced just as it is. When self-compassion arises in response to suffering, however, you also feel care and concern for the fact that you are having knee pain. This means that at the same time your present-moment experience is mindfully accepted without resistance, the wish for yourself as the experiencer to be free of suffering in future moments is also present.

Mindfulness and self-compassion involve a sort of paradox. Mindfulness invites us to just "be" with experience, whereas self-compassion involves more "doing." Self-compassion motivates us to soothe, comfort, and support ourselves to the extent possible when our experience is difficult (e.g., maybe standing up and stretching would help alleviate your knee pain). The reason why we can hold "being" and "doing" together simultaneously is that the "doing" is a special way of relating to the *sentient being* having that experience. When we are self-compassionate, we fully embrace ourselves with compassion *because* we are suffering, rather than holding the attitude that "I'll be kind to myself to get rid of this pain!" If self-compassion is misused in the service of resistance, it will add to our suffering rather than alleviate it. Mindfulness helps us to maintain the spacious attitude of acceptance.

The same process can occur in relating to the suffering of others. When someone tells you about a painful situation and you don't truly listen and empathize with this person's pain, but immediately jump to giving advice to fix the problem (and to make your own discomfort go away), you aren't really being compassionate. Compassion requires mindfulness to turn toward pain and accept its existence without resistance. While compassion is focused on the alleviation of suffering, it is not attached or dependent on the outcome of compassion (i.e., "I'll still be kind and understanding even if the pain doesn't lessen"). Conversely, compassion provides the emotional safety needed to fully feel, be open to, and accept the presence of pain—to be mindful. Thus mindfulness and compassion mutually enhance one another and are integrally intertwined.

The Yin and Yang of Self-Compassion

When we explore the attributes that are at play in self-compassion, we find seemingly opposite qualities that are also complementary and interdependent, like the concepts of yin and yang in traditional Chinese philosophy. The yin of self-compassion contains the attributes of "being" with ourselves in a compassionate way—*comforting, soothing,* and *validating* ourselves. The yang of self-compassion is about "acting" in the world—*protecting, providing,* and *motivating* ourselves.

Yin

- *Comforting.* Comforting is something that we might do for a dear friend who is struggling, and we can do it for ourselves. It means providing support for our *emotional* needs.
- *Soothing.* Soothing is another way to help ourselves feel better, particularly to feel *physically* calmer.
- *Validating.* Validation means that we clearly *understand* our experience, that we can find words for that experience, and that we can talk to ourselves in a kind and tender manner.

Yang

- *Protecting.* The first step toward self-compassion is feeling safe from harm. Protecting means saying "no" to others who are hurting us, or to the harm we inflict on ourselves in various ways.
- *Providing.* Providing means giving ourselves what we genuinely need. First we have to *know* what we need, saying "yes," and then we can go ahead and try to meet our needs.
- *Motivating.* We all have patterns of behavior that are no longer serving us that we need to let go of, as well as dreams and aspirations we want to pursue. Self-compassion motivates like a good coach, with encouragement, support, and understanding, not harsh criticism.

The yin of self-compassion allows us to stop struggling and just be there for ourselves with an open heart. A good metaphor for yin self-compassion is a parent cradling and rocking a crying child. When we feel hurt or inadequate, we can relate to ourselves in a tender way, validating our pain and accepting ourselves for who we are. The yang of self-compassion provides its action energy. A good metaphor is "Momma bear," who protects her cubs when threatened, or catches fish to feed them, or is willing to leave her comfortable home where the resources have been depleted to a find a new territory with more to offer. Yang self-compassion can be *fierce*—we draw our boundaries, say no, stand up for ourselves. We commit to meeting our own emotional, physical, and spiritual needs, knowing that they matter. We use constructive criticism to motivate change because we care about ourselves and don't want to suffer, not because we fear being unworthy.

The question is "What do I need now?" Sometimes we need to stand up and act decisively in the world, and sometimes we need to turn toward ourselves in a soft and tender way. Often we need both. As practitioners of self-compassion, we can keep the different qualities of compassion in mind and use our wisdom to decide what to do when. Most importantly, we need to honor both the fierce and tender sides of self-compassion. When yin and yang self-compassion are balanced and integrated, they manifest as a caring force. Force is more effective when it is caring because it is focused on the alleviation of suffering. This is the message taught by great leaders such as Gandhi, Mother Teresa, or Martin Luther King, Jr., who used compassionate action to effect societal change. We can also turn this power inward, using yin and yang self-compassion to cope with difficulty, build inner strength, and find true peace and happiness.

The Roots of Self-Compassion

Paul Gilbert (2009), who views the development of self-compassion through the lens of evolutionary psychology, proposes that how we relate to ourselves taps into our human physiology. For instance, self-criticism activates the threat defense system (associated with feelings of danger and arousal of the sympathetic nervous system). The amygdala is one of the oldest parts of the brain and was designed to quickly detect threats in the environment. When we feel in danger, the amygdala sends signals that increase blood pressure, adrenaline, and the hormone cortisol, mobilizing the strength and energy we need to confront or avoid a threat. Although this system was designed by evolution to deal with external, physical danger, it is just as readily activated by threats to our self-concept. Self-criticism is an unfortunate way of battling against internal challenges to our self-esteem. And since we are both the attacker and the attacked when we are being self-critical, the sympathetic nervous system can become especially strongly activated.

In contrast, Gilbert (2009) argues that self-compassion is often associated with mammalian caregiving (self-soothing, feelings of affiliation and safety, and activation of the parasympathetic nervous system). The evolutionary advance of mammals over reptiles is that since our young are born very immature, they require a longer developmental period to adapt to their environment. Mammals have the capacity to give and receive support, protection, and nurturance, which means that parents wouldn't abandon their children immediately after birth, and children wouldn't wander off alone into the dangerous wild (Wang, 2005). The capacity to feel affection and interconnection is part of our biological nature. *We are hardwired to care.*

We can frame the various elements of self-compassion in terms of a state of balance between the sympathetic and parasympathetic nervous systems (see Chapter 3), which are known to interact and co-vary continuously (Porges, 2007). Self-judgment, isolation, and over-identification can be seen as the stress response turned inward when our self-concept is threatened. Self-judgment is the fight response in the form of self-criticism and self-attack. Isolation represents the flight response—the desire to flee from others and hide in shame. Over-identification can be seen as the freeze response—becoming self-absorbed and getting stuck in a ruminative cycle of thought about our own unworthiness. At the same time, self-kindness, recognition of common humanity, and mindfulness can be seen to generate feelings of safety in response to threat. Self-kindness involves protecting, nurturing, and supporting ourselves, counteracting the self-critical fight response. Common humanity generates feelings of connection and affiliation, counteracting the isolating flight response. Self-compassion also entails mindfulness, which provides a sense of perspective and psychological flexibility that counteracts the freeze response of over-identification (Creswell, 2015; Tirch, Schoendorff, & Silberstein, 2014). Of course, there is considerable interaction among all the system components, and this model is a simplified one. In fact, research shows that the various components of self-compassion do not substantially differ in terms of their association with markers of decreased sympathetic response (e.g., alpha-amylase, interleukin-6) after a stressful situation (Neff, Long, et al., 2018) or with vagally mediated heart rate variability, a marker of increased parasympathetic response (Svendsen et al., 2016). As Porges (2003) makes clear, the two types of autonomic nervous system responding interact and co-vary as a system.

How Does Self-Compassion Relate to Self-Esteem?

It's important to distinguish self-compassion from self-esteem, especially since the two are easily confused (Neff, 2011b). *Self-esteem* refers to the degree to which we evaluate ourselves positively, and is often based on comparisons with others (Harter, 1999). There is a general consensus that self-esteem is essential for good mental health, while the lack of self-esteem undermines well-being and fosters depression, anxiety, and other pathologies (Leary, 1999). There are potential problems with high self-esteem, however—not in terms of having it, but in terms of getting and keeping it (Crocker & Park, 2004).

In American culture, high self-esteem requires standing out in a crowd—being special and above average (Heine, Lehman, Markus, & Kitayama, 1999). How do *you* feel when someone evaluates your work performance, or parenting skills, or intelligence as simply average? Ouch! The problem, of course, is that it's impossible for everyone to be above average at the same time. While there may be some areas in which we excel, there's always someone more attractive, successful, and popular than we are, meaning that we may feel like failures whenever we compare ourselves to those "better" than ourselves.

The desire to see ourselves as better than average, however, can lead to some downright nasty behavior. Why do early adolescents begin to bully others? If I can be seen as the cool, tough kid in contrast to the wimpy kid I just picked on, I get a self-esteem boost (Salmivalli, Kaukiainen, Kaistaniemi, & Lagerspetz, 1999). Why are we so prejudiced? If I believe that my ethnic, gender, national, or political group is better than yours, I get another self-esteem boost (Fein & Spencer, 1997).

Indeed, the emphasis placed on self-esteem in American society has led to a worrying trend: Researchers Jean Twenge from San Diego State University and Keith Campbell from the University of Georgia, who have tracked the narcissism scores of college students since 1987, find that the narcissism of modern-day students is at the highest level ever recorded (see, e.g., Twenge, Konrath, Foster, Campbell, & Bushman, 2008). Although narcissists have extremely high self-esteem, they also feel self-entitled and have inflated, unrealistic conceptions of themselves, which tend to drive people away over time (Twenge & Campbell, 2009). The researchers attribute the rise in narcissism to well-meaning but misguided parents and teachers who tell kids how special and great they are in an attempt to raise their self-esteem.

Self-compassion is different from self-esteem. Although they're both strongly linked to psychological well-being, self-esteem is a positive evaluation of self-worth, while self-compassion isn't a judgment or an evaluation at all. Instead, self-compassion is a way of *relating* to the ever-changing landscape of who we are with kindness and acceptance—especially when we fail or feel inadequate.

Self-esteem is inherently fragile, bouncing up and down according to our latest success or failure (Crocker, Luhtanen, Cooper, & Bouvrette, 2003). Self-esteem is a fair-weather friend, there for us in good times, deserting us when our luck turns. But self-compassion is always there for us, a reliable source of support even when our worldly stock has crashed.

It still hurts when our pride is dashed, but we can be kind to ourselves precisely *because* it hurts: "Wow, that was pretty humiliating. I'm so sorry. It's okay, though; these things happen."

Self-esteem requires feeling better than others, whereas self-compassion requires simply acknowledging that we share the human condition of imperfection. This means that we don't have to feel better than others to feel good about ourselves. Self-compassion also offers more emotional stability than self-esteem because it is always there for us—when we're on top of the world, and when we fall flat on our faces. Self-compassion is a portable friend we can always rely on, in good times and bad.

Common Misgivings about Self-Compassion

There are many blocks to self-compassion in Western culture, often resulting from misconceptions about its meaning and consequences (Robinson et al., 2016). Research dispelling these misconceptions is presented in Chapter 3, but it is worth considering here what the most common misgivings about self-compassion are.

One common misconception is that self-compassion is *selfish*. Many people assume that spending time and energy being kind and caring toward themselves means automatically that they must be neglecting everybody else for their own self-focused ends. But is compassion really a zero-sum game? Think about the times you've been lost in the throes of self-criticism. Are you self-focused or other-focused in the moment? Do you have more or fewer resources to give to others? Most people find that when they're absorbed in self-judgment, they actually have little bandwidth left over to think about anything other than their inadequate, worthless selves.

Unfortunately, the ideal of being modest, self-effacing, and caring for the welfare of others often comes with the corollary tendency to treat ourselves badly. This is especially true for women, who have been found to have slightly lower levels of self-compassion than men, even while they tend to be more caring, empathetic, and giving toward others (Yarnell et al., 2015). Perhaps this isn't so surprising, given that women are socialized to care selflessly for their partners, children, friends, and elderly parents, but may not have been taught to care for themselves. While the feminist revolution helped expand the roles available to women, and we now see more female leaders in business and politics than ever before, the idea that women should be selfless caregivers really hasn't gone away. It's just that women are now supposed to be successful at their careers, *in addition to* being the ultimate nurturers at home.

The irony is that being good to yourself actually gives you the emotional resources to be good to others, while being harsh with yourself only gets in the way. For instance, research shows that self-compassionate people are rated by their partners as being more caring and giving in their relationships (Neff & Beretvas, 2013). This makes sense. If I'm cold toward myself and rely on my partner to meet all my emotional needs, I'm going to behave badly when they're not met. But if I'm able to give myself care and support, and thus to meet many of my own needs directly, I'll have more emotional resources available to give to my partner.

Another common misconception about self-compassion is that it means feeling sorry for yourself—that it's just a dressed-up form of self-pity. In fact, self-compassion is an *antidote* to self-pity and the tendency to complain about bad luck. This isn't because self-compassion means tuning out the bad stuff; in fact, self-compassion makes us more willing to accept, experience, and acknowledge difficult feelings with kindness, which paradoxically helps us digest what happened to us and move on. Self-compassionate people are less likely to get swallowed up by self-pitying thoughts about how bad things are (Raes, 2010). That seems to be one of the reasons self-compassionate people have better mental health. Whereas self-pity emphasizes egocentric feelings of separation and exaggerates the extent of personal distress, self-compassion allows us to connect our own suffering to that of others. It softens rather than strengthens the internal boundaries between ourselves and others. Moreover, the recognition of common humanity helps put our own situations into perspective. This doesn't mean denying the validity of our own suffering, but when we consider the bigger picture, our problems may not be as bad as we think.

Some people fear that self-compassion is weak or cowardly, or at least passive. In this case, feelings of compassion are confused with "being nice" all the time. However, as mentioned earlier, self-compassion in its yang form can be fierce, taking a strong and resolute stand against anything that causes harm. Instead of being a weakness, self-compassion is an important source of coping and resilience. When we go through major life crises, such as divorce, major illness, or trauma, self-compassion makes all the difference in our ability to survive and even thrive in the face of adversity (Brion, Leary, & Drabkin, 2014; Hiraoka et al., 2015; Sbarra, Smith, & Mehl, 2012). It's not just what we face in life, but how we relate to ourselves when the going gets tough—as inner allies or enemies—that determines our ability to get through successfully.

Another common misgiving about self-compassion is that it will lead to *self-indulgence*. Doesn't being kind to ourselves mean giving ourselves whatever we want? ("I'm feeling sad. Hmmm. That tub of chocolate ice cream is looking pretty good right now.") It must be remembered that self-compassion has its eye on the prize—the alleviation of suffering. Self-indulgence, on the other hand, involves giving ourselves short-term pleasure at the cost of long-term harm. A compassionate mother wouldn't give her daughter endless bowls of ice cream and let her skip school whenever she wanted, would she? That would be indulgent. Instead, a compassionate mother tells her child to do her homework and eat her vegetables. Self-compassion avoids self-indulgence because it harms us, whereas long-term health and well-being often require delaying gratification.

Many people doubt the value of self-compassion by asking, "But don't we *need* to be critical of ourselves sometimes?" In this case, there is confusion between harsh self-judgment and constructive criticism. Self-compassion lets go of belittling, demeaning self-judgments such as "I'm a lazy, good-for-nothing loser." When we care about ourselves, however, we will constructively point out ways we could do things better. This criticism is always aimed at concrete behaviors, however, and does not involve global self-evaluation. For instance, a self-compassionate inner voice might say, "The fact that you haven't been to the gym in 6 months has made you feel tired and unhealthy. Maybe you should make a change." This is a more constructive form of feedback than "You're a lazy slob!" (and certainly less painful). Often the tone of the message determines whether a critique is constructive or destructive.

Because many people assume self-compassion just involves self-acceptance (yin) without understanding that it also involves taking action (yang), they fear that self-compassion will undermine their *motivation* to improve. The idea is that if they don't criticize themselves for failing to live up to their standards, they will automatically succumb to slothful defeatism. Unfortunately, this is a major block to self-compassion. But let's think for a moment how compassionate parents successfully motivate their children. If your teenage son comes home one day with a failing English grade, you could look disgusted and hiss, "Stupid boy. You'll never amount to anything. I'm ashamed of you." (Makes you cringe, doesn't it? Yet that's exactly the type of thing we tell ourselves when we fail to meet our own high expectations.) Most likely, rather than motivating your son, this torrent of shame will just make him lose faith in himself, blame outside factors ("the test was unfair"), and eventually stop trying altogether.

Alternatively, you could adopt a compassionate approach by saying, "Oh, bummer, you must be so upset. Hey, give me a hug. It happens to all of us. But we need to get your English grades up because I know you want to get into a good college. What can I do to help and support you to do better next time? I believe in you." Notice that there's honest recognition of the failure, sympathy for your son's unhappiness, *and* encouragement to go beyond or around this momentary bump in the road. Ideally, this type of caring response will help him maintain his self-confidence and feel emotionally supported. It will also provide the sense of safety needed for him to look closely at where things went wrong (maybe he should have studied more and played fewer video games), so he can learn from his mistakes.

It seems easy to see this when we're thinking about healthy parenting, but it's not so easy to apply this same logic to ourselves. We're deeply attached to our self-criticism, and at some level we think the pain is helpful.

To the extent that self-criticism *does* work as a motivator, it's because we're driven by the desire to avoid self-judgment when we fail. But if we know that failure will be met with a barrage of self-criticism, sometimes it can be too frightening even to try. This is why self-criticism is associated with underachievement and self-handicapping strategies like procrastination (Powers, Koestner, & Zuroff, 2007). We also use self-criticism as a means of shaming ourselves into action when confronting personal weaknesses. However, this approach backfires if weaknesses remain unacknowledged in an attempt to avoid self-censure (Horney, 1950). With self-compassion, however, we strive to achieve for a very different reason—because we *care*. You might say that the motivation behind self-compassion is love, whereas the motivation behind self-criticism is fear. If we truly care about ourselves, we'll do things to make ourselves happy, such as taking on challenging new projects or learning new skills. And because self-compassion gives us the safety we need to acknowledge our weaknesses, we'll be in a better position to change them for the better.

A Pathway to Happiness

As the overview of research presented in the next chapter demonstrates, self-compassion is a powerful way to achieve well-being and contentment in our lives. By giving ourselves unconditional kindness and support, and by accepting our imperfections as part of the human condition, we help to alleviate difficult psychological states such as depression, anxiety, and stress, while fostering positive mind-states such as happiness and optimism (Zessin et al., 2015). The nurturing quality of self-compassion allows us to thrive and prosper, and to appreciate the beauty of life, even in hard times. Rather than trying to control life and our emotional reactions to it, or getting angry and frustrated when things don't go exactly the way we want them to, we can take a different path. We can soothe our agitated minds with yin self-compassion, and draw on the power of yang self-compassion, so that we're better able to cope with the challenges that come our way.

Self-compassion provides a refuge from the stormy seas of positive and negative self-judgment, so that we can finally stop asking, "Am I as good as they are? Am I good enough?" The happiness of self-compassion isn't based on being better than anyone else, or on achieving success in our endeavors. The happiness of self-compassion comes from relating to the imperfection of life, and our imperfect selves, with open hearts and minds.

We have the means to provide ourselves with the type of warm, supportive care that we deeply yearn for. When we tap into our deep inner wellsprings of kindness, acknowledge the shared nature of the human experience, and open to the reality of the present moment, we feel more fulfilled and alive. Self-compassion is an alchemical process that can transform suffering into joy. As our colleague Michelle Becker has pointed out, when we embrace our pain with an open heart, a new state emerges—a state of "loving, connected presence"—corresponding to the three components of self-compassion. Especially when the tender healing power of self-compassion is combined with the fierce commitment to alleviate suffering, we can *thrive* in the midst of challenge and change.

POINTS TO REMEMBER

* Self-compassion is simply compassion turned inward. It can be applied to any moment of suffering, large or small.

* Self-compassion has three main components: (1) self-kindness versus self-judgment, (2) common humanity versus isolation, and (3) mindfulness versus over-identification.

* Mindfulness is typically associated with loving awareness of *experience*. Self-compassion is loving awareness of the *experiencer*.

* The *yin* of self-compassion involves *being* with ourselves in an accepting way—comforting, soothing, and validating our pain. The *yang* of self-compassion involves *action* to alleviate our suffering—protecting, providing, and motivating ourselves, when needed.

* Self-compassion and self-esteem are both positive ways of relating to oneself, but self-esteem is an evaluation of self-worth that is conditional and based on success, whereas self-compassion involves unconditional self-acceptance even in moments of failure.

* Common myths about self-compassion can be dispelled:

  ◆ Self-compassion is not selfish or self-centered. It gives us the emotional resources needed to care for others.

  ◆ Self-compassion is not a form of self-pity. It allows us to see the interconnected experiences of self and others without exaggeration.

  ◆ Self-compassion is not weak, but can be fiercely self-protective and self-supporting. It is a source of strength and resilience in challenging situations.

  ◆ Self-compassion is not self-indulgent. Because it is ultimately aimed at the alleviation of suffering, self-compassion chooses long-term well-being over short-term pleasure.

  ◆ Self-compassion involves constructive criticism and discernment, not harsh, belittling self-judgment.

  ◆ Self-compassion enhances rather than undermines motivation. Unlike self-criticism, self-compassion motivates with care, support, and encouragement, rather than fear and shame.

Chapter 3

The Science
of Self-Compassion

We live in a time when science is validating what humans have
known throughout the ages: that compassion is not a luxury;
it is a necessity for our well-being, resilience, and survival.
—JOAN HALIFAX (2012b)

In our increasingly secular, diverse world, scientific research is an important way to make sense of our lives and separate fact from fiction. Research
also gives us the confidence to try something new, such as embarking on the
challenging path to self-compassion. Self-compassion research is expanding exponentially (see Figure 3.1), following a trajectory similar to that
of mindfulness research, and both mindfulness and self-compassion are
currently being integrated into all aspects of modern society. This chapter
reviews existing scientific studies on self-compassion and describes con-
verging trends in the research.

The Methodology of Self-Compassion Research

So far, the majority of studies on self-compassion have been conducted
using the Self-Compassion Scale (SCS; Neff, 2003a), a 26-item self-report
measure that is designed to measure self-compassion as defined by Neff
(2003b). The 12-item short form of the SCS (SCS-SF) is also frequently used
in research, given that it has a near-perfect correlation with the long form
(Raes, Pommier, Neff, & Van Gucht, 2011). The SCS is a straightforward
assessment of how often people engage in the various thoughts, emotions,
and behaviors that align with the different dimensions of self-compassion.
It is designed to measure self-compassion as a holistic construct, but the
six subscales of the SCS can be used individually to examine the aspects of
self-compassion associated with increased positive and decreased negative

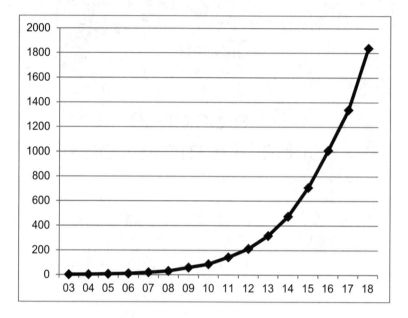

FIGURE 3.1. Research publications on self-compassion, 2003–2017. (N = 1,840, based on a Google Scholar search of entries with the term *self-compassion* in the title.)

self-responding in times of struggle. Sample items for the subscales are as follows: Self-Kindness ("I try to be loving towards myself when I'm feeling emotional pain"), Self-Judgment ("I'm disapproving and judgmental about my own flaws and inadequacies"), Common Humanity ("When things are going badly for me, I see the difficulties as part of life that everyone goes through"), Isolation ("When I think about my inadequacies, it tends to make me feel more separate and cut off from the rest of the world"), Mindfulness ("When I'm feeling down I try to approach my feelings with curiosity and openness"), and Over-identification ("When something upsets me I get carried away with my feelings") (see also Chapter 2). Negative items are reverse-coded, so that higher scores indicate a relative lack of uncompassionate self-responding.

The SCS has high internal reliability (Neff, 2003a) and also taps into behaviors that can be readily observed by others. For instance, self-assessments of self-compassion are highly correlated (0.70) with assessments made by partners in long-term relationships (Neff & Beretvas, 2013). Individuals can take the SCS and have their scores automatically calculated at *https://self-compassion.org*. This can be a useful way to track progress in learning the skill of self-compassion in settings such as in psychotherapy, mindfulness, and compassion training, or generally throughout our lives.

Some authors have suggested that the SCS should be used to measure compassionate and uncompassionate self-responding separately, and that positive and negative SCS scores rather than a total SCS score should be used (e.g., Costa, Marôco, Pinto-Gouveia, Ferreira, & Castilho, 2015; Gilbert, McEwan, Matos, & Rivis, 2011; Muris, 2015). Support for a two-factor solution to the SCS has been inconsistent, however (e.g., Cleare, Gumley, Cleare, & O'Connor, 2018; Neff, Whittaker, & Karl, 2017). Neff, Tóth-Király, Yarnell, and colleagues (2018) argue that a bifactor approach combined with exploratory structural equation modeling (ESEM) offers the most theoretically consistent way to examine the SCS, given that the six components are thought to operate as a dynamic system. In a large international collaboration, they used bifactor ESEM to examine the factor structure of the SCS in 20 diverse samples ($N = 11,685$); support was found in every sample for use of six subscale scores or a total score, but not for use of separate scores representing positive versus negative self-responding. Moreover, 95% of the reliable variance could be attributed to a general factor.

Support for the view that self-compassion is best thought of as a system composed of six interacting elements can be found in the fact that the vast majority of intervention studies examining change in self-compassion have found a simultaneous increase in scores on the three positive subscales and a decrease on the three negative subscales of the SCS of roughly the same magnitude. This is true for studies using a wide variety of methodologies, such as self-compassion meditation training (Albertson, Neff, & Dill-Shackleford, 2015; Toole & Craighead, 2016; Wallmark, Safarzadeh, Daukantaite, & Maddux, 2012), online psychoeducation (Finlay-Jones, Kane, & Rees, 2017; Krieger, Martig, van den Brink, & Berger, 2016), compassion-focused therapy (Beaumont, Irons, Rayner, & Dagnall, 2016; Kelly & Carter, 2015; Kelly, Wisniewski, Martin-Wagar, & Hoffman, 2017), or MSC training (Finlay-Jones, Xie, Huang, Ma, & Guo, 2018; Neff, 2016a). Mindfulness-based interventions also yield a simultaneous increase in positive and decrease in negative SCS subscale scores (Birnie, Speca, & Carlson, 2010; Greeson, Juberg, Maytan, James, & Rogers, 2014; Raab, Sogge, Parker, & Flament, 2015; Whitesman & Mash, 2016). The fact that all six components of self-compassion change simultaneously suggest that self-compassion operates holistically.

It should be noted that other measures of self-compassion also exist and are employed in research. For instance, Gilbert, Clarke, Hempel, Miles, and Irons (2004) created the Forms of Self-Criticism and Self-Reassuring Scale to measure these two ways of relating to oneself. More recently, Gilbert and colleagues (2017) developed the Compassion Engagement and Action Scales (CEAS), based on the broadly used definition of compassion as sensitivity to suffering with a commitment to try to alleviate it (Goetz, Keltner, & Simon-Thomas, 2010). The CEAS includes a self-compassion subscale with items tapping into engagement with distress (e.g., tolerating and being sensitive to distress) and the motivation to alleviate that distress (e.g., thinking about and taking actions to help). Notably, the CEAS does not include warmth, kindness, concern, or feelings of shared humanity as a feature of compassion, so it represents a quite different conceptualization of self-compassion than that proposed by Neff (2003b).

Increasingly, researchers are using alternative methods that don't involve self-report to empirically examine the impact of self-compassion on well-being. These methods include experimental induction of a self-compassionate state of mind through writing (e.g., Breines & Chen, 2012); observations of the degree of self-compassion displayed in written or oral dialogues (e.g., Sbarra et al., 2012); and both short-term and long-term self-compassion interventions (e.g., Neff & Germer, 2013; Smeets, Neff, Alberts, & Peters, 2014). Findings converge, whether self-compassion is examined with the SCS or other methodological approaches, providing confidence in the general body of self-compassion research (Neff et al., 2017).

For example, higher scores on the SCS have been associated with greater levels of happiness, optimism, life satisfaction, body appreciation, perceived competence, and motivation (Hollis-Walker & Colosimo, 2011; Neff, Hsieh, & Dejitterat, 2005; Neff, Pisitsungkagarn, & Hsieh, 2008; Neff, Rude, & Kirkpatrick, 2007); lower levels of depression, anxiety, stress, rumination, self-criticism, perfectionism, body shame, and fear of failure (Breines, Toole, Tu, & Chen, 2014; Finlay-Jones, Rees, & Kane, 2015; Neff, 2003a; Neff et al., 2005; Raes, 2010); and healthier physiological responses to stress (Breines, Thoma, et al., 2014; Friis, Johnson, Cutfield, & Consedine, 2016). This same pattern of results has been obtained with experimental methods involving behavioral interventions or mood manipulations designed to increase self-compassion (Albertson et al., 2015; Arch et al., 2014; Breines & Chen, 2012; Diedrich, Grant, Hofmann, Hiller, & Berking, 2014; Johnson & O'Brien, 2013; Leary, Tate, Adams, Allen, & Hancock, 2007; Mosewich, Crocker, Kowalski, & DeLongis, 2013; Neff & Germer, 2013; Odou & Brinker, 2014; Shapira & Mongrain, 2010; Smeets et al., 2014).

Self-Compassion and Emotional Well-Being

The empirical literature overwhelmingly supports the link between self-compassion and well-being (MacBeth & Gumley, 2012; Neff, Long, et al., 2018; Zessin et al., 2015). One of the most consistent findings is that greater self-compassion is linked to less depression, anxiety, and stress. In fact, a meta-analysis (MacBeth & Gumley, 2012) examining the link between self-compassion and psychopathology across 20 studies found a large effect size. While most of the research on the link between self-compassion and psychopathology has been conducted with adults, a meta-analysis also supported this negative link between self-compassion and psychological distress among adolescents, again with a large effect size (Marsh, Chan, & MacBeth, 2018). Of course, a key feature of self-compassion is the lack of self-criticism, and self-criticism is known to be an important predictor of anxiety and depression (Blatt, 1995). However, self-compassion still offers protection against anxiety and depression when self-criticism and negative affect are controlled for (Neff, 2003a; Neff, Kirkpatrick, & Rude, 2007). Moreover, self-compassion predicts well-being when neuroticism is controlled for (Neff, Tóth-Királ, & Colisomo, 2018; Stutts, Leary, Zeveney, & Hufnagle, 2018).

Various research studies have examined the protective effects of self-compassion against psychopathology. For example, inducing a self-compassionate mood has been found to reduce socially anxious students' anticipatory anxiety before giving a speech (Harwood & Kocovski, 2017). Stutts and colleagues (2018) found that self-compassion levels at baseline predicted lower depression, anxiety, and negative affect after 6 months, and also moderated the effects of stress so that it was less strongly related to negative outcomes. Similarly, self-compassion was found to protect against the deleterious effects of mind wandering in a depressed sample (Greenberg et al., 2018). Importantly, self-compassion has been linked to reduced suicidal ideation and nonsuicidal self-injury in nonclinical populations (Chang et al., 2016; Jiang et al., 2016; Kelliher Rabon, Sirois, & Hirsch, 2018; Xavier, Gouveia, & Cunha, 2016).

Although self-compassion reduces negative thinking (Arimitsu & Hofmann, 2015), it is not merely a matter of looking on the bright side of things or avoiding painful emotions (Krieger, Altenstein, Baettig, Doerig, & Holtforth, 2013). Self-compassionate people recognize when they are suffering, but are kind toward themselves in these moments, acknowledging their connectedness with the rest of humanity. For instance, one study investigated the ways in which self-compassionate people deal with negative life events by asking participants to report about problems experienced over a 20-day period (Leary et al., 2007). Individuals with higher levels of self-compassion had a better perspective on their problems and were less likely to feel isolated by them. They also experienced less anxiety and self-consciousness when thinking about their difficulties. Similarly, self-compassionate individuals have been found to use more connected language when writing about their weakness; to use fewer first-person singular pronouns such as *I*; to use more first-person plural pronouns such as *we*; and to make more social references to friends, family, and other humans (Neff, Kirkpatrick, & Rude, 2007).

Self-compassion is associated with greater emotional intelligence (Heffernan, Griffin, McNulty, & Fitzpatrick, 2010; Neff, 2003a; Neff, Long, et al., 2018), suggesting that self-compassion represents a wiser way of dealing with difficult feelings. For example, self-compassionate people are less likely to ruminate on their negative thoughts and emotions than are those low in self-compassion (Fresnics & Borders, 2017; Odou & Brinker, 2015; Raes, 2010), meaning that they don't get stuck in the quagmire of negative thinking. They report better emotional coping skills, including greater ability to bounce back from negative moods (Diedrich, Burger, Kirchner, & Berking, 2017; Neely, Schallert, Mohammed, Roberts, & Chen, 2009; Neff et al., 2005; Sirois, Molnar, & Hirsch, 2015).

Self-compassion also appears to help people deal with shame. One study asked participants to think of an episode from their past in which they were ashamed of themselves, and then asked them to write about the incident self-compassionately (Johnson & O'Brien, 2013). For instance, they were instructed to "Write a paragraph expressing understanding, kindness, and concern to yourself the way you might express concern to a friend who had undergone the experience." Those in the self-compassionate writing condition (compared to an expressive writing control condition) reported significant decreases in shame and negative affect. Self-compassionate individuals who were asked to do a difficult task (subtracting the number 17 starting from a given four-digit number as fast as possible) were less likely to feel shame about their performance after being socially evaluated (Ewert, Gaube, & Geisler, 2018). Similarly, parents who were helped to feel self-compassionate about a shame-provoking parenting event felt less guilt and shame than those in a control condition did (Sirois, Bogels, & Emerson, 2018). Among African Americans who had recently attempted suicide, self-compassion provided a buffer between feelings of shame and depression (Zhang et al., 2018).

In addition to reducing negative mind-states, self-compassion appears to bolster positive mind-states. For example, higher self-compassion levels are associated with greater feelings of psychological well-being, life satisfaction, hope, happiness, optimism, gratitude, curiosity, vitality, and positive affect (Breen, Kashdan, Lenser, & Fincham, 2010; Gunnell, Mosewich, McEwen, Eklund, & Crocker, 2017; Hollis-Walker & Colosimo, 2011; Hope, Koestner, & Milyavskaya, 2014; Neff, Long, et al., 2018; Neff, Rude, & Kirkpatrick, 2007; Umphrey & Sherblom, 2014; Yang, Zhang, & Kou, 2016). Self-compassion is also linked to greater feelings of authenticity (Zhang et al., 2019). Self-compassion is associated with more autonomy, competence, and relatedness (Neff, 2003a; Gunnell et al., 2017), suggesting that this supportive self-stance helps meet the basic psychological needs that Deci and Ryan (1995) argue are fundamental to well-being. A longitudinal study examined the impact of writing a self-compassionate letter to oneself for 5 days, and found that this activity not only decreased depression levels for 3 months, but increased happiness for 6 months (Shapira & Mongrain, 2010). This is the beauty of self-compassion: By wrapping our pain in the warm embrace of self-compassion, we can generate positive feelings of loving, connected presence at the same time that we can ameliorate negative emotions.

Self-Compassion versus Self-Esteem

Research suggests that while self-compassion yields mental health benefits similar to those of self-esteem, it does not have the same pitfalls. In a survey involving a large community sample in the Netherlands (Neff & Vonk, 2009), for example, higher SCS scores were associated with more stability in state feelings of self-worth over an 8-month period (assessed 12 different times) than trait self-esteem was. This may be related to the fact that self-compassion was also found to be less contingent on personal traits like physical attractiveness or successful performance than self-esteem was. Results indicated that self-compassion was associated with lower levels of social comparison, public self-consciousness, self-rumination, anger, and closed-mindedness than self-esteem. Also, self-esteem had a robust association with narcissism, while self-compassion had no association with narcissism. These findings indicate that in contrast to those with high self-esteem, self-compassionate people are less focused on evaluating themselves, feeling superior to others, defending their viewpoints, or angrily reacting against those who disagree with them.

Self-compassion also appears to provide greater ability to cope with stress than self-esteem does. One study asked participants to report their stress levels and mood twice a day for 14 days on their smartphones (Krieger, Hermann, Zimmermann, & Holtforth, 2015), and found their general levels of self-compassion, but not global self-esteem, predicted less negative affect in the midst of stressful situations. Self-compassion may also buffer the impact of low self-esteem on well-being. For instance, a longitudinal study with adolescents found that ninth-grade students with low self-esteem but high self-compassion were more psychologically healthy 1 year later than those who were also low in self-compassion (Marshall et al., 2015).

Leary and colleagues (2007) conducted a study that compared self-compassion and self-esteem in terms of accepting feedback. Participants were asked to make a videotape that would introduce and describe themselves. They were then told that someone would watch their tape and give them feedback in terms of how warm, friendly, intelligent, likeable, and mature they appeared (the feedback was given by a study confederate). Half the participants received positive feedback, the other neutral feedback. Self-compassionate people were relatively unflustered regardless of whether the feedback was positive or neutral, and were willing to say that the feedback was based on their own personality either way. People with high levels of self-esteem, however, tended to get upset when they received neutral feedback ("What, I'm just *average?*"). They were also more likely to deny that the neutral feedback was due to their own personality, but rather to attribute it to factors such as the observer's mood. This suggests that self-compassionate people are better able to accept who they are, regardless of the degree of praise they receive from others. Self-esteem, on the other hand, only thrives when the reviews are good, and may lead to evasive tactics when there's a possibility of facing unpleasant truths about oneself (Swann, 1996).

Self-Compassion Compared to Mindfulness

Some researchers have been interested in exploring whether self-compassion and mindfulness have different relationships to well-being outcomes. Although self-compassion includes mindfulness of negative self-related thoughts, it adds the components of self-kindness and common humanity, which can make an additional contribution to mental health. When the links among mindfulness, self-compassion, and well-being in people with moderate to severe anxiety and/or depression were examined, for instance, it was found that self-compassion explained significantly more variance in terms of anxiety, worry, depression, and quality of life than did mindfulness alone (Van Dam, Sheppard, Forsyth, & Earleywine, 2011). Similarly, self-compassion appears to be a stronger predictor than mindfulness of depression, anxiety, happiness, positive and negative affect, and life satisfaction among college undergraduates (Woodruff et al., 2014). Researchers have also found that inducing a self-compassionate response to sad emotions is more effective for decreasing depressed mood in currently and formerly depressed individuals than is a strategy of mindful acceptance (Ehret, Joormann, & Berking, 2018).

Interestingly, self-compassion negatively predicts shame-proneness, but mindfulness does not (Woods & Proeve, 2014), suggesting that kindness and connectedness are needed to prevent negative self-related thoughts from manifesting as shame. Moreover, mindfulness and self-compassion appear to play distinct roles in the link between self-stigma and well-being among people with mental illness and people living with HIV (Yang & Mak, 2016). Mindfulness primarily moderates the link between the automaticity of self-stigma among people with mental illness, and self-compassion primarily moderates the link between stigma identity and well-being among people living with HIV.

Several researchers have compared the role of mindfulness and self-compassion in terms of well-being gains associated with meditation. Although increased mindfulness and self-compassion both help explain the link between meditation and happiness (Campos et al., 2016), self-compassion predicts psychological well-being more strongly than mindfulness does among meditators, even after meditation experience is controlled for (Baer, Lykins, & Peters, 2012). In a study of adolescents who took a 5-day meditation retreat (Galla, 2016), gains in self-compassion were a stronger predictor of well-being in terms of perceived stress, rumination, depressive symptoms, life satisfaction, and positive and negative affect than gains in mindfulness were. Researchers have also found that giving participants brief instructions to be warm and compassionate to themselves prior to a mindfulness meditation session made them more willing to continue the training (Rowe, Shepstone, Carnelley, Cavanagh, & Millings, 2016), suggesting that self-support as people learn the difficult skill of mindfulness meditation helps prevent them from becoming discouraged and giving up.

Self-Compassion and Motivation

Although some people worry that self-compassion leads to complacency, there is ample empirical evidence to support the idea that self-compassion enhances rather than undermines motivation. For instance, while self-compassion is negatively related to perfectionism, it has no association with the level of performance standards adopted for the self (Neff, 2003a). Self-compassionate people aim just as high, but also recognize and accept that they can't always reach their goals. Brief self-compassion training has been shown to increase personal initiative—that is, the desire to reach one's full potential (Dundas, Binder, Hansen, & Stige, 2017). Self-compassionate people have been found to have less motivational anxiety and engage in fewer self-handicapping behaviors such as procrastination than those who lack self-compassion (Sirois, 2014; Williams, Stark, & Foster, 2008). They are less likely to suffer from the so-called "imposter phenomenon," which can inhibit achievement motivation in academic contexts (Patzak, Kollmayer, & Schober, 2017). They are also more likely to remain positive when encountering difficulties in job searches (Kreemers, van Hooft, & van Vianen, 2018). In addition, Neff and colleagues (2005) found that self-compassion is positively associated with mastery goals (the intrinsic motivation to learn and grow) and negatively associated with performance goals (the desire to enhance one's self-image; Dweck, 1986). Thus self-compassionate people are motivated to achieve, but for intrinsic reasons, not because they want to garner social approval. A longitudinal study examined the impact of incoming college freshmen's self-compassion on their reactions to thwarted goal progress over their first school year (Hope et al., 2014). They found that higher levels of self-compassion predicted lower levels of negative affect on days when goals weren't achieved. The study also found that self-compassionate students were more concerned with whether their goals were personally meaningful than with goal success. Thus self-compassion appears to help individuals relate to goals wisely, with less attachment to outcomes.

Self-compassionate people have been found to have less fear of failure (Neff et al., 2005), and when they do fail, they're more likely to try again

(Neely et al., 2009). In this way, self-compassion allows people to learn from failure rather than being debilitated by it. For instance, a series of studies were conducted to examine the impact of self-compassion on the way that people think about past behavior that they regret (Zhang & Chen, 2016). One study coded the level of self-compassion displayed in spontaneous descriptions of regret experiences on a blog, and found that those who described their experience with greater self-compassion were also judged as having expressed more personal improvement. A second study found that higher trait self-compassion predicted greater self-reported and observer-rated personal improvement derived from recalled regret experiences. The third study helped people to take a compassionate and understanding perspective toward a recalled regret experience, and found that they reported more personal improvement than those in two control conditions ("Validate your positive qualities" or "Think about a hobby you enjoy"). Overall, these results suggested that self-compassion spurs positive growth in the face of regrets.

Another study examined how self-compassion would affect motivation to learn after failure (Breines & Chen, 2012). Students were given a difficult vocabulary test that they all did poorly on. One group of students were told to be self-compassionate about the failure; one group was given a self-esteem boost (e.g., "You must be smart if you got into this university"); and one group was given no instructions. The students were next told that they would receive a second vocabulary test, and were given a list of words and definitions they could study for as long as they wanted before taking it. Study time was used as a measure of improvement motivation. The students who were told to be self-compassionate after failing the first test spent more time studying than those in the other two conditions. And study time was linked to how well participants actually performed on the test. These findings suggest that being kind to ourselves when we fail or make mistakes gives us the emotional support needed to try our best, and to keep trying even when discouraged. They also suggest that self-compassion helps foster the type of grit and resilience in the face of failure that researchers are learning is key to life success (Duckworth, 2016).

Research indicates that self-compassion also increases motivation in athletic contexts. Self-compassionate individuals have been found to be more intrinsically motivated to exercise, and their goals for exercising are more related to health than to ego-linked concerns such as being better than others (Magnus, Kowalski, & McHugh, 2010; Mosewich, Kowalski, Sabiston, Sedgwick, & Tracy, 2011). Research has also found that self-compassionate athletes have more constructive reactions (i.e., positive, perseverant, and responsible) and fewer maladaptive reactions (i.e., ruminative, passive, and self-critical) to emotionally difficult sport situations (Ferguson, Kowalski, Mack, & Sabiston, 2015). Moreover, Mosewich and colleagues (2013) found that 1 week of self-compassion training was effective in helping athletes to react in more productive ways (less self-criticism, rumination, and concern over mistakes) to sport setback experiences.

Although some may worry that self-compassion means "letting ourselves off the hook," research suggests that self-compassion also increases the motivation to take personal responsibility for our actions. In one study, for instance, participants were asked to recall a recent action they felt guilty about (e.g., cheating on an exam, lying to a romantic partner, saying something harmful) that *still* made them feel bad about themselves when they thought about it (Breines & Chen, 2012). The researchers found that participants who were helped to be self-compassionate about their recent transgression reported being more motivated to apologize for the harm done and more committed to not repeating the behavior than those in two control conditions reported themselves as being. A similar study examined the link between students' self-compassion and acceptance of their own moral transgressions in two cultures—China and the United States (Wang, Chen, Poon, Teng, & Jin, 2017). Results indicated that in both cultures, increased self-compassion was linked to a lessened tendency to be accepting of actions such as stealing or plagiarism, or else displaying selfish behavior in a game task. So while self-compassion increases acceptance of the self, it does not result in accepting bad behavior.

Only one set of studies found an exception to this pattern (Baker & McNulty, 2011). The researchers were interested in examining the links among gender, conscientiousness, self-compassion, and the tendency to repair interpersonal mistakes in romantic relationships (e.g., to figure out solutions to problems). While conscientious men who were self-compassionate were more likely to repair mistakes, unconscientious men who were self-compassionate were less likely to do so. This suggests that these men used self-compassion as an excuse for not doing the right thing. It should be noted that self-compassionate people are typically more conscientious. Thus, given that this is a unique finding with an unusual subset of individuals (men high in self-compassion and low in conscientiousness), caution should be used in generalizing results. Still, it is a useful reminder that anything can be misused if one's intentions are not true.

Self-Compassion and Health

The commonly held fear that self-compassion may lead to self-indulgence is countered by research showing that self-compassion promotes health-related behaviors (Biber & Ellis, 2017; Homan & Sirois, 2017). For instance, research suggests that self-compassion is an important feature of healthy aging (Allen & Leary, 2014; Brown, Huffman, Bryant, 2018), and that elderly people who are self-compassionate are more likely to seek medical treatment when needed (Terry & Leary, 2011) or to use assistive devices such as walkers (Allen, Goldwasser, & Leary, 2012). In a series of three studies, researchers found that self-compassionate individuals were more motivated to stay healthy and to seek medical attention for health problems than were those who lacked self-compassion (Terry, Leary, Mehta, & Henderson, 2013). Moreover, they found that motivated self-kindness and benevolent self-talk mediated the link between self-compassion and proactive health behaviors. Self-compassion is linked to greater feelings of health self-efficacy (i.e., confidence in being able to carry out actions important for taking care of one's health), as well as actual healthy behaviors such as eating balanced meals, regular physical activity, and getting enough sleep (Sirois & Hirsch, 2019; Sirois, Kitner, & Hirsch, 2015). Self-compassion is associated with greater dietary adherence among those with celiac disease (Dowd & Jung, 2017), and greater self-care among those with diabetes (Ferrari, Dal Cin, & Steele, 2017). In fact, a large multinational study of individuals living with HIV/AIDS found that those with greater self-compassion were less likely to engage in risky behaviors such as having unprotected sex (Rose et al., 2014).

Self-compassion also appears to help people stop or reduce smoking. Individuals who were taught to be compassionate about the difficulties of giving up smoking through 3 weeks of compassion-focused therapy reduced their smoking to a greater extent than those trained to reflect upon and monitor their smoking (Kelly, Zuroff, Foa, & Gilbert, 2009). The self-compassion intervention was especially effective among those who were highly self-critical or resistant to change. Other research suggests that self-compassionate individuals are less likely to be addicted to chocolate (Diac, Constantinescu, Sefter, Raşia, & Târgoveçu, 2017), and that increasing self-compassion helps alcohol-dependent individuals drink less (Brooks, Kay-Lambkin, Bowman, & Childs, 2012).

Self-Compassion, Stress, and Coping

Self-compassion has been shown to be an effective way to cope with difficult and stressful emotional experiences (Allen & Leary, 2010). For instance, self-compassion appears to be key in helping people adjust after divorce. Researchers asked divorcing adults to complete a 4-minute stream-of-consciousness recording about their separation experience, and independent judges rated how self-compassionate their dialogues were. Those who displayed greater self-compassion when talking about their breakups evidenced better psychological adjustment not only at the time, but over 9 months (Sbarra et al., 2012). Self-compassion has also been found to aid adjustment to university life: Undergraduates with higher levels of self-compassion have been shown to experience less psychological distress when confronted with academic pressure and social difficulties (Kyeong, 2013), and also have fewer feelings of homesickness during their first semester at college (Terry, Leary, & Metta, 2013). A longitudinal study (Gunnell et al., 2017) found that changes in self-compassion among college freshmen were associated with changes in well-being, in part because self-compassion was linked to greater psychological need satisfaction.

Research indicates that self-compassion is also a powerful tool for successfully coping with a variety of health challenges. For instance, self-compassionate individuals have been shown to maintain more emotional balance, function better in daily life, and subjectively perceive less pain as a result of chronic pain (Costa & Pinto-Gouveia, 2011; Wren et al., 2012). Similarly, self-compassion was related to better adjustment, including lower stress, anxiety, and shame, among individuals living with HIV (Brion et al., 2014) and those diagnosed with cancer (Gillanders, Sinclair, MacLean, & Jardine, 2015). In fact, research indicates that self-compassion helps women deal with their breast cancer treatment, including less psychological distress and greater adjustment to cancer-related body changes (Przez-dziecki et al., 2013). Self-compassion has also been linked to resilience in adults with spina bifida (Hayter & Dorstyn, 2013) and multiple sclerosis (Nery-Hurwit, Yun, & Ebbeck, 2017). Similarly, self-compassion appears to be a buffer against infertility-related stress (Galhardo, Cunha, Pinto-Gouveia, & Matos, 2013). Sirois, Molnar, and Hirsch (2015) found that individuals with chronic illness with more self-compassion experienced less stress because they had more adaptive coping styles (e.g., positively reframing or accepting the situation) and fewer maladaptive coping styles (e.g., giving up or blaming oneself). Self-compassion has also been shown to benefit couples coping with volvodynia in terms of their psychological, sexual, and relationship adjustment (Santerre-Baillargeon et al., 2018).

Perhaps not surprisingly, self-compassion appears to be an important protective factor for posttraumatic stress (Beaumont, Galpin, & Jenkins, 2012; Thompson & Waltz, 2008). For instance, when the mental health functioning of combat veterans returning from their tours in Iraq or Afghanistan was examined, researchers found that more self-compassionate veterans had better functioning in daily life, including fewer symptoms of posttraumatic stress disorder (PTSD) as a result of combat exposure (Dahm et al., 2015). In fact, having low levels of self-compassion was found to be a stronger predictor of developing PTSD symptoms than experiencing high levels of combat exposure itself was (Hiraoka et al., 2015). Encouragingly, it was found that a 12-week loving-kindness training course reduced depression and PTSD symptoms in veterans, and that the increased self-compassion associated with the training helped to explain these improvements (Kearney et al., 2013). One study examined the mental health of adolescents shortly after a major forest fire that destroyed part of their community, and found that youths with more self-compassion had fewer symptoms of PTSD, panic, depression, and suicidality 6 months later (Zeller, Yuval, Nitzan-Assayag, & Bernstein, 2015). Finally, greater emotional regulation skills appeared to be the mechanism by which self-compassion predicted lessened PTSD symptoms among women who had experienced severe and repeated interpersonal trauma (Scoglio et al., 2018). Taken as a whole, this body of research confirms that self-compassion is a strength that helps one cope with life's biggest challenges.

Self-Compassion, Body Image, and Disordered Eating

A systematic review of the literature found evidence that self-compassion is associated with more positive body image and reduced disordered eating symptomatology (Braun et al., 2016). Studies have found that higher levels of self-compassion are associated with less body dissatisfaction, less body shame, and fewer body image concerns (Daye, Webb, & Jafari, 2014; Ferreira, Pinto-Gouveia, & Duarte, 2013; Mosewich et al., 2011; Przedzziecki et al., 2013; Wasylkiw, MacKinnon, & MacLellan, 2012; Webb, Fiery, & Jafari, 2016). Self-compassion also appears to be negatively related to social appearance comparisons—that is, the tendency to assess social attractiveness by comparing one's physical appearance to others (Duarte, Ferreira, Trindade, & Pinto-Gouveia, 2015; Homan & Tylka, 2015). Moreover, self-compassion appears to be a more adaptive response than self-esteem to appearance concerns. Moffitt, Neumann, and Williamson (2018) found that enhancing self-compassion after a body image threat reduced body dissatisfaction and increased self-improvement motivation, compared to a self-esteem enhancement condition. In addition to reducing body dissatisfaction, self-compassion appears to enhance women's ability to appreciate their bodies (Homan & Tylka, 2015; Marta-Simões, Ferreira, & Mendes, 2016; Pisitsungkagarn, Taephant, & Attasaranya, 2013; Wasylkiw et al., 2012). *Body appreciation* refers to the extent to which women like, accept, and respect their bodies despite weight, shape, and imperfections and is a positive psychological strength that has been linked to optimism and life satisfaction (Avalos, Tylka, & Wood-Barcalow, 2005). By embracing an imperfect body with compassion, an individual has more ability to be grateful for its gifts.

It appears that people can be taught to be more self-compassionate toward their bodies. For instance, a brief self-compassion writing intervention was found to help breast cancer survivors have a more self-compassionate attitude to a memory of a distressing body image–related event and experience less negative affect as a result (Przedzziecki & Sherman, 2016). A 3-week period of self-compassion meditation training was found to improve body satisfaction in a multigenerational group of women

(Albertson et al., 2015). Results suggested that compared to a wait-list control group, intervention participants experienced significantly greater reductions in body dissatisfaction, body shame, and self-worth contingent on appearance, as well as greater gains in body appreciation. All improvements were maintained when participants were assessed 3 months later. A study examining the impact of self-compassion meditation on body image (using the same methods as Albertson et al., 2015) found that only 1 week of training increased body appreciation and lessened appearance-contingent self-worth and body surveillance, compared to findings for wait-list controls (Toole & Craighead, 2016). Use of a cellphone app called BodiMojo designed to help adolescents have self-compassion toward their bodies increased appearance-related self-esteem (Rodgers et al., 2018).

Self-compassion is also a buffer against eating pathology. It has been linked to less severe binge eating (Webb & Forman, 2013), as well as lower levels of disordered eating in women with clinical eating disorders (Ferreira et al., 2013). A series of longitudinal studies (Kelly & Carter, 2014; Kelly, Carter, & Borairi, 2014; Kelly, Carter, Zuroff, & Borairi, 2013) found that gains in self-compassion early in eating disorder treatment predicted subsequent reduction in disordered eating. A daily diary designed to examine the link between self-compassion and disordered eating in college students found that less disordered eating behaviors were observed on days when participants reported higher levels of self-compassion toward their appearance (Breines, Toole, et al., 2014). Thus self-compassion appears to help individuals adopt healthier eating behaviors. Moreover, this skill can be taught.

In one study, patients with binge-eating disorder were randomly assigned to a treatment condition based on self-compassion, to cognitive-behavioral therapy, or to a wait-list control (Kelly & Carter, 2015). The self-compassion intervention was most effective in reducing eating pathology, weight, and eating concerns. Another study helps demonstrate *how* self-compassion encourages healthier eating. Dieters often display a paradoxical tendency: If they break their diet and eat high-calorie foods, they tend to eat more afterward as a way to reduce bad feelings associated with their lapse (Heatherton & Polivy, 1990). Adams and Leary (2007) conducted a study in which female undergraduates had to eat a doughnut (under the guise of eating habits research). After eating the doughnut, half of the participants were given this additional instruction: "Several people have told me that they feel bad about eating doughnuts in this study, so I hope you won't be hard on yourself. Everyone eats unhealthily sometimes, and everyone in this study eats this stuff, so I don't think there's any reason to feel really bad about it." Those in the control condition weren't told anything. The researchers found that among women who were dieting, those who were in the control condition reported feeling guilty, ashamed, and so on. Moreover, when they were later given the opportunity to eat as much candy as they wanted as part of a "taste-testing" session, they ate more than participants in other groups (even more than nondieters). Dieters who were encouraged to be self-compassionate about eating the doughnut, on the other hand, were kinder to themselves and less upset after eating the doughnut. They also ate less candy during the taste-testing session than others. Thus being self-compassionate appears to help people stick to healthy eating goals.

Group Differences in Self-Compassion

It appears that self-compassion levels may vary across people of different ages, genders, and cultures. For instance, a meta-analysis (Yarnell et al., 2015) found that self-compassion increased with age, and that women were less self-compassionate than men. The effect sizes were quite small, however. Although the reasons for these differences are unclear, it could be that at earlier ages (most of the younger populations included in the analyses were college undergraduates), individuals are less accepting of themselves as they strive to find their place in the world. The gender difference might be due to the fact that females tend to be more self-critical and to have a more ruminative coping style than males do (Leadbeater, Kuperminc, Blatt, & Hertzog, 1999; Nolen-Hoeksema, Larson, & Grayson, 1999). The meta-analysis also found a significant interaction between age and gender, however, so that gender differences were apparent at earlier but not older ages. Thus it may be that with increasing age and maturity, women learn skills of self-kindness to counteract their self-criticism. Interestingly, an interaction of age and gender has also been found in self-compassion levels among adolescents (Bluth & Blanton, 2015). Older female adolescents in high school tend to have less self-compassion than younger female adolescents in middle school, and only older females report less self-compassion than males (Bluth, Campo, Futch, & Gaylord, 2016). These findings suggest that late adolescence is particularly challenging for females in terms of self-compassion—a situation perhaps linked to the types of popularity and body image concerns highlighted in the film *Mean Girls* (Michaels & Waters, 2004). Luckily, however, these differences tend to dissipate over time.

Also, it is important to take the complexity of gender into account when sex differences in self-compassion are considered. For instance, it appears that women who endorse more androgynous gender role norms do not suffer from lower levels of self-compassion than men; it is mainly feminine women who account for the difference (Yarnell, Neff, Davidson, & Mullarkey, 2018). It is likely that feminine norms of self-sacrifice lead women to pay less attention to their own needs. Similarly, men who more strongly conform to masculine gender role norms have lower levels of self-compassion, suggesting that adherence to traditional expectations for male behavior such as emotional control and dominance may undermine men's ability to be self-compassionate (Reilly, Rochlen, & Awad, 2014). Heath, Brenner, Vogel, Lannin, and Strass (2017) found that self-compassion moderated the link between masculine norm adherence and barriers for men to seeking mental health counseling, with more self-compassionate men being less likely to experience help-seeking self-stigma or to fear self-disclosure to a counselor. Thus the interaction of self-compassion and gender role norms is complex and likely bidirectional.

There has been very little research examining differences in self-compassion based on other demographic characteristics. A study of college undergraduates seeking services at their college mental health centers (participants came from 10 different universities located in six different states across the United States) found that self-compassion levels did not differ by race/ethnicity, sexual orientation, or year in college (Lockard, Hayes, Neff, & Locke, 2014). However, lesbian, gay, bisexual, transgender, and queer (LGBTQ) individuals who are fully "out" have higher levels of self-compassion (Crews & Crawford, 2015), and self-compassion is linked to greater happiness in this group (Greene & Britton, 2015).

There also appear to be cross-cultural variation in self-compassion, but it is not a simple East–West difference. One study examined self-compassion levels in Thailand, Taiwan, and the United States, and found that self-compassion was highest in Thailand and lowest in Taiwan, with the United States falling in between (Neff et al., 2008). This may be because Thais are strongly influenced by Buddhism, and the value of compassion is emphasized in parenting practices and everyday interactions in Thailand. In contrast, the Taiwanese are more influenced by Confucianism, with shame and self-criticism emphasized as a means of parental and social control. Perhaps Americans in this study had more moderate levels of self-compassion, due to the mixed messages American culture gives in terms of positive self-regard (e.g., a strong emphasis on self-esteem, but also an isolating, competitive ethos). In fact, Americans had significantly higher levels of self-esteem than those in the other two groups. In all three cultures, however, greater self-compassion significantly predicted less depression and greater life satisfaction, suggesting that there may be universal benefits to self-compassion despite cultural differences in its prevalence.

Self-Compassion in Relationships

While there is evidence that self-compassion psychologically benefits the individual, there is also evidence that self-compassion benefits interpersonal relationships. In a study of heterosexual couples (Neff & Beretvas, 2013), self-compassionate individuals were described by their partners as being more emotionally connected, accepting, and autonomy-supporting, and as being less detached, controlling, and verbally or physically aggressive, than those lacking self-compassion. Self-compassion was also associated with greater relationship satisfaction and attachment security. Because self-compassionate people give themselves care and support, they appear to have more emotional resources available to give to their partners. The trait of self-compassion negatively predicts romantic jealousy—an association that is partially explained by a greater willingness to forgive one's partner (Tandler & Petersen, 2018). Self-compassion also appears to help romantic couples in which one partner is diagnosed with lung cancer: One study found that individuals with more self-compassion reported less distress and better communication about the cancer (Schellekens et al., 2016). Moreover, at the dyadic level, self-compassion was less strongly associated with distress if one's partner reported high self-compassion. In other words, when one partner displays less self-compassion, the other partner may compensate by showing more self-compassion, which helps alleviate distress in both partners.

Research has found that self-compassionate college students tend to have more compassionate goals in relationships with friends and roommates, meaning that they tend to provide social support and encourage interpersonal trust with relationship partners (Crocker & Canevello, 2008; Wayment, West, & Craddock, 2016). Other research (Yarnell & Neff, 2013) has found that self-compassionate individuals are more likely to compromise in conflict situations with mothers, fathers, and romantic partners, while those lacking self-compassion tended to subordinate their needs to partners. This pattern makes sense, given that people with high levels of self-compassion say they tend to be as kind to themselves as to others, but people with low levels of self-compassion say they tend to be kinder to others than to themselves (Neff, 2003a). The study also showed that self-compassionate people felt more authentic and experienced less turmoil when resolving relationship conflicts, and reported a greater sense of well-being in their relationships. Similarly, self-compassion is linked to less pathological concern for others, defined as an overinvestment in satisfying others' needs and the tendency to repress or deny one's own needs (Gerber, Tolmacz, & Doron, 2015). Finally, self-compassion has been associated with the tendency to apologize for and repair past relationship harms (Breines & Chen, 2012; Howell, Dopko, Turowski, & Buro, 2011; Vazeou-Nieuwenhuis & Schumann, 2018), which also facilitates harmony within relationships.

A set of two studies further illustrates how self-compassion affects the ways that people make and accept apologies in interpersonal relationships (Allen, Barton, & Stevenson, 2015). The first study examined imagined responses to hypothetical scenarios in which participants unintentionally let someone down (e.g., being 45 minutes late to pick up a close friend's child from school, due to a work emergency); it found that self-compassionate individuals said they would be more likely to make statements to the person they let down that reflected self-compassion for making the mistake (e.g., "Sometimes situations come up that prevent you from doing what you wanted to do") versus self-critical statements (e.g., "I feel like a horrible human being, letting you down when you trusted me"). A second study examined how people would ideally want another to respond if they had been unintentionally let down—with self-compassionate or self-critical statements made about the mistake—using hypothetical scenarios similar to those used in the first study. The researchers found that self-compassionate participants preferred self-compassionate responses and were just as likely to forgive someone, regardless of the type of response offered. Less self-compassionate people, however, preferred and were more likely to forgive someone who made self-critical statements. This suggests that although self-compassion may be an adaptive internal response when letting others down, it may actually be more functional to be *outwardly* self-critical about making mistakes when dealing with others who are self-critical.

Self-Compassion and Other-Focused Concern

An interesting question concerns whether or not self-compassion is linked to compassion for others. Cultivating an openhearted stance toward oneself that recognizes human interconnectedness should theoretically facilitate being kind, forgiving, and empathetic toward others. Although more research on this topic is needed, preliminary findings suggest that self-compassion *is* linked to other-focused concern, but that this link differs somewhat according to age and life experience.

A study by Neff and Pommier (2013) examined the link between self-compassion and other-focused concern among college undergraduates, an older community sample, and individuals practicing Buddhist meditation. In all three groups, self-compassionate people were less likely to experience personal distress, meaning that they were more able to confront others' suffering without being overwhelmed. In addition, self-compassion was significantly associated with greater forgiveness and perspective taking. These behaviors require understanding the vast web of causes and conditions that lead people to act as they do. The ability to forgive and understand one's flawed humanity, therefore, appears also to apply to others. Self-compassion was significantly but weakly linked to compassion for others, empathetic concern, and altruism among the community and Buddhist samples. This association is probably not as robust as might be expected because of the fact that the large majority of people are more compassionate to others than to themselves (Knox et al., 2016), attenuating the association. Interestingly, no link was found between self-compassion and other-focused concern (i.e., compassion, empathetic concern and altruism) among undergraduates. This may be because young adults often struggle to recognize the shared aspects of their life experience, overestimating their distinctiveness from others (Lapsley, FitzGerald, Rice, & Jackson, 1989). Their beliefs about why they are deserving of care and why others are deserving of care are therefore likely to be poorly integrated. The link between self-compassion and other-focused concern was strongest among meditators, which may be the result of practices like loving-kindness meditation that are intentionally designed to cultivate compassion for self and others (Hofmann et al., 2011). In fact, people trained in loving-kindness meditation have been shown to increase in compassion for both themselves and others (Weibel, 2008). Research on the MSC program (see Chapter 4) has also found that training in self-compassion increases compassion for self and others (Neff & Germer, 2013). This suggests that although it is possible to have compassion for others without having compassion for oneself, increasing self-compassion tends to increase compassion for others.

Other research suggests that increasing self-compassion can enhance altruistic behavior. For instance, one study found that increasing self-compassion through a self-affirmation writing procedure led to more helping behavior in response to a laboratory shelf collapse incident (e.g., picking up fallen items after a shelf "accidentally" collapsed when the experimenter was out of the room; Lindsay & Creswell, 2014). Another study found that individuals high in self-compassion were more willing to help others whose predicament was partly their own fault (Welp & Brown, 2014). Perhaps because self-compassionate people see making mistakes as part of the human condition, their willingness to help overrides judgments of blame. Taken as a whole, this body of research suggests that self-compassion helps engender interpersonal concern for others.

Self-Compassion for Caregivers

Research indicates that self-compassion is an important asset for caregivers (Raab, 2014). For instance, greater self-compassion is associated with less *caregiver fatigue* (the negative feelings of stress and burnout that arise when resonating with the pain of patients) and with greater *compassion satisfaction* (the positive feelings experienced from one's work, such as feeling energized, happy, and grateful for being able to make a difference in the world) among caregivers in various professions, such as therapists, nurses, pediatric residents, doctoral trainees, midwives, and clergy (Atkinson, Rodman, Thuras, Shiroma, & Lim, 2017; Barnard & Curry, 2012; Beaumont, Durkin, Hollins Martin, & Carson, 2016a, 2016b; Durkin, Beaumont, Hollins Martin, & Carson, 2016; Olson, Kemper, & Mahan, 2015; Richardson, Trusty, & George, 2018; Ringenbach, 2009). Higher levels of self-compassion were linked to personal resilience among physicians (Trockel,

Hamidi, Murphy, de Vries, & Bohman, 2017) and to less sleep disturbance among health care professionals, even after stress levels were controlled for (Kemper, Mo, & Khayat, 2015). Research indicates that self-compassion is also helpful for informal caregivers. For instance, among those caring for an elderly person with dementia, self-compassion was linked to lessened feelings of caregiver burden and more functional coping strategies for caregiver stress (Lloyd, Muers, Patterson, & Marczak, 2018). Similarly, a study of parents of children with autism found that higher levels of self-compassion were linked to less stress and depression, as well as more life satisfaction and hope (Neff & Faso, 2014). Self-compassion was actually a stronger predictor of parental adjustment than the autism symptom severity itself, suggesting that more important than the degree of the caregiving challenge parents face is how they relate to themselves in the midst of that challenge.

Luckily, research suggests that self-compassion can be trained in caregivers. A study of healthcare professionals found that mindfulness training increased participants' self-compassion, which in turn predicted reductions in their stress levels (Shapiro, Astin, Bishop, & Cordova, 2005). Moreover, 6 weeks of online self-compassion instruction decreased stress and improved emotion regulation and well-being among therapists in training (Finlay-Jones et al., 2015). Thus giving oneself compassion appears to provide the emotional resources needed to care for others.

Caring for others, on the other hand, may help people know *how* to be self-compassionate. Research suggests one way that people learn to be self-compassionate is by modeling inner supportive dialogues on the more familiar experience of giving support to others. In a series of four experiments, Breines and Chen (2013) examined the hypothesis that activating support-giving schemas can increase state self-compassion. In the first two studies, participants first recalled a past negative event or experienced a lab-based test failure; they were then randomly assigned to recall an experience of giving support versus having fun with another person; and, finally, they completed a measure of state self-compassion. Those who remembered giving support were more self-compassionate. The second two experiments examined the effects of actually giving support to another person (via written advice), compared to not giving support or simply reading about another's problem, and found that this also resulted in a greater ability to be self-compassionate.

Self-Compassion and Early Family History

Research suggests that early family experiences may play a key role in the development of self-compassion. Attachment history appears to be associated with self-compassion, for instance; insecure attachment has been linked to lower levels of self-compassion than secure attachment (e.g.,

Joeng et al., 2017; Mackintosh, Power, Schwannauer, & Chan, 2018; Raque-Bogdan, Ericson, Jackson, Martin, & Bryan, 2011; Wei, Liao, Ku, & Shaffer, 2011). Although most of this research is correlational, it has been found that experimentally priming attachment security (e.g., asking individuals to visualize a particular person with whom they feel comfortable and safe, and to whom they can turn when they are upset) increases state self-compassion, suggesting a causal relationship (Pepping, Davis, O'Donovan, & Pal, 2015). Similarly, early memories of warmth and safety are positively linked to self-compassion (Kearney & Hicks, 2016; Marta-Simões, Ferreira, & Mendes, 2018), whereas parental rejection, criticism, overprotection, and stressful family relationships are negatively related to self-compassion (Neff & McGehee, 2010; Pepping et al., 2015).

Not surprisingly, childhood emotional abuse is associated with lower levels of self-compassion (Barlow, Turow, & Gerhart, 2017), and individuals with a trauma history who have low self-compassion experience more emotional distress and are more likely to abuse alcohol or make a serious suicide attempt (Tanaka, Wekerle, Schmuck, Paglia-Boak, & MAP Research Team, 2011). Research suggests that lessened self-compassion is an important pathway by which early trauma creates later dysfunction. For instance, self-compassion has been found to mediate the link between childhood maltreatment and later emotional dysregulation (Vettese, Dyer, Li, & Wekerle, 2011) and PTSD symptoms (Barlow et al., 2017). Similarly, self-compassion was found to mediate the link between perceived parental maltreatment (abuse or indifference) and mental health symptom severity among adults in psychotherapy (Westphal, Leahy, Pala, & Wupperman, 2016). This may indicate that people with trauma histories who learn to have compassion for themselves may be able to deal with their past in a more productive manner. In fact, self-compassion is linked to greater post-traumatic growth and healing (Wong & Yeung, 2017). However, survivors of childhood maltreatment often experience greater fear of self-compassion (Boykin et al., 2018), a concept related to *backdraft* as defined in MSC (see Chapter 11). This can be a significant barrier to developing this resource.

Self-Compassion in Clinical Populations

Compared to self-compassion levels in the general population, these levels tend to be lower among individuals meeting criteria for mental health conditions such as bipolar disorder (Døssing et al., 2015), depression (Krieger et al., 2013), generalized anxiety disorder (Hoge et al., 2013), social anxiety disorder (Werner et al., 2012), substance use disorder (Phelps, Paniagua, Willcockson, & Potter, 2018), or persecutory delusions (Collett, Pugh, Waite, & Freeman, 2016). Research also suggests that variation in self-compassion helps to explain the degree of mental health experienced in clinical populations. For instance, higher levels of self-compassion are associated with lessened symptomatology among individuals with schizophrenia (Eicher, Davis, & Lysaker, 2013), obsessive–compulsive disorder (Wetterneck, Lee, Smith, & Hart, 2013), and generalized anxiety disorder (Hoge et al., 2013). It predicts less fear of negative evaluation among those with social anxiety disorder (Werner et al., 2012), and lessened shame, rumination, and hypersexuality among men diagnosed with hypersexual disorder (Reid, Temko, Moghaddam, & Fong, 2014).

Self-compassion is linked to fewer depressive symptoms in individuals with unipolar depression, and this link is mediated by the ability to tolerate negative emotions (Diedrich et al., 2017). Moreover, it appears that self-compassion can be taught to those with major depressive disorder. In an experimental study, Diedrich and colleagues (2014) induced a depressed mood by having participants read a series of statements (e.g., "I think I am a loser") while sad music played in the background. The participants were then asked to rate their mood. They were next assigned to a waiting condition or to one of three emotion regulation conditions in which they were guided to be self-compassionate, to cognitively reappraise their thinking, or to accept their feelings before rating their mood again. Participants who were initially feeling high levels of depressed mood benefited more from the self-compassion condition than those in either the waiting, cognitive reappraisal, or acceptance condition. Interestingly, a study by the same research group (Diedrich, Hofmann, Cuijpers, & Berking, 2016) found individuals with major depressive disorder who were taught to use self-compassion as a preparatory strategy experienced significantly greater reduction of depressed mood during cognitive reappraisal than those in a waiting control condition, suggesting that these different emotion regulation skills may be mutually supportive.

Change in self-compassion appears to be a key mechanism of therapeutic action (Baer, 2010; Galili-Weinstock et al., 2018; Germer & Neff, 2013). For example, Neff, Kirkpatrick, and Rude (2007) conducted a study that tracked changes in self-compassion experienced by therapy clients over a 1-month interval. Therapists used a Gestalt two-chair technique designed to help clients lessen self-criticism and have greater compassion for themselves (Greenberg, 1983; Safran, 1998). Results indicated that increased self-compassion levels over the month-long period (which were assessed under the guise of an unrelated study) were linked to fewer experiences of self-criticism, depression, rumination, thought suppression, and anxiety. Another study found that self-compassion appeared to play a role in therapeutic outcomes for individuals diagnosed with Cluster C personality disorders (Schanche, Stiles, McCullough, Svartberg, & Nielsen, 2011). Results showed that increases in self-compassion from early to late in therapy significantly predicted pre- to posttreatment decreases in psychiatric symptoms, interpersonal problems, and personality pathology.

An interesting question concerns the directionality of the link between self-compassion and psychopathology over the course of therapy. One study used cross-lagged time analyses to examine the directionality of the link between self-compassion and depressive episodes in outpatients undergoing psychotherapy; this link was assessed directly after therapy, as well as 6 and 12 months later (Krieger, Berger, & Holtforth, 2016). It was found that increases in SCS scores predicted reduced depressive symptoms later, but that depressive symptoms did not predict subsequent levels of self-compassion, suggesting a causal role for self-compassion in reducing depression. Similarly, research has examined whether self-compassion influences the process of change in therapy for patients diagnosed with PTSD (Hoffart, Øktedalen, & Langkaas, 2015). Self-compassion levels were assessed weekly over 10 weeks of treatment, and it was found that changes in self-compassion predicted PTSD symptoms (with gains in self-compassion predicting lessened systems), while the opposite was not true. This suggests that self-compassion may be an important causal agent of therapeutic change.

The Neurophysiology of Self-Compassion

Self-compassion appears to foster physical as well as emotional well-being. For instance, higher levels of self-compassion are linked with fewer self-reported health symptoms such as abdominal pain, skin rashes, earaches, or respiratory problems (Dunne, Sheffield, & Chilcot, 2018; Hall, Row, Wuensch, & Godley, 2013). Higher self-compassion scores are associated with lower levels of hyperarousal—linked to immune dysfunction in the face of stressful events—in individuals diagnosed with the autoimmune disorder scleroderma (Kearney & Hicks, 2016), as well as women diagnosed with breast cancer (Kearney & Hicks, 2017). This latter study also found that self-compassion was linked to later age of onset of the cancer, which the authors suggest may be due to enhanced immune function among self-compassionate individuals. In fact, researchers found that an intervention teaching self-compassion increased immune function as measured by immunoglobulin A (IgA).

An increasing body of research suggests that self-compassion taps into the autonomic nervous system, with self-compassion entailing greater activation of the self-soothing response and lesser activation of the threat response (Kirschner et al., 2019), as proposed by Gilbert (2009). Put another way, self-compassion appears to reduce threat reactions to stress by suppressing sympathetic nervous system activity and increasing parasympathetic activity through the stimulation of the vagus nerve (Porges, 2003). For instance, Rockliff, Gilbert, McEwan, Lightman, and Glover (2008) asked participants to imagine receiving compassion and feeling it in their bodies, and found that this lowered salivary cortisol levels (an indicator of sympathetic nervous system activity) and increased heart rate variability (an indicator of parasympathetic nervous system activity, linked to flexible responding and the ability to self-soothe when stressed; Porges, 2007). Another study (Herriot, Wrosch, & Gouin, 2018) found that higher levels of self-compassion were linked to lower daily cortisol levels among older adults who reported more intense regret, physical health problems, or functional disability. Higher levels of self-compassion are associated with greater vagally mediated heart rate variability (Svendsen et al., 2016), including in response to experimentally induced stress (Luo, Qiao, & Che, 2018). A study that asked participants to think about a recent episode when they were ashamed of or disappointed in themselves, and then to speak to themselves compassionately while looking at a mirror, found that self-compassion increased soothing positive affect and increased heart rate variability (Petrocchi, Ottaviani, & Couyoumdjian, 2016). Higher self-compassion levels have been associated with reduced sympathetic arousal in response to a standard laboratory-based stressor (the Trier Social Stress Test), as assessed via levels of salivary alpha-amylase (Breines et al., 2015) and interleukin-6 (Breines, Thoma, et al., 2014). Similarly, brief training in self-compassion meditation was found to result in diminished salivary alpha-amylase and subjective anxiety responses to stress, while stabilizing heart rate variability compared to control conditions (Arch et al., 2014).

There is preliminary neurological evidence for the link between psychological well-being and self-compassion. Parrish and colleagues (2018) conducted a functional magnetic resonance imaging (fMRI) study and found a negative correlation between ventromedial prefrontal cortex (VMPFC)–amygdala connectivity and overall self-compassion. The VMPFC is thought to directly impact threat-related activity in the amygdala, so VMPFC–amygdala connectivity may be a mechanism by which self-compassion protects against stress and negative emotions. In another fMRI study, Pires and colleagues (2018) found that women managers with greater self-compassion responded to disturbing emotional images with higher activation of the precuneus (a brain region related to self-referential processing), yet were also less stressed and depressed. This suggests that self-compassion may allow individuals to pay greater attention to negative emotions without being overwhelmed by them.

Finally, a study by Friis and colleagues (2015) found that self-compassion levels buffered the negative effect of diabetes-related distress on the hemoglobin A_{1C} (HbA$_{1C}$) test (a test of average blood glucose levels), so that distress did not lead to higher HbA$_{1C}$ levels among those who were more self-compassionate. These same researchers also conducted a randomized controlled trial of the MSC program for patients with diabetes (Friis et al., 2016); they found that participants in MSC had both reduced diabetes-related distress and HbA$_{1C}$ levels compared to a wait-list control group and that these improvements were maintained 3 months later (see Chapter 4). This is the magic of self-compassion: By relating to ourselves in a more supportive manner in times of struggle, we reduce suffering and enhance well-being in both body and mind.

POINTS TO REMEMBER

* The scientific research on self-compassion is expanding at an exponential rate. This body of research is comprised mainly of correlational studies using the SCS, but other research methodologies are increasingly being applied, such as studying self-compassion training outcomes or using experimental mood manipulations. Findings converge across methodologies.

* Research strongly challenges misconceptions about self-compassion. Individuals with high self-compassion tend to:
  * Be more self-confident and motivated to improve after failure.
  * Take greater personal responsibility for mistakes.
  * Engage more readily in health-related behaviors.
  * Have more strength to cope with challenging life circumstances.
  * Experience more caring personal relationships.

* Self-compassion is linked to:
  * Reduced negative states such as depression, anxiety, and shame, and increased positive states like happiness and life satisfaction.
  * Fewer problems related to striving for self-esteem such as narcissism, social comparison, contingent self-worth, and emotional instability.
  * Healthier body image and less disordered eating behaviors.
  * Reduced risk of caregiver burnout.
  * Better physical health and immune function, in part due to increased parasympathetic and reduced sympathetic nervous system activation.

* Women tend to be slightly less self-compassionate than men, though gender role orientation, age, and culture also affect self-compassion.

* While self-compassion is linked to more concern with others, people tend to be more compassionate to others than to themselves.

* Positive early family interactions tend to increase self-compassion, while early trauma tends to reduce self-compassion levels.

* Individuals with clinical disorders tend to have less self-compassion, and increased self-compassion appears to be an important mechanism of change in therapy.

Chapter 4

Teaching Self-Compassion

The individual is capable of both great compassion and great indifference.
We have it within our means to nourish the former and outgrow the latter.
—NORMAN COUSINS (1974/1991, p. 72)

Given that the benefits of self-compassion have been well established, a crucial question concerns whether people can *learn* to be more self-compassionate. The answer is clearly "yes." Research indicates that a variety of methods can enhance self-compassion. This chapter reviews the training research and, wherever possible, the percentage gain in self-compassion (total scores on the SCS) is indicated.

One pathway to self-compassion involves body-based approaches such as yoga. For instance, young adults who participated in a 4-month residential yoga program increased in self-compassion (11%), compared to demographically matched controls, and this increased self-compassion was linked to enhanced quality of life and decreased stress (Gard et al., 2012). A qualitative study of the impact of yoga on self-compassion among victims of sexual abuse (Crews, Stolz-Newton, & Grant, 2016) identified themes indicating that yoga was an important form of self-care. As one participant explained it,

> "Before, I would never do anything for myself. And this is kind of my little time. . . . It's my 'love me' time. It's like relaxing my body and my shoulders and my mind and sometimes it's like I could just take a nap on the mat. You know? It's just that relaxing. . . . You can feel it in your body. . . . So to physically do that and physically see that I'm doing something for my body, it helps me . . . put the band aid on myself. [Yoga] helps me to tell myself that, 'Hey. I'm okay.' " (p. 148)

For these participants, accepting and being gentle with their bodies through yoga was a direct pathway to being accepting and gentle toward themselves as a whole.

Loving-kindness meditation (LKM) also appears to be an effective way to increase self-compassion. LKM involves generating goodwill toward a series of targets—typically the self, a benefactor, a neutral person, a challenging person, and eventually all sentient beings. Phrases such as the following are used to express these good intentions: "May you be safe. May you be happy. May you be peaceful. May you live with ease." LKM may be used to cultivate self-compassion when the object of goodwill is oneself in the midst of suffering (see Chapter 13). In traditional LKM, the "self" is only one of many targets, but time spent wishing oneself well appears to increase self-compassion (see review by Boellinghaus, Jones, & Hutton, 2014). For example, in a pilot study of veterans with PTSD who took a 12-week LKM course, significant increases in self-compassion were found (25%), and these increases helped explain reductions in PTSD symptoms and depression displayed by participants over the course of the training (Kearney et al., 2013). Similarly, a randomized controlled trial (Shahar et al., 2015) found that highly self-critical individuals who took 7 weeks of LKM training showed significant gains in self-compassion (17%), compared to a wait-list control group.

Self-Compassion in Mindfulness- and Acceptance-Based Interventions

Mindfulness-based interventions are another important way to increase self-compassion; this is not surprising, given that mindfulness is a core component of self-compassion. The most widespread mindfulness-based intervention is mindfulness-based stress reduction (MBSR), an experiential learning course that includes eight weekly group sessions, a half-day retreat, and a core curriculum of formal and informal mindfulness meditation practices (Kabat-Zinn, 1990). Mindfulness-based cognitive therapy (MBCT) is an increasingly popular variant on MBSR that has been adapted for clinical use, particularly for the prevention of depressive relapse (Segal et al., 2013). Meta-analytic reviews indicate that MBSR and MBCT lead to significant improvements in physical and psychological functioning in a wide range of populations (Chiesa & Serretti, 2009; Grossman, Niemann, Schmidt, & Walach, 2004; Hofmann, Sawyer, Witt, & Oh, 2010).

There is growing evidence that self-compassion is increased through participation in mindfulness-based interventions. For instance, several studies have found increased scores on the SCS as a result of MBSR (Birnie et al., 2010 [16%]; Evans, Wyka, Blaha, & Allen, 2018 [17%]; Raab et al., 2015 [10%]; Shapiro, Brown, & Biegel, 2007 [16%]) and MBCT (Goodman et al., 2014 [26%]; James & Rimes, 2018 [35%]; Proeve, Anton, & Kenny, 2018 [26%]; Rimes & Wingrove, 2011 [7%]; Taylor, Strauss, Cavanagh, & Jones, 2014 [33%]). Although self-compassion is not a skill explicitly taught in MBSR and MBCT, leaders of these programs often convey implicit messages about the importance of being kind and gentle with oneself, both in responding to participants' questions and by embodying a general quality of emotional warmth. The variability in the amount of self-compassion gained by participants in the above studies may be due partly to variability in teacher warmth, although research is needed to examine this issue. Also, in MBSR, LKM is typically taught on the 1-day silent meditation retreat that is part of the program (Santorelli, Meleo-Meyer, & Koerbel, 2017), and it is known that LKM increases self-compassion. And of course, given that mindfulness is a foundational element of self-compassion, it makes sense that being mindful of negative thoughts and emotions also increases the ability to be self-compassionate.

One of the main ways in which MBSR and MBCT may increase self-compassion is by feeling the care and support of other group members. In a qualitative study of MBCT (Allen, Bromley, Kuyken, & Sonnenberg, 2009), for instance, one participant (p. 420) wrote: "I didn't feel guilty. I think it's a feeling of safety, that everyone else has got the same problems, and that you could go to that group, and know that nobody was going to say 'oh snap out of it', or . . . everybody understood what you felt like."

Some researchers have proposed that self-compassion may be a key mechanism by which mindfulness-based interventions improve well-being (Baer, 2010; Evans et al., 2018; Hölzel et al., 2011; Wyka, Blaha, & Allen, 2018). In support of this idea, health care professionals who took an MBSR program reported significantly increased self-compassion (22%) and reduced stress, compared to a wait-list control group; the gains in self-compassion mediated the reductions in stress associated with the program (Shapiro et al., 2005). A similar study found that people who participated in MBSR reported significant gains in self-compassion (24%) compared to a wait-list control group, and that gains in self-compassion mediated the program's effects on worry and fear of emotion (Keng, Smoski, Robins, Ekblad, & Brantley, 2012). Kuyken and colleagues (2010) compared the effects of MBCT to those of maintenance antidepressants on relapse in depression and found that increases in mindfulness and self-compassion (12%) both mediated the link between MBCT and depressive symptoms at a 15-month follow-up. However, they found that increased self-compassion, but not mindfulness, reduced the link between cognitive reactivity and depressive relapse. Greenberg and colleagues (2018) also found that MBCT increased self-compassion (24%), and that increased self-compassion predicted depressive improvement in MBCT, particularly by protecting against the negative effects of mind wandering.

Self-compassion is also implicitly taught in acceptance and commitment therapy (ACT), a popular, mindfulness-based therapy model (Neff & Tirch, 2013). Many of the main principles of ACT encourage being kind and compassionate to oneself. For instance, the principle of acceptance includes acceptance of one's personal shortcomings and painful experiences; de-fusion includes building awareness of self-critical thinking; the notion of self-as-context leads to more flexible, empathic ways of relating to oneself; and core values often emphasize self-kindness and self-care (Luoma & Platt, 2015). A randomized controlled trial that compared a 6-hour ACT-based workshop targeting self-compassion to a wait-list control found that it significantly increased self-compassion (23%), while reducing general psychological distress and anxiety (Yadavaia, Hayes, & Vilardaga, 2014). Moreover, the increased psychological flexibility that emerged from the ACT training was a significant mediator of changes in self-compassion and other outcomes. Similarly, Web-based ACT training (Viskovich & Pakenham, 2018) was found to increase self-compassion (12%) in college students.

Although mindfulness-based interventions have been shown to increase self-compassion, these programs do not explicitly teach self-compassion skills, focusing primarily on enhancing the skill of mindfulness. In a study by Hildebrandt, McCall, and Singer (2017; raw data provided by first author), researchers found that affect training with an explicit emphasis on compassion led to a greater increase in self-compassion (8%) than did mindfulness training alone (4%). This suggests that explicitly training self-compassion may help to develop this skill.

For this reason, several interventions have been developed that specifically focus on developing compassion for self and others, and research suggests that these compassion-based interventions are effective at raising self-compassion and enhancing well-being (Kirby, 2017; Kirby, Tellegen, & Steindl, 2017; Møller, Sami, & Shapiro, 2019; Wilson, Mackintosh, Power, & Chan, 2018).

Other Compassion Training Programs

In addition to MSC, there are currently three structured, time-limited, empirically supported programs designed specifically to train compassion. They are compassion cultivation training (CCT; Jazaieri et al., 2013), cognitively-based compassion training (CBCT; Pace et al., 2009), and mindfulness-based compassionate living (MBCL; Bartels-Velthuis et al., 2016; van den Brink & Koster, 2015). There is also compassion-focused therapy (CFT; Gilbert, 2009), a model of psychotherapy with a well-articulated theoretical base and an abundance of practical exercises. Each of these compassion-based programs has a different origin and emphasis and they vary in format and target audience, but they all share the goal of cultivating compassion toward self and others. We now compare and contrast MSC with these programs, noting the unique strengths of each, as well as examining their base of empirical support.

Compassion Cultivation Training

The CCT program was developed by Thupten Jinpa, a leading Tibetan scholar, and colleagues at Stanford University. The focus of CCT is on cultivating omnidirectional compassion. One session of the 8-week program is specifically dedicated to cultivating self-kindness, and another session focuses on self-compassion. The training sequence in CCT is as follows: mindfulness; loving-kindness and compassion for a loved one; loving-kindness and compassion for oneself; cultivation of a sense of common humanity; kindness toward challenging and difficult persons; and finally active compassion. Compassion for oneself permeates CCT, although less prominently than in MSC. Conversely, compassion for others permeates MSC (there are seven practices and class exercises that cultivate compassion for *others*), but this emphasis is less prominent than in CCT. This suggests that the two programs are nonredundant and complementary.

In CCT, a variety of meditations build systematically upon one another, culminating in "active compassion," or Tibetan *tonglen* meditation. In traditional *tonglen* practice, the meditator draws in the suffering of others with the in-breath, imagines the suffering dissolving in one's own radiant heart, and then breathes out compassion to the sufferer. *Tonglen* has been adapted for MSC as the Giving and Receiving Compassion meditation, in which compassion is both inhaled and exhaled—"in for me and out for you." In actual practice, both *tonglen* meditation and Giving and Receiving Compassion provide a sense of breathing suffering *and* compassion both in and out, even though the meditations have different emphases. Both of these meditations also soften the sense of a separate self and cultivate an experience of common humanity.

Research has established the beneficial outcomes of CCT. A randomized controlled trial (Jazaieri et al., 2013) found that CCT decreased fear of giving compassion to others, fear of receiving compassion from others, and fear of self-compassion in participants, compared to a wait-list control group. It also increased self-compassion (15%). Examining the same sample, Jazaieri and colleagues (2014) found that participation in CCT increased mindfulness and happiness, and decreased worry and emotional suppression compared to the control group. In both sets of analyses, amount of formal meditation practice was related to improved outcomes. Two more studies examined this same sample of CCT participants. Jazaieri and colleagues (2016) contacted participants twice a day over the course of the 9-week CCT program to determine how often their minds were wandering to pleasant, neutral, or unpleasant topics, as well as to assess any caring behaviors performed toward oneself or others. Results indicated that compassion meditation decreased mind wandering to neutral topics and increased caring behaviors toward oneself. A path analysis also revealed that greater frequency of compassion meditation practice was related to reductions in mind wandering to unpleasant topics and increases in mind wandering to pleasant topics, both of which were related to increases in caring behaviors for oneself and others. Jazaieri and colleagues (2018) found that CCT participants also increased their acceptance of negative mood states like anxiety or stress and experienced increased feelings of calm over time.

A second randomized wait-list-controlled trial of CCT was conducted in Chile (Brito-Pons, Campos, & Cebolla, 2018). Compared to the wait-list group, CCT participants showed significant improvements in compassion-related outcomes: increased self-compassion (28%), empathic concern, compassion for others, and identification with all of humanity, as well as increased life satisfaction, happiness, and mindfulness and decreased depression, stress, and personal distress. Finally, a pilot study of CCT among health care workers (Scarlet, Altmeyer, Knier, & Harpin, 2017) found significant improvements in participants' self-compassion (16%), fear of compassion, mindfulness, and level of interpersonal conflict experienced at work. In addition, the results indicated marginally significant improvements in self-reported job satisfaction. In summary, these studies suggest that although CCT is primarily focused on developing compassion for others, it also enhances the well-being of the person practicing compassion.

Cognitively-Based Compassion Training

CBCT was originally developed by Lobsang Tenzin Negi, a former Tibetan monk, at Emory University to address stress in university students (Reddy et al., 2013). CBCT is a secularized form of Tibetan *lojong* practice designed to reduce narrowly self-oriented thinking and to broaden and strengthen care and consideration for others. CBCT dedicates its introductory sessions to training in attentional stability and openness to moment-to-moment experience (mindfulness). It then teaches analytical meditations in four modules: self-compassion; common humanity; interdependence, appreciation, and affection; and empathic concern and engaged compassion (Negi, 2009, 2016; Ozawa-de Silva & Dodson-Lavelle, 2011). The analytical modules enlist critical thinking to examine automatic emotional and behavioral reactions that may be misleading and harmful to self and others. Noticing and understanding these patterns, supported by increased attentional stability, enables participants to sustain cognitive insights as well as prosocial affect (such as gratitude and kindness) toward self and others. Self-compassion is understood in CBCT as a healthy motivation to develop realistic and positive attitudes toward difficult life circumstances.

At least nine randomized controlled trials have been conducted on the efficacy of CBCT. For example, Gonzalez-Hernandez and colleagues (2018) examined the impact of CBCT among breast cancer survivors, and found that it increased self-compassion (17%) and decreased stress caused by fear of cancer recurrence. LoParo, Mack, Patterson, Negi, and Kaslow (2018) examined CBCT among African Americans who had attempted suicide, and found that self-compassion significantly increased (8%) compared to a peer support control group. Dodds and colleagues (2015) found that CBCT for women with breast cancer increased mindfulness and physical well-being, and decreased functional impairment, avoidance, and fatigue, compared to a wait-list control group. Mascaro and colleagues (2018) found that CBCT enhanced compassion and improved daily functioning in medical students. Compared to a wait-list control group, students randomly assigned to CBCT reported increased compassion, as well as decreased loneliness and depression. Changes in compassion were most robust in individuals reporting high levels of depression at baseline, suggesting that CBCT may benefit those most in need by breaking the link between personal suffering and a concomitant drop in compassion. Other research on CBCT with adolescents in foster care has found that practice time is associated with decreases in anti-inflammatory markers (salivary C-reactive protein concentration; Pace et al., 2013) and with increased hopefulness (Reddy et al., 2013). Finally, CBCT improved outcomes compared to a control group in terms of increased empathetic accuracy and related neural activity (Mascaro, Rilling, Negi, & Raison, 2013). Taken together, these findings indicate that CBCT is an effective method for increasing compassion and improving psychological and physiological health.

Mindfulness-Based Compassionate Living

MBCL was developed by two pioneering mindfulness teachers in the Netherlands—psychiatrist and psychotherapist Erik van den Brink and meditation teacher Frits Koster—at a mental health center to support clients who benefited from mindfulness practice but felt the need to further develop a kind and compassionate attitude toward themselves. The program is increasingly being offered to the general public and is designed as a deepening course for participants who are already familiar with mindfulness practice, preferably by having taken a course in MBSR, MBCT, or an equivalent.

MBCL is a unique blend of Western and Buddhist psychologies, integrating the work of Paul Gilbert (2009), Tara Brach (2003), and ourselves (Germer, 2009; Neff, 2011a). MBCL combines the evolutionary psychology of CFT, especially the CFT model of emotion regulation and compassionate imagery, with positive psychology and secular adaptations of traditional Buddhist contemplative practices such as *metta* and *tonglen* meditation. Important informal practices in MBCL are the Breathing Spaces with Kindness and Compassion, adapted from MBCT's Three-Minute Breathing Space. Similar to MSC, MBCL explicitly cultivates the qualities of kindness, compassion, appreciative joy, and equanimity. Some elements of MSC found in MBCL include the Self-Compassion Break, the Sense and Savor Walk, the Compassionate Body Scan, Self-Compassion in Daily Life, and the concept of *backdraft*. Perhaps the characteristic that most clearly differentiates MSC and MBCL is the special focus on cultivating *self*-compassion in MSC. It is noteworthy that both MBCL and MSC have been mainly influenced by the mindfulness tradition, whereas the other compassion training programs have a stronger Tibetan flavor. Although it used to be a requirement that participants take a course in MBSR or MBCT before taking MBCL, this requirement has now been relaxed.

A pilot study of psychiatric outpatients taking the nine-session MBCL program after having taken MBCT at a local mindfulness training center found that participants reported improved outcomes in terms of increased self-compassion (13%) and mindfulness as well as reduced depression (Bartels-Velthuis et al., 2016). A second pilot study (Schuling et al., 2018) with recurrently depressed participants also found that MBCL increased self-compassion (14%). Early results from a randomized controlled trial (Schuling, 2018; Schuling et al., 2016), moreover, suggest that compared to a treatment-as-usual control group, individuals with recurrent depression who took MBCL after MBCT reported significantly increased self-compassion (15%), mindfulness, and quality of life, as well as decreased depression and rumination.

Compassion-Focused Therapy

CFT was developed by eminent British psychologist Paul Gilbert (2000, 2005, 2009) to address self-criticism and shame in an inpatient psychiatric hospital population. CFT is based on evolutionary psychology, cognitive-behavioral therapy, and Tibetan Buddhist psychology. CFT includes a wide range of practices known as Compassionate Mind Training (CMT; Gilbert & Proctor, 2006: Matos, Duarte, Duarte, Gilbert, & Pinto-Gouveia, 2018) that are primarily aimed at developing self-compassion, as we might expect from a clinical program where alleviating personal distress is the first order of business. In CFT, mindfulness is used to stabilize attention for the work of compassion training and to "shine a spotlight" on how the human mind functions, especially in response to threat. This form of treatment helps clients develop the skills and attributes of a self-compassionate mind, especially when their more habitual form of self-to-self relating involves shame and self-attack.

CFT increases awareness and understanding of automatic emotional reactions such as self-criticism that have evolved in humans over time, and of how these patterns are often reinforced in early childhood. The key principles of CFT involve helping people to extend warmth and understanding toward themselves; motivating them to care for their own well-being; and helping them to become sensitive to their own needs, tolerate personal distress, and reduce tendencies toward self-judgment (Gilbert, 2009). Although CFT is a type of individual therapy, it is sometimes taught in a time-limited group therapy format, which can vary in length from 4 to 16 weeks.

The development of CFT preceded that of MSC chronologically, and a number of elements from CFT have migrated into MSC, such as learning that the physiology of compassion is rooted in the mammalian caregiving system (see Chapter 10), visualizing an ideal compassionate image to activate compassion (Chapter 17, Compassionate Friend meditation), and attuning to the soothing rhythm of the breath (Chapter 11, Affectionate Breathing meditation). CFT has three different approaches to evoking self-compassion that are also in MSC: namely, self-to-other compassion (i.e., "How would you treat a friend?"), other-to-self compassion (i.e., "What would a compassionate friend say to you?"), and self-to-self compassion (i.e., "What would your compassionate self say right now?"). Psychotherapists who teach MSC tend to be familiar with CFT as well.

There is a large empirical literature on CFT that cannot be adequately covered here (for reviews, see Kirby, 2017; Leaviss & Uttley, 2015). This research suggests that CFT is effective at increasing self-compassion and treating individuals with a wide variety of clinical conditions. For instance, a randomized controlled trial conducted with outpatients with eating disorders found that 12 weeks of CFT led to greater increases in self-compassion (34%) and reductions in shame and eating disorder pathology than did treatment as usual (Kelly et al., 2017). Another randomized trial (Gharraee, Tajrishi, Farani, Bolhari, & Farahani, 2018) found that 12 weeks of CFT increased self-compassion (28%) and quality of life while reducing anxiety symptoms among individuals with social anxiety. A study by Parry and Malpus (2017) found that 8 weeks of CFT increased self-compassion (32%) and reduced depression and anxiety among individuals with persistent pain. Brähler and colleagues (2013) conducted a randomized controlled trial comparing 16 sessions of CFT to treatment as usual among individuals with schizophrenia and found that the CFT group displayed more compassion toward painful aspects of their psychosis and greater clinical improvements, in addition to bigger reductions in depression and perceived social marginalization. In summary, CFT shows a great deal of promise for helping people with various clinical disorders to develop self-compassion, even if their more habitual form of relating to themselves is maladaptive.

Research suggests that CMT practices are also effective for nonclinical populations. Beaumont, Rayner, Durkin, and Bowling (2017) found that student psychotherapists in training who took six sessions of CMT experienced increased self-compassion (12%) afterward. Similarly, Matos and colleagues (2018) found that just 2 hours of CMT training plus 2 weeks of practice resulted in significant increases in positive affect, improved heart rate variability, and compassion toward self and others, as well as significant reductions in shame, self-criticism, fears of compassion, and stress (the CEAS rather than SCS was used to measure self-compassion).

Research on the MSC Program

Although the MSC program outlined in this manual is still in its early stages, there is increasing evidence to suggest that it is effective at increasing self-compassion and other aspects of psychological well-being, and that the skills of self-compassion learned in MSC are maintained over time. This body of research is covered here in some detail, since it provides empirical support for the program as described in the rest of this book. We first conducted a small pilot study of the MSC program (Neff & Germer, 2013) with 21 participants (95% female; mean age = 51.26 years). We found program participation significantly increased self-compassion (34%), mindfulness, social connectedness, life satisfaction, and happiness and also decreased depression, anxiety, and stress. Based on these encouraging results, we next conducted a randomized controlled study of the MSC program (Neff & Germer, 2013) that compared outcomes for 51 individuals (77% female; mean age = 50.10 years) randomly assigned to either MSC or a wait-list control group. The large majority of participants (76%) reported having prior experience with mindfulness meditation. Participants from both groups were asked to complete a series of self-report scales 2 weeks before and 2 weeks after the MSC program; MSC participants were also assessed 6 months and 1 year later. The questionnaires assessed self-compassion, mindfulness, compassion for others, life satisfaction, social connectedness, happiness, depression, anxiety, stress, and emotional avoidance.

There were no differences between groups at pretest on any of these measures. At posttest, however, MSC participants demonstrated a significantly greater increase in their self-compassion levels (43%) than controls did, with a large effect size indicated. MSC participants also had significantly larger increases in mindfulness, compassion for others, and life satisfaction, as well as greater decreases in depression, anxiety, stress, and emotional avoidance.

Note that significant group differences were not found in happiness or social connectedness. When examining the results further, however, we found that this lack of group differences occurred because improvements were also observed for the wait-list control group. While MSC participants' scores on all outcome measures increased from pre- to posttest, the control group's levels of self-compassion, mindfulness, happiness, and social connectedness *also* significantly increased. This helps explain why MSC participants' gains in happiness and social connectedness were not significantly greater than those of the control group. The question remains, however: Why did outcomes for the control group improve? To explore the issue further, we contacted control participants after completion of the study to inquire if they had engaged in activities during the study period to increase their self-compassion. Specifically, we asked if they had read books on self-compassion (e.g., Germer, 2009; Neff, 2011a) or visited websites that offered information and downloadable meditations on self-compassion. We also asked if they had tried to bring more self-compassion into their everyday life. Almost all the control participants responded. Fifty percent reported reading books or learning about self-compassion online, and 77% said that they had intentionally tried to practice self-compassion in their lives. This actually strengthens our confidence in the study findings because the members of the waiting-list control group were relatively active in their attempts to increase self-compassion, making comparative gains by the intervention group more marked.

In terms of changes in self-compassion over time, we found that the MSC participants' self-compassion scores increased from pretest to Week 3 of the program, then increased again from Week 3 to Week 6 of the program, but did not significantly increase from Week 6 to posttest. Moreover, there were no changes in self-compassion when the MSC participants were examined 6 months later (with 92% of intervention participants taking the follow-up survey) and 1 year later (only 56% of these participants took the 1-year follow-up). These results suggest that skills of self-compassion imparted in the MSC program are learned gradually, but that once they are learned, they remain relatively stable. We also asked participants how many times per week they practiced formal meditation, or how many times per week they practiced informal self-compassion techniques in daily life. How often participants practiced self-compassion predicted the degree to which their self-compassion increased. There were no differences between formal and informal practice in predicting self-compassion gains. (The importance of informal practice has been corroborated by research on mindfulness training [Elwafi, Witkiewitz, Mallik, Thornhill, & Brewer, 2013].) Overall, our research implies that self-compassion is a teachable skill that is "dose-dependent." That is, the more people practice it, the more they learn it.

Gains in other study outcomes were also maintained at the 6-month and 1-year follow-ups. In fact, life satisfaction actually increased from the time of program completion to the 1-year follow-up, suggesting that the continued practice of self-compassion can continue to enhance participants' quality of life over time. Given there was attrition from the 6-month to the 1-year follow-up, however, these results should be interpreted with caution because those participants who were most satisfied with their lives may also have been the most likely to fill out the 1-year follow-up survey.

The study was further limited by the lack of an active control group—a shortcoming that will need to be addressed in future research. Also, given that most participants had prior mindfulness meditation experience, we can't know for sure whether the practices taught in the program were only effective for those who already knew how to meditate. On the other hand, the fact that MSC participants increased in well-being, even though most had prior meditation experience, suggests that MSC offers tangible benefits over and above meditation alone.

A second randomized controlled trial has been conducted on MSC (Friis et al., 2016). The study included 63 participants (68% female; mean age = 42.87 years) suffering from Type 1 or Type 2 diabetes. It compared outcomes for those randomly assigned to the MSC program (n = 32) or to a wait-list control condition (n = 31). Measures of self-compassion, depressive symptoms, diabetes-specific distress, and glycemic control (indicated by HbA_{1c} values at the three time points) were taken at the start of the program, at the end of the program, and at a 3-month follow-up.

There were no group differences at pretest on any of these measures. At the 3-month follow-up, however, MSC participants demonstrated a significantly greater increase in self-compassion (27%), and decrease in depression and diabetes distress, compared to controls. MSC participants also averaged a clinically and statistically meaningful decrease in HbA_{1c} between baseline and the 3-month follow-up. There were no overall changes for the wait-list control group. These findings suggest that learning to be kinder to oneself (rather than being harshly self-critical) may have both emotional and metabolic benefits among patients with diabetes.

Research has also examined the impact of MSC on health care providers. Delaney (2018) conducted a small mixed-method pilot study of MSC on caregiving fatigue and resilience among nurses. Results indicated that the training increased self-compassion (24%), mindfulness, resilience, and compassion satisfaction, while reducing secondary traumatic stress and burnout. Findings were supported by the qualitative data gathered: Nurses indicated that the training increased their ability to cope, reduced self-criticism, and enhanced positive mental states.

It appears that the benefits of MSC are not limited to Western cultures. A pilot study of MSC was conducted with 44 community females (mean age = 36.6 years) in Beijing, China (Finlay-Jones, Xie, Huang, Ma, & Guo, 2018). Participants were asked to complete a series of self-report scales just before and after the program, and also at a 3-month follow-up. Significant improvements were observed over the course of the program in terms of increased self-compassion (43%), compassion for others, and mindfulness, and reduced fear of self-compassion, rumination, maladaptive perfectionism, depression, anxiety, and stress, with large effect sizes observed. The majority of these improvements were maintained at the 3-month follow-up. This suggests that the MSC program is effective for increasing self-compassion and well-being in non-Western populations.

An adaptation of MSC for adolescents has been created by Lorraine Hobbs and Karen Bluth (2016), called "making friends with yourself" (MFY). Each weekly session in this 8-week course has a specific theme that roughly parallels the themes of the adult program. In general, the program differs from the adult program in that classes are shorter (about 90 minutes) and more activity-based, and guided meditations are shorter, meaning that they are more developmentally appropriate. MFY includes several hands-on activities that encourage participants' self-discovery of mindfulness and self-compassion. For example, one exercise includes a role play to demonstrate understanding of how we relate to ourselves and set the groundwork for self-compassion practice. There is also an art activity that illustrates the value of imperfection. Discussion of the developing adolescent brain is also woven throughout the course.

Bluth, Gaylord, Campo, Mullarkey, and Hobbs (2016) conducted a mixed-methods study of the MFY program with 34 adolescents (74% female; ages 14–17 years). It compared outcomes for those randomly assigned to the MFY program ($n = 16$) versus a wait-list control condition ($n = 18$). Participants from both groups were asked to complete a series of self-report scales at baseline and immediately after the program, assessing self-compassion, mindfulness, life satisfaction, social connection, depression, anxiety, and positive and negative mood. Classes were also audio-recorded and transcribed, and teens gave verbal feedback about the acceptability of the program.

Participants in the MFY program reported significantly greater gains in self-compassion (11%) and life satisfaction, as well as decreases in depression, compared to the wait-list control group, with trends toward significance in terms of increased mindfulness and social connection and decreased anxiety. Given the small sample size, these trends may have been significant with more participants. Teens also generally gave positive feedback about the program. As one teen said,

> "I guess I'm thankful for the tools that I've learned, because I get a lot of anxiety about school, especially. I feel like in the last few weeks my anxiety in the moment has decreased because I'm mindful and compassionate toward myself, and I don't know, I feel much better about a lot of stuff I have to do, because I know it's not the end of the world if I don't do it or whatever." (p. 486)

Bluth and Eisenlohr-Moul (2017) also examined outcomes for adolescents ($N = 47$, 53% female, ages 11–17) enrolled in MFY in five cohorts. Self-report measures were completed at pretest, posttest, and at 6-week follow-up. Multilevel growth analyses indicated that over time participants increased in self-compassion (17%), mindfulness, resilience, curiosity/exploration, and gratitude, as well as decreased in perceived stress. Similarly,

Campo and colleagues (2017) conducted a study of an adapted version of the MFY program taught online to female young adult cancer survivors (*N* = 25, ages 18–29). Not only did participants report enjoying the program and finding it helpful, they evidenced increased self-compassion (29%), mindfulness, improved body image, posttraumatic growth, and decreased social isolation, anxiety, and depression. These findings are encouraging and suggest that it is possible to teach the skills of MSC at an early age, potentially altering the developmental trajectory of youths in a way that could produce benefits over a lifetime.

Finally, research has been conducted on brief self-compassion training based on the MSC protocol. For instance, Smeets, Neff, Alberts, and Peters (2014) conducted a study in which practices adapted from the MSC program were taught (such as the Self-Compassion Break, Compassionate Letter to Myself, and Finding Loving-Kindness Phrases) to female college students over the course of 3 weeks. Participants included 49 female psychology students (mean age = 19.96 years) entering their first or second year at a European university, who were randomly assigned to either the self-compassion intervention group (*n* = 27) or an active time management control group (*n* = 22). Both groups met for three short sessions over 3 consecutive weeks, with two active intervention sessions lasting about 90 minutes and a closing session lasting about 45 minutes. Various self-report scales were administered 1 week before and 1 week after the intervention. It was found that the brief MSC intervention led to significantly greater increases in self-compassion (21%), mindfulness, optimism, and self-efficacy, as well as significantly greater decreases in rumination, compared to the control group.

The success of this brief training is encouraging and suggests that the benefits of self-compassion can be potentially taught without requiring meditation. For this reason, we are currently pilot-testing brief versions of MSC for populations such as teachers, parents of chronically ill children, and health care workers at risk of burnout. Preliminary results of a randomized wait-list-controlled trial of a brief protocol consisting of six 1-hour sessions used with health care workers at a children's hospital suggest that the brief intervention is effective for this population. Not only did participants report enjoying the program, it significantly increased self-compassion (16%), mindfulness, compassion for others, and compassion satisfaction and decreased stress. There was also a moderator effect so that participants initially low in self-compassion experienced significant reductions in depression (those initially high in self-compassion did not). Moreover, all gains were maintained at 3-month follow-up. These brief interventions are promising given that they require less of a time commitment, and they may be more appropriate for those who are disinclined to adopt a meditation practice and who prefer to simply integrate self-compassion practice into their daily life. Research is in its early stages, however, and it remains to be seen how much practice is needed to learn the new habit of self-compassion in a way that makes an impact over the long term.

Implicit versus Explicit Training in Self-Compassion

Although mindfulness-based interventions such as MBSR and MBCT have been shown to raise self-compassion, and although increased self-compassion appears to be a key mechanism of these interventions, there is some disagreement about whether self-compassion is best taught implicitly or explicitly. Jon Kabat-Zinn (2005) writes that MBSR teachers have "always attempted to embody lovingkindness. . . . So to my mind, nothing ever needed to be said explicitly about it. Better to be loving and kind, as best we could, in everything that we were and everything that we did, and leave it at that" (p. 285). This argument is echoed by Segal and colleagues (2013) in their MBCT training manual, where they argue that self-compassion is best taught through implicit means:

> If self-compassion in MBCT develops through pervasive indirect, even implicit instruction, then much of the responsibility for embodying this rests with the instructor. Kindness, initially conveyed by the instructor's personal warmth, attentiveness, and welcoming stance, is reinforced throughout the program, by the gentle approach taken with participants, especially in the presence of negative affect such as sadness or anger. In this way, mindfulness and compassion are caught and not taught. (p. 140)

This approach implies that self-compassion skills are sufficiently bolstered through such implicit approaches as teacher warmth and responses to participants' questions and comments.

The question of whether self-compassion is taught more effectively through implicit or explicit means is ultimately an empirical one. To our knowledge, only one study has tackled this question. Brito-Pons and colleagues (2018) compared outcomes for participants who enrolled in a CCT course (n = 26) versus an MBSR course (n = 32) at the same university in Chile, although it should be noted that participants were not randomized between the two conditions. Still, the study offers preliminary insights into potential differences between the explicit versus implicit teaching of compassion. Both groups gained significantly in self-compassion (CCT = 28%, MBSR = 15%). Although gains were larger in CCT, they were not significantly different from MBSR. CCT participants also reported significant increases in compassion for others (8%), empathic concern (14%), and identification with humanity (15%). Participants taking MBSR did not show significant increases in these outcomes (3%, 2%, and –1%, respectively). Interestingly, both groups had nearly identical significant gains in mindfulness (CCT = 17%, MBSR = 16%), suggesting that results were not solely due to the topic of each program.

More research that directly compares the relative impact of programs such as MBSR, MBCT, and MSC will be needed before the overlapping and unique benefits of each are understood. It is likely that each program is effective at enhancing some skills more than others. For instance, MBSR and MBCT may be more likely to impact phenomena such as cognitive flexibility, attentional functioning, and interoception (Keng et al., 2012), whereas compassion-based programs may be more likely to increase self-compassion and concern with others. Thus compassion-based programs are likely to be complementary to MBSR or MBCT and a useful supplement, especially for those who tend to be self-critical.

Some attempts have been made at creating interventions that *combine* explicit mindfulness and self-compassion training to address particular disorders. For instance, Palmeira, Pinto-Gouveia, and Cunha (2017) created a 12-week program for weight loss called Kg-Free that draws on mindfulness, ACT, and compassion-based approaches. A randomized controlled trial found KG-Free significantly increased self-compassion (13%), healthy behaviors, psychological functioning, and quality of life and decreased weight-related negative experiences compared to a treatment-as-usual control group. It is unclear whether this one-size-fits-all approach is more or less effective than approaches that focus on one type of training at a time, but results suggest that more research is warranted.

In fact, an important area for future research will be to determine whether individual difference variables play a role in the relative impact of each type of program on well-being. MBSR and MBCT may be more effective in improving well-being for those who have low preexisting levels of mindfulness, for instance, while MSC may be more effective for those with lower levels of self-compassion. Research might also fruitfully explore whether well-being is maximized when both types of programs are taken, and, if so, in what order. Intuitively, it would seem optimal to learn mindfulness before self-compassion, given that mindfulness of suffering forms the foundation for self-compassion. However, people suffering from severe shame or self-criticism may need to cultivate self-compassion first, in order to have the sense of emotional safety needed to fully turn toward their pain with mindfulness. Either way, it is likely that interventions explicitly teaching mindfulness and ones explicitly teaching self-compassion are both needed. In the Buddhist tradition, mindfulness and compassion are considered to be two wings of a bird (Kraus & Sears, 2009), and both are necessary to fly.

Another important area of future research is on teaching self-compassion outside of live in-person settings. As mentioned previously,

Campo and colleagues (2017) found that live online self-compassion training appeared to be effective with cancer survivors. McEwan and Gilbert (2016) found that practicing compassionate imagery online for 5 minutes daily over 2 weeks increased self-compassion (17%) and that the effect was even stronger among those initially high in self-criticism. The online exercises also reduced feelings of inadequacy, depression, anxiety, and stress, and most gains were maintained at a 6-month follow-up assessment.

It appears that self-compassion may be learned in a variety of formats. Sommers-Spijkerman, Trompetter, Schreurs, and Bohlmeijer (2018) examined the impact of using a self-help book to learn self-compassion. They conducted a randomized controlled trial of Dutch participants with low to moderate levels of well-being ($N = 120$) who were sent a self-help book based on CFT principles to read at home, compared to a wait-list control group ($N = 122$). Intervention participants received weekly email guidance for practice. The group who read the self-help book gained significantly more self-compassion (25%), as well as enhanced emotional, psychological, and social well-being (assessed with a variety of measures) compared to the control group. Moreover, the intervention group continued to show improvement on many of the well-being measures at 9-month follow-up, including self-compassion (30%). Given the convenience (and ubiquity) of self-help books, these results are highly promising.

Another way to deliver self-compassion training is through mobile apps. Mak and colleagues (2018) conducted a randomized controlled trial in Hong Kong in which participants were given an app based on mindfulness ($n = 703$), cognitive-behavioral-based psychoeducation ($n = 753$), or an app called "Living with Heart" based on MSC ($n = 705$). Participants were asked to use the app for 28 days, although usage dropped off steeply after 1 week. Participants who completed the training were evenly distributed across groups: self-compassion ($n = 112$), mindfulness ($n = 104$), and cognitive behavioral ($n = 126$). Significantly greater gains in self-compassion were reported by those using the self-compassion (12%) and cognitive-behavioral (7%) apps than those using the mindfulness app (2%). The groups did not differ in terms of other well-being outcomes, however.

Finally, Falconer and colleagues (2014) used virtual reality to teach self-compassion, with apparent success. Participants with recurrent depression were shown a virtual image of a distressed child and then were recorded giving compassion to the child. Participants were then randomly assigned to two groups: either they saw their own virtual reality image giving compassion to themselves in a first-person perspective ($n = 22$) or else saw the event from a third-person perspective ($n = 21$). This method resulted in significantly greater increases in self-compassion for those with a first-person perspective (28%) compared to a third-person perspective (–1%). Both conditions experienced decreased self-criticism to the same extent and condition did not differentially impact mood.

Given the ease and affordability of many of these various technologies, these results are highly encouraging. The development and refinement of new ways to help people to learn self-compassion from the comfort of their own homes—whether through online interventions, self-help books, mobile apps, or virtual reality—means that the number of individuals who are potentially able to learn this important life skill could be in the millions.

POINTS TO REMEMBER

* Self-compassion can be learned through a variety of methods, including yoga and LKM.

* Mindfulness- and acceptance-based interventions, such as MBSR, MBCT, and ACT, have also been shown to increase self-compassion. Although self-compassion is taught implicitly in mindfulness approaches, it appears to be a key mechanism of program effectiveness.

* Two compassion training programs that focus primarily on compassion for *others,* CCT and CBCT, also appear to enhance self-compassion and personal well-being.

* Another structured compassion program, MBCL, teaches compassion and self-compassion and has received preliminary empirical support.

* CFT is a model of psychotherapy specifically designed to cultivate compassion and self-compassion. Research has demonstrated beneficial outcomes of CFT in a variety of clinical populations.

* Two randomized controlled trials of MSC indicate that it leads to enhanced self-compassion as well as mental and physical well-being, and a pilot study from China suggests that MSC is effective in non-Western populations.

* The MSC program has been adapted for adolescents in the MFY program, and the efficacy of this program has also been supported in a randomized controlled trial and two pilot studies.

* Future research is needed to compare explicit versus implicit approaches to enhancing self-compassion, and to determine whether individual differences between participants have an impact on outcome. Another fruitful area of research is the relative benefit to participants of the order in which they learn mindfulness, compassion for others, and/or self-compassion.

* Other technologies may be used to teach self-compassion, such as online training, self-help books, mobile apps, or virtual reality. These various methods show promise and should be explored further.

PART II

On Teaching Mindful Self-Compassion

True intuitive expertise is learned from prolonged experience
with good feedback on mistakes.
—DANIEL KAHNEMAN (2011)

The MSC program is an experiential learning process (Kolb, 2015). Each classroom is a laboratory, and each exercise an experiment. We introduce a variety of practices to our participants, such as savoring the breath or repeating loving-kindness phrases, and then explore through collaborative inquiry and group discussion what transpired in each student's experience. MSC participants are encouraged to discover what works for them—what opens their awareness to present-moment experience (mindfulness), and what allows them to respond with kindness and understanding (self-compassion). One participant summarized her experience of the MSC program thus: "It's really quite simple: Sit down. See what arises. Give yourself love." Notwithstanding, it can be quite tricky to *teach* self-compassion, especially because we know relatively little about our students. There is no simple recipe.

Particular skills, or *domains of competence,* are necessary to teach MSC. Rebecca Crane and colleagues (2013) carefully articulated and validated six domains of competence for leading mindfulness-based interventions such as MBSR and MBCT. Those domains largely pertain to MSC as well, but since the focus of MSC is specifically on training self-compassion rather than mindfulness, the domains have been slightly modified. For example, teaching didactic topics and engaging in inquiry are considered the same domain of competence in the Crane and colleagues model but are considered different domains in MSC because MSC inquiry is primarily an exercise in nonverbal, emotional resonance and has less to do with conveying course themes. The domains of competence will surely continue to evolve as we understand and refine, experientially and empirically, what is needed to teach MSC.

The six domains of competence presented in this part of the book are:

1. Understanding the curriculum.
2. Teaching topics and guiding practices.
3. Embodying self-compassion.
4. Relating compassionately to others.
5. Facilitating group process.
6. Engaging in inquiry.

A review of these teaching domains can provide a sense of the skills and attitude required to teach self-compassion, even if a reader is not planning to teach MSC itself.

Individuals are required to take an MSC course before taking MSC teacher training, and we also advise readers to do so before they teach self-compassion in any professional context. Personal experience of self-compassion is necessary for a lasting change in understanding to happen (Kang, Gray, & Dovidio, 2015). Personal experience also helps teachers to understand obstacles that inevitably arise during the learning process and ways to overcome them. To find more information on where to take the MSC program online or in person, please click the "Train" tab at *http://centerformsc.org*. In order to teach the 8-week MSC program, formal teacher training is required. As mentioned previously, self-compassion can be emotionally activating and training is necessary in order to know how to teach the program safely and effectively. Ruijgrok-Lupton, Crane, and Dorjee (2017) showed that the level of a teacher's *training,* compared to the teacher's meditation or mindfulness teaching *experience,* had a greater impact on the well-being of participants who took a mindfulness course. For information about MSC teacher training, please click the "Teach" tab at *http://.centerformsc.org*.

The first of the following chapters, Chapter 5, reviews the structure and curriculum of MSC. Chapter 6 summarizes how to teach didactic topics and guide meditations and class exercises. Chapter 7 focuses on two related domains of competence: embodying self-compassion and being a compassionate teacher. Chapter 8 offers insights and suggestions for facilitating group process, and Chapter 9 begins the journey into inquiry-based learning and teaching.

Chapter 5

Understanding the Curriculum

I never teach my pupils; I only attempt to provide
the conditions in which they can learn.
—ALBERT EINSTEIN (quoted in King, 1964, p. 126)

The first domain of competence for MSC teachers is *understanding the curriculum*. This chapter first provides an overview of the practical details of conducting an 8-week MSC course. We describe the basic structure of the program, including co-teaching and participant selection; the physical setting and materials required to conduct a course; and the components of each session (e.g., topics, meditations, informal practices, exercises, inquiry). We conclude the chapter with a discussion of adaptations to the MSC curriculum.

After completing the MSC teacher training and before teaching their first MSC course, teachers often feel intimidated by the comprehensiveness of the curriculum and the diverse skills required to teach MSC. There is indeed a lot to do, but the curriculum has been carefully honed over the years to guide participants step by step into a deeper understanding of self-compassion through talks, class exercises, meditation, poetry, films, movement, and group discussion. Teachers usually need to teach the MSC course three or four times before they feel relaxed with a group. Teachers should therefore be patient with their own trajectories as teachers, allowing themselves to be at their own particular levels of competence. Everyone has to start somewhere. The curriculum does a lot of the work, and novice teachers simply need to unfold the curriculum—that is, to reveal its contents to students one element at a time—in a way that feels natural and spacious for all concerned.

Basic Structure of MSC

The MSC program includes eight weekly sessions of 2¾ hours each (including a 15-minute break during each session), plus an additional 4-hour retreat, for a total of about 24 teaching hours. A separate orientation session can be offered to prospective participants before the 8-week course begins. The recommended group size is 8–25 participants with two co-teachers.

Co-Teaching

Ideally, MSC is taught by two trained teachers. The main tasks of MSC teachers are delivering the curriculum and attending to the emotional needs of the group. Co-teaching is recommended because it can be difficult to do both these activities at the same time. For example, while one teacher is leading a challenging exercise, a co-teacher can walk over to a participant who is crying and offer a tissue as an expression of caring.

Co-teachers also provide emotional support to one another. Compassion training is emotionally activating, and teachers will inevitably experience their students' struggles as their own. Some students communicate their struggles in behaviors that interfere with the group process. When that happens, for example, it's a comfort to have a co-teacher who may be able to connect with the student in a different way and help maintain a positive attitude in the classroom.

It is not always possible to work with a co-teacher. For instance, there may not be two trained MSC teachers in the same geographic area, or a course may be too small to financially support two teachers. In that case, an MSC teacher may choose to work with a *teaching assistant*. A teaching assistant is a person who has skills related to teaching MSC, such as teaching mindfulness, but has not yet been formally trained to teach MSC. Often the assistant has already taken an MSC course as a participant. A teaching assistant can occasionally lead a meditation, facilitate small-group discussions, or help with administration of the course. The trained MSC teacher maintains responsibility for the content and quality of the course.

We also recommend that one of the two MSC teachers be a trained mental health professional. An assistant who is also a trained mental health professional is called a *mental health assistant*. Mental health assistants may or may not have taken the MSC course already. Sometimes they participate as group members in exchange for free tuition, but they also keep an eye on the needs of the other group members and step forward in the rare case of an emergency. For example, if a participant is emotionally triggered in class and has difficulty calming down, a mental health assistant can accompany the student outside the classroom for a private conversation, while the teacher continues leading the group. The need for a mental health assistant depends largely on the emotional resilience of individual group members.

Selection of Participants

The best way to select participants for an MSC course is to help them select themselves. The program description should contain accurate information, so prospective group members can match their expectations with the course itself. The description should point out, for example, that MSC is an experiential workshop and not a retreat (although it *includes* a half-day retreat); people generally expect a retreat to be quieter, more relaxing, and less emotionally activating than a workshop. The description should also state that MSC is primarily self-compassion training, not mindfulness training. Finally, the course description should make it clear that while MSC is therapeutic, it is not group therapy. MSC is a structured program designed to cultivate the resources of mindfulness and self-compassion, not to heal old wounds.

Some participants are not entirely self-selected; they are referred by health care providers or persuasive family members. As MSC grows in popularity, professional referrals are occurring with greater frequency. Teachers need to make sure that these applicants understand the nature of the program and are committed to full participation. If not, a participant's ambivalence will have an impact on other group members. It is best for MSC teachers to start with a group of committed individuals who are willing to meet emotional challenges as the course unfolds.

When participants register for MSC, they complete a background information form. Typically, this form includes:

- Contact information.
- Why the applicant wishes to take the course.
- Prior and current meditation practice.
- Physical health and limitations.
- Psychological history:
  - Current stressors, and how the applicant is coping with them.
  - Current treatment, including any medications.
  - Contact information for treatment providers.

Applicants are expected to sign the background information form, acknowledging that they plan to attend every session of the course; that they are prepared to practice mindfulness and self-compassion for 30 minutes each day (formal and informal practices combined); and that they are responsible for their own safety and well-being throughout the program. Some teachers ask applicants to sign a more detailed informed consent form outlining emotional risks and benefits associated with the program (see also Santorelli et al., 2017).

Teachers use the background information to help determine whether each prospective student will benefit from the program. MSC is designed for teaching members of the general population, not for treating clinical conditions. This means that prospective applicants must be able to engage in self-reflection and explore their inner landscapes without becoming easily overwhelmed. If the teachers have concerns about an applicant, they may contact the applicant and discuss whether this is the right time for this person to participate in the program. Teachers should not accept applicants who make them feel uneasy, and teachers should consult with colleagues if they are uncertain whether to accept an applicant.

Exclusion Criteria

The main reason to exclude an applicant is emotional dysregulation. An emotionally dysregulated participant is likely to require too much attention from the teachers and to have difficulty progressing through the course with the rest of the students. Individuals who are prone to reexperiencing traumatic memories that interfere with their daily functioning should postpone their participation until a time when they are more emotionally stable. Another reason to exclude an applicant is a person's likelihood of interfering with the group learning experience. For example, a participant who might have a tendency to split the group into factions or compete with the teachers for control should be discouraged from participating.

A psychiatric diagnosis should not, in and of itself, stand in the way of participating in an MSC course. This is because people with a history of mental illness who have learned to manage their symptoms can benefit a great deal from learning self-compassion. However, MSC is probably not suitable for people who are in an acute phase of mental illness (e.g., depression, anxiety, suicidality, psychosis), are actively addicted to drugs or alcohol, or are only recently clean and sober. Those who have experienced recent trauma (e.g., divorce, violence, death of a loved one) should first become emotionally stable, perhaps in individual therapy, before starting an MSC course. People going through an acute health crisis (e.g., chemotherapy, recovery from severe physical injury) are also advised to wait until they can fully participate in the course. For more on screening applicants and ensuring safety, we suggest reviewing the Brown University meditation safety toolbox (*https://www.brown.edu/research/labs/britton/resources/meditation-safety-toolbox*).

All candidates should be considered on the basis of their individual strengths and weaknesses. The suggestions given above refer to the standard MSC curriculum and to typical MSC teachers. Some teachers have expertise with particular populations (e.g., borderline personality disorder, trauma, substance abuse), and adaptations of the MSC program are currently being developed to address the needs of specialized groups.

Forming a Group

Teachers should carefully consider the *combination* of participants in their classes. For example, MSC teachers who are psychotherapists may or may not want to include their clients in their MSC group if some other group members are not clients. Teachers with participants from the same workplace need to consider whether it makes sense to include people with different levels of authority (bosses and employees) in the same group. It is important that all participants feel safe and willing to share with others. Generally speaking, homogeneous groups (e.g., participants of similar age, ethnicity, gender identity, socioeconomic status, and/or intellectual capacity) are easier to lead than heterogeneous groups, but heterogeneous groups are likely to offer a deeper experience of common humanity.

The *location* of a group matters. The ideal setting is private, neutral, safe, and attractive. Teachers try to create a special culture—a culture of kindness—in MSC courses. Groups that are held at a workplace, for example, are likely to be influenced by the workplace culture and to evoke familiar work interactions.

Group size is another consideration. The MSC curriculum has been designed for groups of 8–25, but it is scalable because the curriculum provides many opportunities for small-group interactions. Large groups (20+ participants) may be challenging for introverted or shy participants. A group of six or fewer participants is probably too small because absences are acutely felt by the remaining group members. Small groups may actually be more work for teachers because group members are more likely to pull for individual attention. When considering group size, as well as the constellation of participants in the group, teachers should be sure to check in with themselves and decide whether they feel comfortable with the arrangements.

Physical Setting and Materials

Typically, MSC takes place in a classroom with chairs arranged in a circle. This seating arrangement allows people to see each other and fosters group cohesion. If there are more than 25 participants, a half-circle of chairs can be arranged within the outer circle. Some experienced meditators prefer to sit on cushions on the floor, or to alternate between cushions and chairs as the course proceeds.

There is usually a table in the room with materials related to the session. The typical materials are these:

- *Nametags.* Nametags are usually worn at each session to facilitate connections between members, especially in large groups.
- *Attendance sheet.* This sheet helps teachers to keep track of attendance for a variety of purposes, such as knowing who may be missing sessions and needing special attention, providing continuing education credit for professionals, or confirming that participants who wish to apply for MSC teacher training have attended 80% of the course.
- *Workbook.* It is highly recommended that teachers provide students with copies of *The Mindful Self-Compassion Workbook* (Neff & Germer, 2018), which serves as a companion to the course.
- *Weekly feedback.* Students are asked to provide weekly written feedback to teachers about their experience of the course, particularly key insights or challenges, practices that were particularly helpful or unhelpful, and any confidential information that a student may wish the teachers to know.
- *Bell.* Teachers can ring a bell to alert participants to time during exercises and after breaks, to signal the end of a practice, or to conclude the session itself.
- *Refreshments.* Snacks are offered at the break to help group members stay nourished, both physically and emotionally.
- *Flipchart or whiteboard.* Poster paper or a whiteboard is used as a visual aid by teachers when delivering short talks; this practice also helps participants to write down conceptual questions and comments for later discussion.
- *Paper and pens.* Participants are encouraged to take notes during talks and to record what they experienced during practices and exercises.
- *Flowers.* Some teachers like to beautify the room by placing a bouquet of flowers on a side table or the floor.

Overview of Session Content

The MSC curriculum has been carefully scaffolded so that the content of each session builds upon the previous session.

- *Session 1* is a welcome session, introducing the participants to the course and to one another. Session 1 also provides a conceptual introduction to self-compassion, with informal practices that can be practiced during the week.

- *Session 2* anchors the program in mindfulness. Formal and informal mindfulness practices are taught to participants, as well as the rationale for mindfulness in MSC. Participants also learn about *backdraft* (when self-compassion activates difficult emotions) and how to manage backdraft with mindfulness practice. Sessions 1 and 2 include more didactic material than subsequent sessions, in order to establish a conceptual foundation for the entire course.

- *Session 3* introduces loving-kindness and the intentional practice of warming up awareness. Loving-kindness is cultivated before compassion because loving-kindness is not directly aimed at suffering and is therefore less challenging. Participants get a chance to discover their own loving-kindness phrases for use in meditation. An interpersonal exercise helps develop intimacy, safety, and trust in the group.

- *Session 4* broadens loving-kindness meditation into a compassionate conversation with ourselves and focuses how to motivate ourselves with kindness rather than self-criticism. By Session 4, many participants discover that self-compassion is more challenging than expected, so the teachers explore what *progress* means and encourage participants to practice compassion for themselves when they stumble or feel that they are inadequate to the task of learning self-compassion.

- *Session 5* focuses on core values and the skill of compassionate listening. These topics and practices are less emotionally challenging than others and are introduced in the middle of the program, to give participants an emotional break while still deepening the practice of self-compassion.

- The *retreat (Session R)* comes after Session 5. It is a chance for students to immerse themselves in the practices already learned and to apply mindfulness and self-compassion to whatever arises in their minds during 4 hours of silence. Some new practices that require physical activity are also introduced during the retreat—walking, stretching, and going outside.

- *Session 6* gives students an opportunity to apply their mindfulness and self-compassion skills to difficult emotions. Students also learn a new informal practice for working with difficult emotions. The emotion of shame is described and demystified in this session because shame is so often associated with self-criticism and is entangled with "sticky" emotions such as guilt and anger.

- *Session 7* addresses challenging relationships. Relationships are the source of most emotional pain. This is an emotionally activating session, but most students are ready for it after practicing mindfulness and self-compassion for 6 weeks. Themes of Session 7 are anger in relationships, caregiver fatigue, and forgiveness.

- *Session 8* brings the course to a close with positive psychology and the practices of savoring, gratitude, and self-appreciation—three interrelated ways to embrace the good in our lives. Students are also invited to review what they have learned, what they would like to remember, and what they would like to practice after the course has ended.

Table 5.1 gives an overview of the entire MSC program, with the specific topics, meditations, informal practices, and exercises covered in each session.

Components of Each Session

Each MSC session follows a particular sequence of activities. (Icons are used below to identify the activity categories, and these icons are used again in Part III, when each session is presented in detail.)

Opening Meditation

Classes begin on time, allowing latecomers to take their seats quietly and join in the opening meditation as they arrive. The opening meditation is about 20–30 minutes long, including the settling/reflection period and inquiry that follow it (see below). The purpose of starting each session with meditation is to emphasize the importance of personal practice and also to evoke a mindful and compassionate state of mind in preparation for learning. All meditations during class time are guided by a teacher. (For more about meditations, see the following pages.)

Settling and Reflection

A few minutes of silence are provided to participants at the end of each meditation, to permit them to settle down and to reflect on what they have experienced. Many participants also like to write down their observations.

Inquiry

The settling-and-reflection period is followed by a brief period of inquiry between a teacher and a few students, one at a time, during which each student's direct experience of the meditation is shared with the whole group. Inquiry often begins with the question "What did you notice?", or it may start with a more specific question about the preceding practice. The inquiry process is described in detail in Chapter 9. Important insights often arise during inquiry or are validated by the teacher during inquiry.

Practice Discussion

After inquiry on the opening meditation, students are invited to comment on their home practice during the past week. The practice discussion may begin with "one-word shares," in which each participant offers a word that captures something of her experience, such as "distracted," "relief," "tears," or "curious." One-word shares are an easy way for teachers to take the pulse of the group.

Teachers then typically open up the floor for discussion, perhaps by asking, "Did anything noteworthy happen when you practiced last week?" or "Did any challenges come up for you?" As always, participants are encouraged to describe their direct experience of practice, rather than to tell stories about their personal lives. The practice discussion takes 10–15 minutes, but it may last longer if a student is struggling with an issue that is of interest to the whole group.

Session Theme

Following the home practice discussion, the title/theme of the new session is given, along with a brief explanation of why this theme comes at this point in the program.

Topic

MSC contains 34 topics and each session usually has two or more main topics. Each topic is taught as succinctly as possible, ideally in an enjoyable, interactive manner. Since MSC is an experiential learning program, the main purpose of teaching topics is to prepare students for the meditations, informal practices, or class exercises that follow.

Practices

The term *practices* in the MSC program refers to three *formal (core) meditations*, four *other meditations*, 20 *informal practices*, and 14 *class exercises*.

MEDITATION

Meditation (or *formal meditation, formal meditation practice,* or *formal practice*) refers to practicing in a specific way for a dedicated period, up to 30 minutes at a time. Formal practice is a laboratory

TABLE 5.1. Overview of the MSC Curriculum

Session no.	Title	Topics	Meditations (M) and informal practices (IP)	Exercises
1	Discovering Mindful Self-Compassion	• Welcome • Practical Details • How to Approach MSC • What Is Self-Compassion? • Misgivings about Self-Compassion • Research on Self-Compassion (Optional)	• Soothing Touch (IP) • Self-Compassion Break (IP)	• Why Am I Here? • Guiding Principles • How Would I Treat a Friend? • Gestures of Self-Compassion (Optional)
2	Practicing Mindfulness	• Wandering Mind • What Is Mindfulness? • Resistance • Backdraft • Mindfulness and Self-Compassion	• Affectionate Breathing (M; Core) • Soles of the Feet (IP) • Mindfulness in Daily Life (IP) • Self-Compassion in Daily Life (IP) • Here-and-Now Stone (IP; Optional)	• How We Cause Ourselves Unnecessary Suffering
3	Practicing Loving-Kindness	• Loving-Kindness and Compassion • Loving-Kindness Meditation • Practicing with Phrases	• Affectionate Breathing (M; Core) • Loving-Kindness for a Loved One (M) • Compassionate Movement (IP; Optional) • Finding Loving-Kindness Phrases (IP)	• Awakening Our Hearts
4	Discovering Your Compassionate Voice	• Stages of Progress • Self-Criticism and Safety	• Loving-Kindness for Ourselves (M; Core) • Compassionate Letter to Myself (IP)	• How Is MSC Going for Me? • Motivating Ourselves with Compassion
5	Living Deeply	• Core Values • Finding Hidden Value in Suffering • Listening with Compassion	• Giving and Receiving Compassion (M; Core) • Living with a Vow (IP) • Compassionate Listening (IP)	• Discovering Our Core Values • Silver Linings

86

Retreat	Retreat		
		• Introduction to the Retreat • Posture Instructions	• Compassionate Body Scan (M) • Sense and Savor Walk (IP) • Affectionate Breathing (M; Core) • Savoring Food (IP) • Soles of the Feet (IP) • Loving-Kindness for Ourselves (M; Core) • Compassionate Movement (IP) • Giving and Receiving Compassion (M; Core) • Compassionate Walking (IP; Optional)	• Coming Out of Silence
6	Meeting Difficult Emotions	• Stages of Acceptance • Strategies for Meeting Difficult Emotions • Shame	• Loving-Kindness for Ourselves (M; Core) • Working with Difficult Emotions (IP) • Working with Shame (IP; Optional)	
7	Exploring Challenging Relationships	• Challenging Relationships • Pain of Disconnection • Forgiveness (Optional) • Pain of Connection • Caregiving Fatigue	• Compassionate Friend (M) • Self-Compassion Break in Relationships (IP) • Compassion with Equanimity (IP)	• Meeting Unmet Needs • Silly Movement (Optional)
8	Embracing Your Life	• Cultivating Happiness • Savoring and Gratitude • Self-Appreciation • Tips for Maintaining a Practice	• Compassion for Self and Others (M) • Gratitude for Small Things (IP) • Appreciating Our Good Qualities (IP)	• What Would I Like to Remember?

to discover what happens in the field of our awareness when, for example, we savor the rhythm of the breath, offer ourselves loving-kindness phrases, send kindness and appreciation to different parts of the body, and so forth. We can do formal meditation practice in a variety of postures, such as sitting, lying down, standing, or walking. Sitting meditation is the most common type of formal meditation, but practicing in other postures should not be considered a lesser form of practice. The three *core* meditations in MSC are Affectionate Breathing, Loving-Kindness for Ourselves, and Giving and Receiving Compassion. The core meditations are taught two to three times (usually for 20–30 minutes, including inquiry) during the program and form the practice base of the MSC program. The other four meditations are Loving-Kindness for a Loved One, Compassionate Body Scan, Compassionate Friend, and Compassion for Self and Others.

INFORMAL PRACTICE

Informal practice refers to an application of mindfulness or self-compassion skills in everyday life—for instance, while driving, at the workplace, or during conversation with others. Each of the 20 informal practices in MSC is taught only once during the program, but can be applied anywhere, at any time. The seven formal meditations can also be distilled into informal practices, such as converting Affectionate Breathing into a few minutes of savoring the rhythm of the breath.

Informal practices have an important role in MSC training because we need suffering to evoke compassion, and suffering is more likely to occur when we're going about our daily lives. Ideally, MSC students will practice *both* formally and informally because these approaches reinforce one another. Preliminary research (Neff & Germer, 2013) showed that formal and informal practices were equally effective in helping MSC participants become more self-compassionate, a finding corroborated by mindfulness research (Elwafi et al., 2013).

EXERCISE

Class exercises are designed to provide a visceral experience of concepts discussed in class. An exercise is often guided in a semi-meditative manner and involves recalling a past or present difficulty in a participant's life as an occasion to evoke self-compassion. In some exercises, participants use pen and paper to write down what they are experiencing.

Class exercises are *not* intended for home practice because they tend to be emotionally activating and are thus best delivered in the relative safety of the classroom. After an exercise, participants usually get a chance to discuss in dyads or triads what they have experienced, which helps to integrate any residual emotions. Some elements of the class exercises can be applied as informal practices in daily life, but participants are not typically encouraged to go home and practice an entire exercise.

Break

A refreshment break comes halfway through each session. Breaks are an opportunity for group members to interact with each other, use the bathroom, eat a snack, or just relax. All sessions should include a break to create an atmosphere of ease, even if teachers feel pressed for time. Teachers need to give themselves a break as well.

Soft Landing

After the break, teachers usually lead a 1- or 2-minute *soft landing*. This practice helps participants settle back into the classroom, and it shows students how to apply mindfulness and self-compassion very briefly, on the spot, in their daily lives. Examples of soft landings are placing a hand over one's heart, feeling the solid ground under one's feet, savoring the movement of the breath, offering oneself an inner smile, physical movement, or whispering a few words of encouragement to oneself.

More Topics and Practices

Before the break, one or two topics are usually presented along with accompanying practices, and after the break there are another one or two topics with practices. The energy of the group tends to decline in the second half of a session, so the latter topics should be delivered in an especially engaging manner, perhaps with more interaction between participants to keep them alert and engaged. As mentioned earlier, covering all the topics and practices in a given session is less essential than maintaining an enjoyable atmosphere in the classroom.

Home Practice

A key task of MSC teachers is to help students develop a daily practice of mindfulness and self-compassion. Toward that end, 5 minutes are allocated at the end of each session to review the practices that the students have just learned. Participants are invited to try these new practices at home, as well as any previously learned practices that they have found enjoyable or beneficial. The recommended length of time for daily practice is 30 minutes per day in any combination of formal and informal practices; again, any of the practices learned during the course can be used. All participants are encouraged to be their own best teachers, applying those practices that fit or resonate most deeply.

Teachers usually stay in touch with their students between sessions to support home practice. Most teachers use emails to send practice reminders, articles, quotes, or web links that students might find inspiring or intriguing. Students also use emails or other online platforms to connect with one another between sessions.

Closing

Sessions usually close with a moment of silence, a poem that reflects the theme of the session, or mindfully listening to the sound of a bell. Closing time is also an opportunity for teachers to express their gratitude to the participants for supporting one another and for their courage and commitment to the practices. Before the session ends, students are also reminded to bring their weekly feedback sheets to the next class.

MSC Adaptations

In the hands of trained and seasoned teachers, the basic MSC program has been shown to be safe and effective for a wide range of people. However, some groups and populations may benefit even more when the MSC program is adapted for them. For example, the MFY program developed for teens (see Chapter 4) includes more personal interactions and fewer reflection exercises than the standard MSC program; art projects have been added; and the sessions are shortened to 1½ hours. Other populations for whom MSC can be adapted to make it more physically or emotionally accessible are professional groups (e.g., health care providers, educators, business professionals, or military personnel) and clinical groups (e.g., clients with anxiety, depression, trauma, cancer, or chronic pain).

MSC can be tailored for most groups without significantly altering the content of the program. An example is the study by Friis and colleagues (2016), described in Chapter 3, in which MSC was taught to patients with diabetes. The intervention took place without special reference to diabetes (although it was clear why everyone was taking the course), and MSC positively affected the participants' glucose levels and reduced their diabetes-related distress.

Experienced teachers often find that they express themselves differently, depending on who is in a particular group. For example, since the majority of MSC participants are women, the language of MSC tends to reflect the sensibilities of women. A group of men, however, may want to hear more scientific evidence, focus on self-compassion as an inner strength, discuss self-compassion as an instrumental value (i.e., as a means to enhance emotional resilience, promote physical and mental health, and/or improve relationships), and focus more on self-coaching (yang quality) than self-soothing (yin quality). These adjustments are usually made by experienced teachers without modifying the basic content of the program.

Teachers should also remain attentive to the cultural needs of their group members. For example, some Christians may take offense if Buddhist sources are disproportionately cited during the course. People of color may perceive racial injury that is invisible to teachers from the dominant culture. If cultural missteps occur, as they inevitably will, teachers can humbly acknowledge their mistakes and make necessary adjustments. The purpose of MSC is to teach the universal resources of mindfulness and compassion, not to indoctrinate anyone into a particular culture.

What's in a Name?

The Center for MSC (CMSC) owns the trademark for the MSC program and is responsible for disseminating MSC in a way that maintains its integrity, consistency, and quality. If a specialized program contains 85% of the MSC curriculum, it is considered an "application" of MSC and may have "MSC" or "Mindful Self-Compassion" in the main title even when it focuses on a specific population, such as "MSC for Men" or "MSC for Diabetes." An "adaptation" contains less than 85% of the curriculum and can use "MSC" in the *subtitle* when approved by CMSC; an example is "Resiliency Training: MSC for Physicians." Not every adaptation requires approval from the CMSC; only those adaptations that bear the acronym "MSC" in the title require approval. Applications and adaptations of MSC should only be developed by trained or certified MSC teachers, respectively.

Notwithstanding, readers are heartily encouraged to use any materials from this book in the context of their professional activities, such as teaching a course on parenting, offering mindfulness instruction to organizations, or conducting psychotherapy. That is primarily why this book was written. Excerpted materials should be cited in the usual way, and publishing of original or adapted text from this book requires permission from Guilford Press. Furthermore, bulk use of the MSC curriculum (eight or more topics or practices) in a structured training program requires permission from CMSC. Receiving permission from CMSC is a relatively easy process since the mission of CMSC is to support the dissemination of mindfulness and self-compassion practice in diverse populations and contexts. Detailed and updated guidelines for permissions and approval of adaptations are provided on the CMSC website.

POINTS TO REMEMBER

* MSC consists of eight sessions (each 2¾ hours long), plus a 4-hour retreat and an optional orientation session. Sessions include talks, meditations, class exercises, informal practices, inquiry, discussions, movement, videos, and poems. The ideal group size is 8–25 participants.

* Whenever possible, it is advisable for an MSC teacher to have a co-teacher or a teaching assistant, to help deliver the curriculum and address the emotional needs of the participants. It is further recommended to have a trained mental health professional in the room at all times.

* The best way to select participants for a course is to provide accurate information for participants to select themselves. They should be chosen on the basis of their ability to participate fully in the program. Since MSC can be emotionally activating, students with acute physical or emotional conditions should postpone their participation to a later date.

* The topics and practices in each session are carefully organized to build upon one another. Learning is primarily experiential. Didactic topics open the door to practices, followed by inquiry into the students' direct experience of the practices.

* Students are encouraged to practice mindfulness and self-compassion at home for 30 minutes per day, formal and informal practice combined. Practice during daily life is no less valuable than formal meditation.

* The MSC program and practices can be customized to meet the needs of different populations. Adaptations that bear the name Mindful Self-Compassion (capitalized) letters) or the acronym MSC require the approval of the Center for MSC. Otherwise, adaptations do not require CMSC approval, but they still require permission if eight or more MSC topics or practices are included in the adaptation.

* Professionals are highly encouraged to integrate the principles and practices of MSC (found in this book) into their ongoing work activities. Permission is rarely required for such professional applications as long as the work is unpublished and the source of the materials is properly cited.

Chapter 6

Teaching Topics
and Guiding Practices

That all our knowledge begins with experience
there can be no doubt.
—IMMANUEL KANT (1781/2016)

The second domain of competence for MSC teachers is skill at *teaching didactic topics and guiding practices,* including leading class exercises and reading poetry. These skills all require "teaching from within." Mindfulness and self-compassion are essentially preconceptual experiential states, and helping students to cultivate them is like pointing a finger at the moon. However, when teachers speak from their inner experience and follow their passion for the subject, the students' minds and bodies are likely to resonate with the teachers' minds and bodies, and the students will get a deeper sense of what the teachers are trying to communicate.

Triangle of Awareness

The MSC course curriculum has been carefully articulated so that teachers have a solid platform on which to base their teaching. The curriculum should be considered a launching pad, not a resting place. Nonetheless, some components of the curriculum require greater fidelity to the written text than others. For example, it is important to adhere closely to the instructions for class exercises, since class exercises tend to activate strong emotions, and the instructions have been refined over the years to be both safe and effective. Didactic topics require less fidelity to the text; it's more important for teachers to teach topics in their own words. Formal and informal meditation practices offer the greatest opportunities for teachers to speak spontaneously, transmitting in tone, cadence, and content what they wish their students to discover within themselves.

There are three fields of awareness among which teachers need to divide their attention during teaching: (1) *inner awareness,* (2) the *text,* and (3) the *group.* (See Figure 6.1.) This "triangle of awareness" has been adapted from the mindfulness teaching model of MSC teacher Rob Brandsma (2017, p. 65). How much emphasis a teacher places on each of these areas depends on what is being taught. For example, when a teacher is reading poetry, it is helpful to get a sense of the audience (the group), but that's not as important as speaking the actual words of the poet (text) from within (inner awareness). When a teacher is teaching a didactic topic, it is especially important to connect with group members in interactive dialogue (group), but the actual text is secondary to conveying the ideas with passion and interest. Inner awareness only matters while delivering a topic insofar as teachers need to find their own voices.

Table 6.1 indicates how much to focus on each aspect of the triangle of awareness while teaching the five modalities—meditations, informal practices, didactic topics, class exercises, and poetry. (Meditations and informal practices are combined in this discussion, since they are taught in the same, meditative manner.) This model is offered as a guide rather than a prescription for how to teach. As noted earlier, all modes of teaching require some degree of "teaching from within." For example, even if a teacher has to recite the exact words of a poem or exercise, the teacher should allow the words to be felt inside and then give voice to what he is feeling while reading. When teaching didactic topics, teachers are more likely to teach from within when they liberate themselves from the script. Rather than reading verbatim from their notes, teachers are encouraged to prioritize in advance

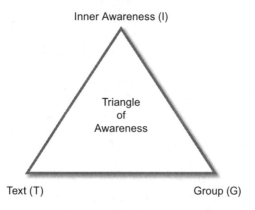

FIGURE 6.1. Triangle of awareness. Based on Brandsma (2017, p. 65).

TABLE 6.1. Focus of Attention in Teaching Modalities

Teaching modalities	Priority[a]		
	Inner awareness	Text	Group
Meditations/informal practices	H	M	L
Didactic topics	L	M	H
Class exercises	M	H	M
Poetry	M	H	L

[a]H, high; M, medium; L, low.

what they want to say, find their own manner of communicating, and then glance at their notes to stay on track while teaching. Some class exercises, however, necessitate reading from the script. One such exercise is Awakening Our Hearts (Session 3). Even we (Chris and Kristin), the developers of MSC, still read over 90% of the instructions for this exercise because the instructions been carefully edited to maximize participants' safety. Following are some points to consider in teaching didactic topics, guiding meditations and informal practices, leading class exercises, and reading poetry.

Didactic Topics

An important goal of the MSC program is for students to become their own best teachers. Toward that end, before they engage in any new practice, students are given the rationale for doing it. For example, before teaching the Self-Compassion Break, we define the components of self-compassion (which constitute that practice). Any didactic points that a teacher does not have time to cover before a practice can always be covered *after* the practice. Direct experience usually speaks for itself.

There are 34 didactic topics contained in the MSC program. Here are some suggestions for delivering topics:

• *Keeping it concise.* Didactic topics are usually taught in up to 15 minutes, especially by experienced teachers. Topics should be considered "teasers" rather than formal lectures, appetizers rather than main courses. Most learning occurs during the practice itself.

• *Following your energy and passion.* Students will learn the most about topics that a teacher is passionate about. Teachers should decide for themselves what points in a topic area energize or excite them, and then build their presentation around those points.

• *Making it interactive.* Whenever possible, teachers should use leading questions, connect students to their own experience, and solicit responses. A didactic topic should feel like a *mutual* learning experience.

• *Letting it be fun.* Everyone is grateful for a good laugh, especially when self-compassion (which requires contact with emotional pain) is being taught. Teachers should feel free to relate humorous anecdotes, tell jokes, and share personal foibles. Talks do not need to be serious to be meaningful.

• *Using examples.* Teachers should have a brief, personal anecdote handy for each topic area that they teach. Ideally, personal examples from a teacher's life will enhance or validate a student's experience. Teachers can also collect stories to illustrate their points. The idea is to "show" with vivid images rather than expound on concepts.

• *Varying the delivery.* Students generally appreciate it when a teacher uses different teaching methods, such as lecture, videos, poetry, movement, music, readings, discussion, research, and Q&A. Unless a topic is very brief, teachers should try to vary their methods of delivery.

The MSC curriculum offered in this book contains more information and supporting materials for each topic than can be delivered in the available time. Beginning teachers often feel compelled to include all the information that they find. However, maintaining an enjoyable, connected atmosphere in the room is more important than delivering all the points in the curriculum. Students are more likely to remember how they *felt* rather than what they heard. Over time, teachers discover how to deliver each topic in an interesting and succinct manner, often without notes. The focus of MSC is transformation, not information.

Meditations and Informal Practices

Guiding formal meditations and informal practices is a subtle art that develops with time. Both formal and informal practices are taught in a meditative way in MSC to give students a felt sense of the practice. Teachers are encouraged to make audio recordings of the three core meditations, to help their students get started with the practices. Alternatively, recordings of the core meditations and selected other MSC practices can be streamed or downloaded from this book's companion website (see the box at the end of the table of contents). *The Mindful Self-Compassion Workbook* (Neff & Germer, 2018) also has a companion website where students can access the audio recordings.

The following points may be helpful to keep in mind while guiding meditations and informal practices.

• *Understanding the intention.* Teachers must know the purpose of each meditation or informal practice they are guiding. For example, Affectionate Breathing is not only a concentration practice in which participants return attention to the breath, again and again; it is also a savoring practice in which they allow themselves to be gently rocked and caressed by the rhythmic motion of breathing. The right words for guided meditations and informal practices are likely to arise when teachers understand their purpose. The intention of every meditation and informal practice is given in Part III.

• *Self-guiding.* Teachers are encouraged to "go inside" and connect with their meditative awareness. A teacher's eyes are partially or fully closed most of the time while guiding meditations and practices. When teachers give themselves sufficient time to hear their own instructions and to experience what they are inviting others to do, they will probably have good pacing.

• *Taking a breath.* Sometimes it helps for teachers to take one or more breaths between instructions, to allow themselves and others a chance to experience the instructions more fully.

• *Finding your own voice.* The printed instructions of a meditation or informal practice should only be used as a guide for teachers. It is okay to peek at the instructions from time to time, but teachers should deliver the instructions in the words that flow spontaneously from their own meditative experience. Students are likely to mentally disengage from the meditation if the instructions sound as if the teacher is reading from the text.

• *Speaking in a natural voice.* Compassion meditations and practices are likely to sound more soothing than mindfulness practices, but teachers also don't want to make their instructions hypnotic or syrupy-sweet. Teachers are encouraged to speak in a natural voice, as they might with a good friend. When teachers are in a compassionate state of mind—in loving, connected presence—the tone takes care of itself, and students naturally absorb what they're trying to communicate.

• *Inviting the listener.* Teachers welcome their listeners into the meditative experience, rather than trying to induce a particular mood or state of mind. In the English language, a simple grammatical way to cultivate an invitational style is to use the present participle of a verb, ending with *-ing.* For example, instead of giving the instruction "Feel your breath," a teacher can say, "Feel*ing* your breath." The present participle implies ongoing activity and also conveys a sense of practicing together.

A teacher's *tone* of voice can also reflect an invitational style. For example, consider the difference between giving directions to the driver of a car ("Make a left turn at the light") and inviting a friend over for dinner ("Are you free on Friday evening to come for dinner?"). An invitational style is likely to be communicated through subtle inflections in the voice.

• *Balancing awareness.* While leading meditations and practices, teachers primarily want to maintain inner awareness, only occasionally looking to see how the group is responding or consulting the written instructions.

• *Stepping back.* Teachers are responsible for guiding the meditation process, not the outcome. In a class of 10 people, there may be 10 different reactions to the same meditation or practice. Therefore, it helps when teachers "take a small backward step." Teachers cannot control what happens to everybody, but they can *respond* in a mindful and compassionate manner.

• *Consolidating the experience.* As noted in Chapter 5, there is almost always a period for settling and reflection after each meditation. During this time, participants can be encouraged to absorb what they experienced (Hanson, 2013). Settling and reflection help to broaden a meditative state into a trait and to create lasting change (Fredrickson, 2004a; Garland et al., 2010).

Class Exercises

Whereas meditations and informal practices are taught in class and practiced at home, class exercises are designed specifically for the classroom. Some *elements* of class exercises may be practiced at home, but students should not go home and practice an entire exercise because class exercises tend to be emotionally activating and need skilled guidance. Class exercises often begin with this instruction: "Bring to mind a situation in which you felt emotional discomfort." There is enough emotional pain that arrives unbidden in students' (and teachers') lives that no one needs to go looking for more to practice self-compassion.

When teachers are leading class exercises, the text and the group (in the triangle of awareness) have top priority. Teachers should stick closely to the written instructions of an exercise. They also need to watch the group to be sure everyone is okay. A teacher's inner awareness is less important in exercises than in meditations because exercises evoke personally challenging situations, and the teacher is not recalling an actual life situation in her own life while leading the exercise. Instead, it is enough for the teacher to connect with the emotional tone of the exercise.

There are 14 class exercises in MSC. Teaching class exercises requires more preparation and attention to detail than guiding meditation or teaching topics does. Class exercises have many elements, such as opening and closing one's eyes, writing and reflecting, sensing, and using memory. Several of the class exercises require pen or pencil and paper. A teacher can sometimes feel like a stage director when leading an exercise.

Three class exercises that may be particularly emotionally activating for participants are as follows:

- Awakening Our Hearts (Session 3)
- Motivating Ourselves with Compassion (Session 4)
- Meeting Unmet Needs (Session 7)

The support of the teachers and fellow students enables these practices to be safe and effective for most people.

There are also some informal practices that are introduced in the same safety-conscious manner as class exercises because these informal practices can be emotionally challenging. They are:

- Finding Loving-Kindness Phrases (Session 3)
- Compassionate Walking (Optional) (Session R, the retreat)
- Working with Shame (Optional) (Session 6)
- Appreciating Our Good Qualities (Session 8)

Class exercises and informal practices tend to be safe, and often a great relief, when practiced in *response* to daily challenges rather than as contemplative practices that evoke difficulties. Furthermore, *components* of class exercises, rather than class exercises in their entirety, can be applied in daily life.

Ensuring Safety

Teachers' first priority is to ensure the safety of their group members (see also Chapter 8). There is always a balance between feeling safe and taking risks to learn something new. When participants know they can return to safety, they are more willing to challenge themselves. Too much challenge, however, may make students feel emotionally overwhelmed and diminish their capacity to learn.

When students choose a problem in their lives to address in a class exercise or informal practice, they often choose a problem that is too challenging, despite cautions to the contrary. When a problem is too difficult, students will lose focus or shut down, rather than learning anything about self-compassion. Therefore, teachers should encourage their students to monitor their own safety levels; they can challenge themselves when they wish, but they should avoid feeling overwhelmed. Students are primarily responsible for their own emotional safety.

Figure 6.2 is offered to students in Session 1 to help them monitor their safety levels. This model is based on the Yerkes–Dodson law (Yerkes & Dodson, 1908), which points to an optimal level of arousal for habit formation, and is used in education (Luckner & Nadler, 1997) and business consulting (Senge et al., 1999). The optimal zone for learning is the *challenged* zone, which is between the comfort zone of feeling *safe* and the danger zone of being *overwhelmed*. The challenged zone is also referred to as the "window of tolerance" in the trauma literature (Ogden, Minton, & Pain, 2006; Siegel, 2012).

Most students err on the side of pushing themselves too hard—*striving* to learn self-compassion by pushing through emotional discomfort—which often leaves them in the overwhelmed zone. For the sake of safety, students of self-compassion are encouraged to become "slow learners."

Before teaching a challenging class exercise, teachers need to assess if everyone in the group is emotionally ready and able to benefit from it. If so, the following safety caveats can also be offered to group members:

- "Feel free *not* to participate in the exercise. That, too, is self-compassion."
- "Choose a mild to moderately difficult situation for the exercise, not a serious or major problem."

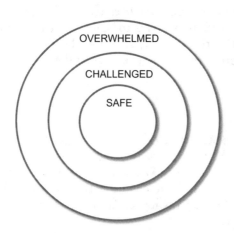

FIGURE 6.2. Monitoring safety.

- "Open or close your eyes at any time."
- "Feel free to mentally disengage from the instructions."
- "Anchor your attention in your breath, the soles of your feet, or any sense object."
- "Practice wholesome distraction, like making up this week's shopping list."
- "Signal for support as needed, and also feel free to leave the room."
- "Ask a teacher for support *after* the exercise, or after the session ends."

While leading an exercise, teachers can also weave these safety suggestions into their instructions.

Teachers can regulate the intensity of an exercise by modulating the tempo and tone of their instructions. Long pauses encourage students to delve more deeply into their inner experience. The softer the tone of a teacher's voice, the more deeply students will go as well. When a teacher speeds up the tempo with more information and adds a lighter touch, students enter into their experience more superficially. Teachers can sense the energy and mood of the group to ascertain how to guide each exercise.

Students process information at different rates, too. Some students are naturally introverted and think slowly and deeply, whereas others like to bounce around their inner landscapes. During a writing exercise, some students finish writing before others have even begun. It's difficult to find a pace that perfectly suits everyone in a group, so teachers aim for a median length of time and invite slower participants to continue the exercise at home if they wish.

Poetry

Each chapter in Part III outlining an MSC session contains suggestions for poems that illustrate topics from the session. Poetry has a unique capacity to evoke subtle states of mind within the listeners. Poems can be recited at the end of a guided meditation or after the break (as a Soft Landing) or can be used to illustrate a topic, shift the mood of a group, or close the session.

Poetry is nothing more than ink on a page until a living, breathing reader makes the words come alive. The best poems to recite are poems that a teacher finds inspiring. Students will be moved by a poem when they feel passion in the teacher's voice. Therefore, it's important for teachers to stay in connection with their inner awareness while reading—to read from within.

Some poems, even short ones, may take years for a poet to write. Therefore, the text of the poem is very important. Before reading a poem, teachers are encouraged to discover which words they would like to emphasize.

The meaning of a line of poetry can change radically, depending on which words the reader considers important.

The structure of a poem, including how the words are aligned on the page, offers additional clues on how to read the poem. Teachers should rehearse their poems before trying them out on their students. Poems should be read slowly enough so that listeners can hear each word and feel what is evoked inside. The pace of a poem is usually about right when teachers give time for the words to land within themselves. Finally, when a poem is presented to others as a gift, it is generally received with appreciation.

Cultivating Yin and Yang

MSC contains a wide variety of practices and exercises for each person to explore. Some practices tend to cultivate yin qualities ("being" with our pain) and emphasize soothing, comforting, and validating. Other practices tend to cultivate yang qualities ("acting" in the world) and emphasize protecting, providing, and motivating (see Chapter 2). Table 6.2 gives examples of practices in MSC that tend to tap into the yin or yang qualities of self-compassion, although most MSC practices contain both yin and yang.

Different attributes of self-compassion are required in different situations, but the ultimate goal is to honor and integrate both yin and yang. The instructions for various practices can be tailored so that participants can emphasize yin or yang depending on their answer to the question "What do I need right now?" A common thread through the yin and yang aspects of self-compassion is the attitude of caring.

TABLE 6.2. Practices Cultivating the Yin and Yang Qualities of Self-Compassion

Yin (session no.)	Yang (session no.)
Self-Compassion Break—yin language (1)	Self-Compassion Break—yang language (1)
Soothing Touch (1)	Self-Compassion in Daily Life (2)
Affectionate Breathing (2)	Motivating Ourselves with Compassion (4)
Compassionate Movement (3)	Compassionate Letter to Myself (4)
Finding Loving-Kindness Phrases (3)	Giving and Receiving Compassion (5)
Loving-Kindness for Ourselves (4)	Discovering Our Core Values (5)
Compassionate Body Scan (Retreat)	Living with a Vow (5)
Working with Difficult Emotions (6)	Self-Compassion Break in Relationships (7)
Compassionate Friend (7)	Meeting Unmet Needs (7)
Appreciating Our Good Qualities (8)	Compassion with Equanimity (7)

POINTS TO REMEMBER

* MSC teachers are encouraged to "teach from within" in all five teaching modalities—meditations, informal practices, didactic topics, class exercises, and poetry.

* Teachers divide their attention among their inner awareness, the written text, and the group members' experience. How much a teacher focuses on each component of the "triangle of awareness" depends on the teaching modality.

* Both formal meditation and informal practices are taught in a meditative way, to give students a felt sense of the practice. The key to guiding meditations and practices is to guide oneself.

* Teachers are encouraged to find their own voices when teaching didactic topics. Other suggestions for teaching topics are to keep talks concise, interactive, and fun; to follow one's passion; to use personal examples; and to vary the teaching with videos, poems, research, movement, and so on.

* Class exercises are the most complicated modality to teach because they are designed to activate difficult emotions and have a variety of components (e.g., reflecting, writing, opening and closing eyes).

* Teachers need to monitor the level of difficulty that students experience during an MSC class. Teachers should help students feel safe or challenged, but stay out of the overwhelmed zone.

* Poetry is an opportunity to give students the felt sense of a topic with relatively few words. Teachers should only recite poems that they find personally meaningful and allow themselves to be emotionally moved by a poem as they read it.

* Self-compassion practices contain tender yin and fierce yang qualities, all of which reflect an attitude of care. Students can explore which attributes and practices appeal to them in different situations and at different times.

Chapter 7

Being a
Compassionate Teacher

> When we honestly ask ourselves which person in
> our lives means the most to us, we often find that
> it is those who, instead of giving advice, solutions,
> or cures, have chosen rather to share our pain and
> touch our wounds with a warm and tender hand.
> —HENRI NOUWEN (2004, p. 38)

The best way to teach self-compassion is to *be* compassionate—toward ourselves and others. Students usually need to feel compassion from their teachers before they can feel it for themselves. Therefore, the third and fourth domains of competence for MSC teachers are *embodying self-compassion* and *relating compassionately to others*; both of these domains are discussed in this chapter. We consider obstacles to being a compassionate teacher, as well as ways for teachers to support themselves in this endeavor.

Embodying Self-Compassion

The three components of self-compassion—kindness, common humanity, and mindfulness—have been described as *loving, connected presence.* When we are in a state of loving, connected presence, we embody self-compassion. In MSC, self-compassion becomes a *way of being* when it is expressed in what a teacher says, how the teacher relates to others, and what type of atmosphere is created in the classroom.

MSC teachers do not have to be perfect to embody self-compassion. As Eugene Gendlin (1990, p. 205) said, "The essence of working with another person is to be present as a living being. And that is lucky because if we had to be smart, or good, or mature, or wise, then we would probably be in trouble." Actually, the teaching of self-compassion can *benefit* from a teacher's mistakes.

> A beginning MSC teacher, Jennifer, once shared with us that she had meticulously prepared for her first MSC class, only to discover shortly before her class began that she had left her notes at home. Caught in a moment of confusion and anxiety, she recognized, "This is indeed a moment of suffering!" She then shared her quandary, including her embarrassment, with the participants in her group. They were greatly amused, but also impressed by how openly and self-compassionately Jennifer responded to her predicament. Jennifer then used her real-time predicament to illustrate the meaning of self-compassion in Session 1. In their post-course evaluations, a few of Jennifer's students wrote that her handling of this situation was the most powerful lesson of the entire course.

A key obstacle to embodying self-compassion is shame. Teachers who want to do their job perfectly are more likely to feel shame when they run into difficulties. Shame is the sense of "I'm not good enough," and may arise in response to ordinary challenges such as misunderstanding what a student is trying to say, having one's authority questioned by a student, or having a student drop out of a course. Fortunately, self-compassion is an antidote to shame (see Chapter 16). When MSC teachers recognize the arising of shame (mindfulness), they may also have the ability to realize that others would feel similarly in such situations (common humanity), and they can be sympathetic with their plight (self-kindness). Teachers who hold moments of shame in this way, especially in front of their students, can set an example of embodied self-compassion.

One reason why MSC teachers are encouraged to embody self-compassion is that human minds neurologically resonate with each other. This makes embodiment an important teaching modality. When the teacher is in an accepting, warm, peaceful, and receptive frame of mind, that attitude will pervade the classroom. When a teacher feels anxious, students will also feel anxious. There is no escaping the influence we have on others by our emotions and attitudes. Resonance is a key topic in the field of social neuroscience (Bernhardt & Singer, 2012; Decety & Cacioppo, 2011; Singer & Lamm, 2009).

A teacher's embodiment of self-compassion also affects the decisions they make in class. For example, a common mistake of beginning teachers is to try to do too much in a session (make too many teaching points, allow too many students to speak, etc.). However, when teachers are self-compassionate, they are likely to notice when they put themselves under unnecessary pressure. Self-compassionate teachers will ensure that all members of the group, including themselves, are operating in a warm, spacious learning environment.

Personal Practice

Of course, we teachers are just human beings, and we embody mindfulness and self-compassion to varying degrees throughout the day. What does it take to increase the possibility that we'll be mindful and self-compassionate while teaching MSC? Personal practice! Jennifer, our beginning teacher described on the previous page, had been practicing mindfulness and self-compassion for over 2 years before her first MSC course, so she was primed to respond accordingly in her moment of distress. Mindfulness and self-compassion had already become habits by the time she entered the classroom.

Research on mindfulness meditation shows that the more we practice, the more mindful we're likely to become (Lazar et al., 2005; Pace et al., 2009; Rubia, 2009). However, simply sitting down to meditate doesn't mean that we're actually meditating. It's possible that we could have been meditating for years and primarily reinforced the habit of daydreaming. It's equally possible to practice meditation for brief periods of time with whole-hearted attention and discover that our lives are transformed by it. People who manage to practice consistently have usually found a balance between quantity and quality of practice.

Formal meditation is especially challenging to practice on a regular basis. Who has time for it? Furthermore, behavior change is usually more elusive than we originally anticipate. Just remember the last time you tried to change your eating or exercise habits, or how quickly you gave up on a New Year's resolution. As an MSC teacher, you'll first need to figure out what it takes to maintain a consistent practice of your own before you can advise others. Next are some tips for maintaining a daily, formal meditation practice.

Making It Pleasant

To encourage you to practice regularly, meditation has to be pleasant. That does not mean *always* pleasant, but sufficiently pleasant for you to want to do it again. What would it take you to make your meditation as easy as breathing or as enjoyable as being loved? When meditation starts to feel like work, you can ask yourself, "Is there any unnecessary striving that I can let go of?" Perhaps meditation *is* work because you are doing it primarily for extrinsic reasons, such as to reduce stress, train your brain, or become a happier person. Instead, can you just let yourself be rocked by the gentle rhythm of your breathing, or whisper kind words into your ear, over and over? That, too, is meditation.

Feeling Comfortable

Make sure that you are physically comfortable when you meditate. Adjust your posture to support your body without effort. You will not want to meditate if it's physically painful. Meditation can be practiced sitting, standing, or lying down. Folded legs are not essential. Find a posture that allows your mind to be tranquil yet alert.

Letting Go of Expectations

While practicing meditation, it's important to let go of expectations, especially the expectation that you will feel good. Unpleasant states of mind will arise and pass during meditation, and your task is simply to meet them all with spacious, loving awareness. Unpleasant states do not necessarily mean that you're practicing incorrectly. Please evaluate the effectiveness of your practice *after* you have meditated, or every few months, rather than during meditation itself.

Starting Small

Preconceived ideas about how long you should be meditating can be an obstacle to practice. The main thing is to *begin.* Can you arrange your schedule so that you sit for just a few minutes and see what happens? Simply stopping the forward tumble of your life, such as sitting down to meditate before opening emails in the morning, overcomes the greatest obstacle. After you begin to meditate, you may want to continue, even though you were previously convinced that you didn't have enough time.

Connecting to Core Values

Does meditation have a meaningful place in your life? Does it support your core values, such as living in love and compassion, or waking up to the preciousness of every moment? Connecting daily meditation to a larger life purpose infuses the practice with energy and meaning.

Finding Social Support

Some people lose interest in meditation because it feels too lonely. If that's the case for you, try finding a teacher, joining a meditation group, listening to guided meditations, seeking online support, or going on a retreat. Social support is a key factor in behavior change (Gallant, 2014), and it is perhaps even more important for developing the habit of meditation because with meditation the rewards are less tangible. Connecting with teachers and fellow meditators shines a light on the meditation process, supports the value of it, and provides inspiration for further practice.

Motivating Yourself with Self-Compassion

Self-compassion is a handy tool for motivating yourself to practice. When your meditation practice lapses, as it will from time to time, take notice of any self-criticism or shame (e.g., "I'm a fraudulent teacher!"). Shame is an emotional burden that interferes with resuming meditation practice. Instead, remind yourself of your core values; think of the pleasure and benefit you derive from practicing; have understanding for how complicated your life is; and then offer yourself the gift of meditation—a time to know what it means to be alive and to receive the love you need.

Going on a Retreat

A retreat is an opportunity to experience the transformative potential of meditation. For example, you might identify unconscious habits of mind, such as a tendency toward perfectionism or self-judgment, and begin to let it go. Sometimes radical new insights emerge from sustained practice, such as firsthand experience of the impermanent nature of experience or a sense of connection to all beings. Taking a deeper dive into meditation on a retreat is likely to inspire you to practice more regularly when you return home.

Insights from Practice

Various insights may emerge from sustained personal practice. These insights help us to embody self-compassion as teachers; they support ongoing practice; and they put us in a better position to respond compassionately when our students encounter similar obstacles on the path.

I'm not very good at self-compassion. One of the earliest discoveries of MSC students is that they are less self-compassionate than they ever imagined. This can be quite disheartening, but it's a useful insight. Most of us usually don't hear the negative chatter in our minds, and we don't realize how much we disregard our needs. When we open to loving-kindness and compassion, we notice the discrepancy between what has been going on all along and what we're hoping to achieve. Discovering that we're not particularly self-compassionate signifies that we're starting to hear the inner conversation more clearly. The pain of this discovery is yet another opportunity to respond with self-compassion.

I feel uneasy about self-compassion. Most of us have misgivings about self-compassion. For example, when we take time to focus on our inner experience and give ourselves kindness, we fear that we might become self-centered or self-indulgent. Ironically, the research points in the opposite direction: It indicates that misgivings are actually mis*conceptions* (see Chapter 2). Misgivings may persist long after we have rationally debunked them because they rub against early childhood or cultural norms. It helps to remember that self-compassion is humble art; we are simply *including* ourselves in the circle of our compassion.

Self-compassion is about doing less, not more. We spend most of our waking hours struggling to achieve one thing or another, such as approval, connection, fame, wealth, or comfort. This attitude of striving naturally carries over to the task of learning to become a more self-compassionate person. We are not actually learning self-compassion; we are learning to embrace our imperfections. When we find ourselves struggling to become more self-compassionate, that's not self-compassion. Self-compassion itself feels like a long, delicious sigh of relief. It's subtraction, not addition.

Love reveals everything unlike itself. Self-compassion plugs us into the relational matrix of our lives—our attachment history. Giving ourselves unconditional love typically reveals the conditions under which we felt unloved in the past (i.e., interactions with early caregivers, current relationships, or cultural biases). This is called *backdraft* and is an essential part of the healing process (see Chapter 11). When we develop the skill of self-compassion, our minds naturally open to old relational pain. As MSC teachers, we and our students learn to expect backdraft and to meet it with the resources of mindfulness and self-compassion.

Practice makes *im*perfect. When some people first hear about self-compassion, they believe that self-compassion will solve all their problems—emotional difficulties, challenging relationships, and so forth. Eventually they discover that despite their best efforts, life remains difficult, and they are the same persons as before. This can be rather disappointing, but it's actually a sign of progress. Meditation teacher Rob Nairn (2009) probably said it best: "The goal of practice is to become a compassionate mess." Being a compassionate mess means being fully human, often struggling, with great compassion.

What we can feel, we can heal. Self-compassion involves opening to pain, not bypassing it. Otherwise, it's just sugar-coating—a vain attempt to manipulate moment-to-moment experience by trying to feel good. Love and sorrow commingle in compassion. Fortunately, we don't need to experience the fullness of our pain to train ourselves in self-compassion; we just need to touch it, as we would touch the flame of a candle with moist fingers.

When we suffer, we practice not to feel better, but because we feel bad. This is the central paradox of self-compassion. Everyone starts on the path to self-compassion to feel better and there is a tendency to apply self-compassion techniques like a magic pill to alleviate human suffering. This approach is destined to fail because it is in the service of resisting moment-to-moment experience (see Chapter 11). We cannot try to manipulate our moment-to-moment experience without making matters worse. A healthy alternative is to allow our hearts to melt in the heat of suffering, spontaneously, without a strategy.

When all else fails, self-compassion! Offering ourselves compassion can trigger three kinds of emotional reactions: We can feel good, bad, or nothing at all. The wish to feel good is a common source of frustration for MSC students because emotions have a life of their own. However, we can practice goodwill toward ourselves, no matter what we're feeling. That is a pivotal insight for MSC practitioners—practicing self-compassion precisely when the practice fails to make us feel better.

Self-compassion is a path, not a destination. As we become seasoned practitioners, we understand more clearly that the journey never ends. Life includes pain. Have we increased our capacity to receive it, and let it go? Have we learned to accept *ourselves* more wholeheartedly, especially when we suffer? With consistent practice, our emotional pain will definitely decrease and our hearts will stay open more continually, but there will always be the need to practice. We never arrive.

Insights such as these are signposts on the map of self-compassion training. They are not the territory itself. As teachers (and students), we need to understand them directly—in our own practice and through our own struggles—before the insights become real and authentic enough to support our teaching.

Relating Compassionately to Others

Relating compassionately to others is the fourth domain of teaching competence. It overlaps with the third domain, embodying self-compassion, but also involves different skills. Compassion for others, for example, has the added complexity of relating to other human beings whom we may hardly know. Students need to *receive* compassion in order to learn *self*-compassion because the learning process can be quite difficult at times. When our students sense that we are *with* them in their struggles, they are more likely to open to the possibility of self-compassion.

Embodying self-compassion, especially the component of common humanity, includes awareness of how a teacher's own identity has been shaped by cultural factors (see also pp. 116–118). It is impossible to be an authentic person in this world and have never experienced bias from culturally determined messages (e.g., body shape, skin color, gender), and members of some marginalized groups experience blatant oppression throughout their lives. To be truly compassionate, teachers need to be open to this source of pain within themselves, to have begun to address it with self-compassion, and to have a commitment to recognizing and alleviating cultural identity pain in others.

Compassionate relating during MSC often occurs during the inquiry process (see Chapter 9). Consider the following inquiry that occurred during a discussion of home practice.

JOSHUA: I'm afraid I'm not very good at self-compassion. When I look inside, I just see so much I don't like, and it isn't going away. I just can't feel good about myself. I'm feeling pretty lost in this program, to tell you the truth.

TEACHER: I can see that you're working really hard at it. Could you describe the feeling that you are struggling with . . . what it's like?

JOSHUA: Yes, it's like a big hole inside. One I could fall into if I'm not careful. It's not a new feeling, but it's here. I hate it.

TEACHER: May I ask where exactly in your body you feel the big hole?

JOSHUA: Sure. It's right in the pit of my stomach.

TEACHER: And is there an emotion tied up with it?

JOSHUA: I'm not sure. Well, mostly *afraid*, I guess. Afraid of something going wrong because I don't know what I'm doing. That's really it. Like being *lost* . . . lost, and frightened about being lost.

TEACHER: Yes, it is scary to feel lost and wonder if you'll ever get it. . . . I'm sure you're not alone in that feeling. (*Pause*) Would you be willing to just let those feelings be there for a moment? (*Pause*) I wonder what you might need when you feel like this—not to fix it, but simply as a comfort? For instance, how would it feel to put a gentle hand where you're feeling the discomfort? (*Joshua puts a hand on his stomach.*)

JOSHUA: It feels pretty nice actually. It also feels good just to be talking about it. It wasn't easy to speak up, I can tell you that.

TEACHER: Then perhaps you're already being compassionate with yourself?

JOSHUA: (*Smiling*) You mean I'm not so bad at this after all?

In this inquiry, the teacher connected with Joshua's struggle to be more self-compassionate and didn't try to fix the problem. Instead, the teacher entered into Joshua's distress. Then, together, they anchored his discomfort in his body, labeled the corresponding emotion, and considered this question: "What do I need?" The supportive interaction with the teacher confirmed for Joshua that he was on the right track in the program.

Qualities of Compassion

When a teacher is being compassionate toward a student, a host of related qualities may arise in the interaction:

- *Curiosity*—genuine interest in what a student is experiencing.
- *Kindness*—a hospitable, nonjudging attitude.
- *Warmth*—a tender inclination of heart toward the individual.
- *Respect*—appreciating the uniqueness of each individual.
- *Allowing*—not fixing and allowing each person to be whole and complete now.
- *Humility*—assuming that one person doesn't know what is best for another.
- *Mutuality*—sense of commonality with others in struggles and aspirations.
- *Confidentiality*—willingness to protect the privacy of others.
- *Receptivity*—ability to listen and learn from others.
- *Flexibility*—capacity to be moved in a new direction by the student.
- *Authenticity*—readiness to be open and honest in a helpful way.
- *Appreciation*—recognizing the inherent strengths in each individual.
- *Attentiveness*—ability to focus on the experience of another.
- *Generosity*—willingness to go beyond one's usual limitations.
- *Empathy*—feeling another's world as one's own.
- *Equanimity*—perspective and steadiness in the midst of strong emotions.
- *Wisdom*—understanding complexity and seeing a way through.
- *Confidence*—inner strength that arises from goodwill.

Teachers who want to increase their capacity for compassion toward others can focus on enhancing any of these compassion-related qualities. For example, intentionally cultivating the quality of "not fixing" might be helpful for psychotherapists who have a habit of trying to fix what's broken. Or for a self-compassion teacher who tends to be a striving and impatient type (commonly called "Type A"), the qualities of mutuality and receptivity might be worth nourishing. By focusing on one personal quality at a time, MSC teachers can widen the spectrum of their compassionate attributes and skills.

Teachers need wisdom to temper how they *express* these qualities of compassion. For example, if a teacher speaks in a warm, motherly tone, one student might enjoy the soothing effect, whereas another may have memories of maternal disapproval or betrayal and feel uneasy. What is medicine for one student could be poison for another. Similarly, one student may need teachers to maintain respectful distance so the student can freely explore his inner world, whereas another might experience the same distance as isolating and lonely. As we grow as MSC teachers, we are likely to recognize our own teaching styles and be able to adjust our favored style to the needs of individual students, or at least to recognize the effect our manner of teaching might have on our students. It also helps to have a co-teacher with a different temperament or teaching style.

Emotion Regulation

Despite our best efforts, sometimes we just don't feel much compassion for our students. Imagine, for example, that you have scheduled an MSC class at the end of the day. One of your students comes to class feeling hungry and angry, and blurts out that the course feels like a total waste of time. How would you react? You might instinctively feel just as angry as your student. You might also conclude that the student is incapable of comprehending what the course is all about. Underneath it all, you might feel ashamed and worry that you are a poor teacher. Where's the compassion now? How do you return to a state of compassion?

Emotion regulation is an important skill for all of us as MSC teachers. It is the capacity to be with emotional pain—ours and that of others—with courage and an open heart. The resources of mindfulness and self-compassion can help. For example, when a teacher is verbally attacked by a participant, the ideal scenario might be to identify shame or anger arising in the body; to allow oneself a moment to breathe gently in for oneself and out for the student (see Chapter 14); and then to explore in a thoughtful manner what the student needs and is hoping to achieve in the course. This approach is likely to induce a shift in physiology from threat to care (see Chapter 2). Of course, it may take a while to rebound after being verbally attacked. That, too, is an opportunity for self-compassion—and for co-teaching.

Co-Teaching

We recommend that MSC be taught, whenever possible, by two teachers (see Chapter 5). A helpful guideline for selecting a co-teacher is whether the person evokes an inner smile when you consider working together. A co-teacher should also be a person whom you genuinely appreciate and respect, and with whom you feel safe. It helps to choose a co-teacher (or an assistant) whose personality or skills complement your own. For example, if you are a woman, you might consider teaching with a man. If you are intellectual by nature, you might wish to work with a more heart-centered person. Every teacher represents a different angle of practice, and diversity in teaching styles opens a wider range of possibilities for students to connect with their teachers and learn from them. Ideally, co-teachers should also have a wish to learn from one another.

MSC students carefully observe the relationship between their co-teachers, often more closely than the teachers are willing to recognize or accept. The relationship between co-teachers inevitably sets the tone for how others in the room relate to one another. When teachers honor and appreciate each other, and enjoy teaching together, this attitude ripples outward to everyone in the room.

Here are some questions that CMSC Executive Director, Steve Hickman, suggests potential co-teachers ask as part of getting to know one another:

- "What most drew you to this program?"
- "Who are some teachers who have impressed or inspired you, and why?"
- "What are you most looking forward to in co-teaching?"
- "What are you most hesitant about when you think of co-teaching?"
- "How do you prefer to receive feedback?"
- "What is one thing that your co-teacher is likely to really appreciate about you?"
- "What is one 'quirk' or 'character flaw' that you possess and that your co-teacher might just have to learn to live with?"
- "What are some of your 'growth edges' in teaching and co-teaching [e.g., trusting the curriculum, not speaking too much, the inquiry process] that you would like to improve?"
- "What are some nonteaching skills or talents that you bring to the table [e.g., organization, marketing/social media, accounting]?"
- "What is your view of the use of humor in teaching the program? How would you characterize your sense of humor?"
- "What is your preferred mode of communication [email, telephone, text message], and what do you consider a reasonable response time for a communication from your co-teacher or participants?"
- "What is your deepest intention for doing this work?"

Course leaders should also be clear from the outset about their respective roles and expectations. Hickman suggests that co-teachers sketch out a memorandum of understanding between them that addresses finances (e.g., splitting profits, handling expenses, scholarships), responsibilities (e.g., marketing, administration, room preparation, class emails), teaching roles (e.g., leadership issues), and plans (e.g., long-term teaching vision). This conversation may seem awkward at first, but it will also prevent future conflicts.

Most co-teaching relationships are neither smooth nor effortless. For example, there may be differences of opinion regarding how to deliver the curriculum or how to work with particular students. Sometimes co-teachers find themselves competing for the affection of students or trying to impress each other. Often one teacher is more experienced or skilled than the other, which inadvertently leads to the less skilled teacher's feeling diminished. It is best to assume *in*compatibility, and plan to accommodate to one another as the course proceeds. Like any relationship, a co-teaching relationship changes over time (Dugo & Beck, 1997).

Co-teachers should also schedule time *after* each session to discuss what they have experienced and learned, ideally when both persons feel relaxed and open to feedback. Teachers can also use the so-called "sandwich method" of giving feedback. The sandwich method reinforces good-will and has three parts: (1) "What I found *most helpful* was . . ."; (2) "What I *might* have found more helpful was . . ."; and (3) "*Another* thing I found helpful was . . ." In other words, a constructive suggestion for improvement is sandwiched between two affirming statements, so that the feedback starts and ends on a positive note. Teachers might also ask each other, "How do you think our group members see us?" With thoughtful preparation and follow-up, co-teaching can be a rewarding experience for everyone.

Ethics

MSC is an inherently ethical program, insofar as compassion is at the heart of most ethical systems (Armstrong, 2010). MSC teachers' authority depends on their ethical integrity. Ethical guidelines have been drafted to remind MSC teachers of the caregiving relationship they have with their students, and to support teachers' efforts to behave compassionately (see Appendix A). Three of those guidelines are the needs to protect the emotional safety of participants, to preserve financial integrity, and to maintain respect for diversity.

Emotional Safety

Since the relationship between teachers and students is asymmetrical, especially in regard to power, it is important for teachers to maintain safe boundaries with and for their students. MSC teachers are required to maintain professional teacher–student relationships with all students during the course, to refrain from seeking additional material or immaterial rewards, and to protect the emotional and psychological safety of their participants.

It is especially important for teachers to maintain safe boundaries regarding sexuality. Students can idealize teachers when the teachers represent something special to the students, and with idealization may come physical attraction. Teachers who have the need to be idealized, or who are lonely in their personal lives, may be inclined to initiate sexual contact with students or comply with sexual invitations. A teacher's capacity to recognize these situations as they arise, as well as discussing them with a co-teacher (and maybe the student), will go a long way toward maintaining psychological safety in the classroom. Teachers may also discover that students become attracted to one another as they grow in emotional intimacy during the course. Teachers should ask students to be mindful of romantic attraction and the harm it may cause to others in their lives, outside the classroom, if they cross physical boundaries.

Financial Integrity

Teaching MSC requires an expenditure of resources—time, energy, money—and teachers need to be fairly compensated for their efforts. Many MSC teachers would teach free of charge if they could, but everyone has bills to pay. We generally recommend that teachers charge for their courses what is being charged in their area for similar 8-week training programs, such as MBSR or MBCT.

A teacher's financial needs may have an impact on how a course is conducted. For example, it may not be financially viable to have a co-teacher if a group is small, or teachers may also be less selective of participants if they need to fill a course for financial reasons. Monetary concerns can also affect how flexible a teacher is when a participant wants to drop out of the program. A teacher who is financially secure might be willing, for example, to offer a student free attendance at a later course. Teachers are encouraged to offer scholarships to less privileged applicants, but this is not always a viable option for teachers. Ideally, teachers make financial decisions from a position of respect both for themselves and for the students.

Embracing Diversity

Our capacity as MSC teachers to respond to others with compassion is limited by our capacity to see our common humanity and our ability to understand the context of people's lives. There are human differences that we may be able to see (e.g., age, skin color, and body type) and differences that might be less visible (e.g., sexual orientation, gender identity, socioeconomic status, early childhood experience, mental or physical illness, religion, politics, literacy, and intellectual abilities) (see Chapter 10). Members of some marginalized groups, such as people of color, and even people in groups that are not a minority, such as women, experience ongoing, systemic oppression.

Our differences can be a source of pride, shame, or a host of other emotions, depending largely on cultural factors, such as how much oppression we experience as our identity develops and how much that oppression is internalized. It is also important to remember that some marginalized individuals have been able to develop strength and resilience in the face of cultural oppression and adversity, such as Susan B. Anthony or Nelson Mandela or Martin Luther King, Jr. (Burt, Lei, & Simons, 2017; Singh, Hays, & Watson, 2011; Spence, Wells, Graham, & George, 2016).

Whatever form oppression takes, the result is *cultural identity pain.* As MSC teachers, we need to be aware and open to our students' cultural identity pain and be ready to validate it and respond with compassion. Creating a space in an MSC class that supports inclusion, diversity, and equity may be a new competency for some MSC teachers, especially for teachers who identify with the dominant culture or have social privilege of one kind or another. Suffering is universal, but not all suffering is equal. Although MSC is ultimately an exercise in common humanity, we get there by validating the uniqueness of each person's experience, especially the experience of pain. Cultural identity pain is a sensitive topic that can evoke feelings of shame, guilt, or anger in just about everyone. Fortunately, self-compassion is a powerful resource for working with such feelings.

When participants arrive at an MSC class for the first time, they often ask themselves, "What is here for me?" as they look around the room for people like themselves. When none are to be found, students at least need to know that the group norms include genuine respect for individual differences and appreciation of the impact of culture on a person's life. Most importantly, the MSC classroom should not be a place where the pain caused by oppression on a personal and systemic level is ignored in an effort to see our common humanity.

MSC teachers are strongly encouraged to develop greater awareness and sensitivity toward the worldviews of those who are culturally diverse. Gaining this type of understanding helps us to view participants' cultural identities as representations of various dimensions and degrees of the self in relation to social disadvantage and/or social privilege. Therefore, we must always be sensitive to the impact of multiple, interacting cultural identities rather than perceiving participants' diverse ways of being as purely one-dimensional. In other words, there is always "diversity within diversity."

Toward that end, teachers may need to take additional training in cultural self-awareness to recognize their own cultural conditioning, uncover unconscious biases, and more closely examine how they are situated in the culture regarding access to power and privilege. This process supports the cultivation of cultural humility, which means acknowledging our limitations, learning to explore social differences despite our discomfort, and remaining open to the reality that cultural identity pain has a profound impact on one's sense of self and lived experience.

MSC teachers from relatively homogeneous cultures may feel that diversity, equity, and inclusion are less applicable to their teaching, but there are marginalized groups that exist within every culture. Expanding our sensitivity to the impact of culture in our lives, especially the impact on those who are subject to daily injury *within* a particular culture, is an important gateway to living and teaching more compassionately.

Additional Supports for Compassion

Sometimes our inner worlds are cauldrons of conflicting impulses, and it is difficult to be compassionate. Some supports for compassion have been mentioned already, such as maintaining a personal practice of mindfulness and self-compassion, a commitment to being compassionate, and ethical standards. Two additional supports are (1) considering ourselves primarily as students rather than as teachers and (2) staying connected to a community of teachers.

Considering ourselves as students helps us remain humble and compassionate as teachers. As G. K. Chesterton (1908/2015) wrote, "Angels can fly because they can take themselves lightly" (p. 78). As long as we suffer in life, we will need to practice mindfulness and self-compassion. That means we are all students. The main differences between us as MSC teachers and our students are that as teachers we know the course curriculum; we have probably been practicing longer than their students; and we are occupying the teacher role.

Joining a community of teachers is another support. There are numerous benefits: We can help one another, learn from one another, be reminded that we're not alone, and enjoy the shared purpose of bringing compassion into the world. Toward that end, the Center for MSC is committed to supporting the worldwide community of teachers through online and face-to-face forums such as advanced training seminars, special interest groups, and conferences.

POINTS TO REMEMBER

* The best way to teach self-compassion is to be compassionate. Learning to embody self-compassion and to relate compassionately toward others are overlapping domains of teacher competence.

* Embodiment of mindfulness and self-compassion teaches through the power of emotional resonance between a teacher and student. Teachers can also model for students that no personal error or imperfection is outside the reach of self-compassion.

* Personal practice—formally in meditation, and informally during the day—is fundamental to embodying self-compassion. Personal practice also enables teachers to understand and support their students as they encounter obstacles to practice.

* Tips for maintaining a formal meditation practice include making it pleasant, feeling physically comfortable, letting go of expectations, starting small, connecting with core values, finding social support, motivating oneself with compassion, and going on a retreat.

* Insights from practice, such as realizing that difficult feelings arise during self-compassion training and are part of the transformative process, help teachers to remain steady and compassionate as their students negotiate similar terrain.

* The manner in which co-teachers relate to one another sets the emotional tone of the whole group. Co-teachers will inevitably have differences of opinion, so they should discuss before and after each session how they can support one another.

* Compassion toward others can be maintained by a commitment to compassionate action, self-compassion, respect for diversity, and ethical standards. It is also helpful to consider oneself primarily a student rather than a teacher, and to stay in touch with a teaching community for support, feedback, and continuing education.

Chapter 8

Facilitating Group Process

> Whatever affects one directly, affects all indirectly. . . .
> I can never be what I ought to be until you are what you
> ought to be . . . this is the interrelated structure of reality.
> —MARTIN LUTHER KING, JR. (1965)

The fifth domain of competence for MSC teachers is *facilitating group process*. This means that MSC teachers try to create a culture of kindness in which each participant experiences compassion and support. A cohesive, nurturing environment also fosters a sense of common humanity that enables participants to be more fully themselves, imperfections and all. Research has shown that self-compassionate individuals adapt better to failure when they witness the struggles of others or have a chance to share their own (Waring & Kelly, 2019). This chapter addresses important skills for leading MSC groups, such as creating safety, working with trauma, balancing the mood of a group, encouraging attendance and participation, and managing challenging participants.

There are four "containers" in an MSC course that can give participants a sense of being held and supported: (1) the physical environment, (2) the teachings, (3) the teacher(s), and (4) the group itself. The *physical environment* should be as safe and pleasant as possible. For example, a simple bouquet of flowers can make an ordinary room, and the people in it, feel cared for. The *teachings* are another source of comfort and support; they help participants get through difficult times. The embodied presence of the *teacher* (or co-teachers) evokes confidence in group members that they, too, have the resources of mindfulness and self-compassion. And, finally, the *group* can be a powerful source of inspiration and support. A cohesive group is especially important because most interactions during an MSC class are among participants rather than with teachers.

Creating Safety

Safety is a prerequisite for learning self-compassion. Careful screening of applicants is an important step toward making MSC safe for everyone (Magyari, 2016; see Chapter 5). Before starting the program, all participants are carefully informed about the nature of the program and sign an agreement that they will take responsibility for their own safety and emotional well-being.

The structure and practices of the MSC curriculum are designed to foster a sense of safety in most participants. Starting with Session 1, participants are invited to establish the norms of the group, such as maintaining confidentiality, respecting boundaries, not giving advice, listening compassionately, and embracing diversity. A teacher's first responsibility is to create the external conditions for safety, so that participants can do the challenging inner work of MSC.

Our intention is to make the MSC classroom not only a "safe space," where everyone can feel comfortable, but also a "brave space" (Arao & Clemens, 2003). A brave space is where each individual's personal identity is acknowledged and respected, where differing opinions are accepted, where interpersonal harm can be discussed, and where students can also exercise the option *not* to discuss a challenging interaction.

Participants are introduced in Session 1 to the concept of *opening and closing.* Opening refers to turning *toward* our experience and being receptive to what is happening—positive, negative, or neutral—and closing refers to turning *away* and trying to limit our exposure to what we are experiencing. We all emotionally open and close throughout the day, and participants also do this throughout the MSC course. Adverse effects are most likely to occur when students are too zealous about learning self-compassion and push themselves to practice when they should stop and rest. Forcing themselves to open when they need to close is not self-compassionate. The theme of opening and closing is carried throughout the course, especially when students feel frustrated with their progress and struggle to be more self-compassionate. Teachers often say, "Please ask yourself whether you are opening or closing right now, and if you are closing, please let yourself close." Knowing *how* to close is a key skill for maintaining safety during MSC, and teachers provide suggestions for closing when emotionally activating practices are introduced.

Keeping students focused on the *resource-building* aspect of MSC also fosters an atmosphere of safety in the classroom. That means that students are learning to *meet* their difficulties in a new way—with mindfulness and self-compassion—rather than intentionally opening old wounds and trying to repair them. The subtle difference in intention between "meeting" and "fixing" problems helps students to regulate how much distress they encounter during the program. People only need a small amount of suffering to practice compassion. A useful metaphor is being immunized with an inactive flu virus (or a small amount of stress) to prepare the immune system for an active flu virus (or greater stress).

Backdraft (see Chapter 11) is likely to make participants feel unsafe during MSC, at least until they know more about backdraft and how to respond to it. Backdraft is the emotional pain, old or new, that arises when people give themselves kindness and compassion. For example, when MSC participants say, "May I love myself just as I am," they are likely to reflect on the unlovable parts of themselves and remember times when they were *not* loved for who they were. Difficult thoughts ("I'm all alone," "I'm a failure"), challenging emotions (shame, grief, fear), or painful sensations (aches and pains) may arise with backdraft. Backdraft becomes even more problematic when participants struggle against it by withdrawing, dissociating, intellectualizing, or criticizing oneself and others. Class exercises have a tendency to evoke backdraft when participants are explicitly asked to remember difficult life events. Backdraft is explained to participants in Session 2 and they are reminded throughout the course to "close" when they feel overwhelmed.

As a final safety precaution, MSC participants typically provide emergency contact information when they start the program, including the names of any mental health providers they may be seeing. Students are also told that their MSC teachers and mental health assistants are available for private consultation, as needed. Sometimes teachers need to be proactive and reach out to students who look distressed or may be too shy to speak up.

Working with Trauma

A number of emotional challenges may emerge during contemplative training, ranging from mild distress to functional impairment (Compson, 2014; Lindahl, Fisher, Cooper, Rosen, & Britton, 2017; Magyari, 2016; Treleaven, 2018). At the mild end of the adverse effects continuum, practitioners can experience anxiety, difficulty sleeping, headaches, or social withdrawal. At the severe end, practitioners may develop irrational beliefs, hallucinations, suicidality, or anhedonia. Factors that influence the development of adverse effects are the *practitioner* (e.g., medical and psychological history, personality, motivation), the *practice* (e.g., amount, intensity, consistency, type, and stage of practice), *relationships* (e.g., early life, practice community, cultural context), and *health behaviors* (e.g., diet, exercise, medication, drugs). To reliably assess adverse effects, teachers should ask their participants directly if they are having uncomfortable experiences during their MSC training (Lindahl et al., 2017). MSC teachers are encouraged to take the meditation safety training developed by Willoughby Britton at Brown University (*www.brown.edu/research/labs/britton/news/2018/02/ first-do-no-harm-meditation-safety-training*).

Old traumas are likely to emerge during self-compassion training. This is because trauma is more prevalent than many people realize. In the United States, 89.7% of the population reports having been exposed to a traumatic event (e.g., fire, physical battery, sexual assault, war zone combat, disaster) (Kilpatrick et al., 2013). Furthermore, self-compassion training tends to attract people who are looking for better ways to manage the sequelae of trauma (i.e., shame, self-criticism, hypervigilance, numbing, avoidance, or intrusive memories). This is why we suggest that a mental health professional be in the room at all times and that applicants be carefully screened. MSC was not designed as a clinical program, but since there is so much trauma in the general population, MSC has been continually modified over the years to make it as safe as possible. We sincerely hope that teachers are conscientious about applying the safety measures currently contained in the curriculum.

"Safety first" is a general rule of MSC training and it applies particularly when working with trauma survivors. Like everyone else, trauma survivors like to challenge themselves, but they also need special instruction in how to titrate the intensity of their experience and return to safety. For example, in the Compassionate Body Scan (a meditation in the retreat session; see Chapter 15), teachers can invite trauma survivors to do the practice in a sitting position rather than lying down, or to move their bodies rather than remaining motionless. Most MSC practices are taught with closed eyes, but participants with trauma histories can be invited to keep their eyes open (either partially or fully). Some parts of the body are more likely than others to hold traumatic memories—for example, the pelvic area for women. When teachers are guiding the Compassionate Body Scan, they should provide participants with the option to skip over a difficult body part if it becomes too activating. Explicit options for grounding are also helpful, such as anchoring attention in the soles of the feet, or mindfully exhaling.

Teachers should not assume that participants with a trauma history will be able to access safety strategies when they need them. Some teachers invite participants to write their safety options on a card that they can consult when they feel overwhelmed. When a teacher notices that a participant seems overwhelmed during an exercise, the teacher can add instructions designed to provide support. Here is an example: "If at any time you find yourself edging into the overwhelmed circle [of the three-circle safety model described in Chapter 6], please feel free to ignore my instructions and go back to the rhythm of the breath, or focus on a point where your body makes contact with the chair or cushion. Opening your eyes, or getting up to take a break from the exercise, are other options." Often a sense of being in control is all that a trauma survivor needs to feel safe.

Teachers need to be especially sensitive and discerning when working with trauma survivors. For example, what may appear like willful determination not to participate in group activities could actually be an effort to stay in the room without becoming overwhelmed. A teacher can ask, "What do you need?", but some trauma survivors will not be able to answer that question since they may be dissociated from their bodies. In that case, a more specific question such as "What do you need *to feel safe?*" or "What could be *soothing* to you right now?" might be more helpful. However, when trauma shuts down a survivor's executive functioning, sometimes *any* question becomes unanswerable. Then teachers need to use their intuition, such as suggesting as short walk outside the room (perhaps with a co-teacher) or giving the student space to be comforted by the rhythm of her own breathing.

Trauma can surface at unexpected times, even during periods of rest and ease. If a student experiences persistent flashbacks, a teacher should have a collaborative conversation with the student about ways of coping and, when necessary, consider the option of discontinuing the course and seeking outside help until the participant is more able to safely engage in the course.

Students themselves are usually the best judges of whether the MSC program is safe for them. Some trauma survivors make significant progress during MSC, despite the intensity of their symptoms. For example, a woman who was numb to her body because of childhood sexual abuse discovered that she could feel her breath for the first time when she focused on how her breath rhythmically rocked her body. On many occasions, Soles of the Feet (the practice of feeling the soles of the feet while walking) has been effectively applied by trauma survivors to anchor their attention in the present moment and away from traumatic memories. Sometimes, the further away from the body that participants place their attention—*outside* the body (sights, sounds) or at the *periphery* of the body (touch points, like the soles of the feet)—the safer the participants are likely to feel. Most reliably, *behavioral* self-compassion (ordinary activities, such as listening to music or chatting with friends) is what keeps the MSC program safe for trauma survivors. (For more on teaching self-compassion to trauma survivors, see Part IV of this book; see also Brähler & Neff, in press; Germer & Neff, 2015).

Balancing a Group's Mood

Groups have moods, just as individuals have moods. The mood of a group may depend on a variety of factors, such as the time of day (e.g., almost everyone is tired at the end of the day), the mood of individual participants (e.g., cheerful, disheartened, curious), the energy of the teachers (e.g., delighted or exhausted), the phase of the course (beginning, middle, or end), and the content of the session (e.g., loving-kindness, core values, difficult emotions). One of the tasks of an MSC teacher is to maintain a balance between opening to pain and responding with mindfulness and compassion—the balance between negative and positive emotions. The MSC curriculum was designed to challenge participants and also give them a chance to recover, but teachers still need to remain alert to the shifting moods of their groups.

Since students tend to focus intently on their teachers, they often feel their teachers' moods as their own. A teacher's mood can be amplified by as many times as there are people in the room. When teachers enjoy teaching the MSC course and take delight in their students, students will reflect those sentiments in kind. If a teacher becomes overwhelmed by the suffering in the room and shows that in various ways (e.g., somber tone, fear, uncertainty), the whole group can become discouraged. When that happens and teachers need to shift the mood of the group in a positive direction, they might try practicing compassion for themselves, addressing the pain in the room in an encouraging manner, or telling a lighthearted story related to the topic at hand.

Of course, sometimes a teacher becomes too emotionally entangled in the group mood, or stuck in personal issues (e.g., the teacher's own self-doubt, irritability, or despair), to shift the atmosphere in the room. That's when a co-teacher needs to step up. A co-teacher might, for example, ask participants to connect with one another in small groups (sharing tends to energize a group), engage in physical movement (e.g., Compassionate Movement, Silly Movement), or take a short break.

After teaching a few MSC courses, teachers tend to become more emotionally resilient. They learn to trust their own capacity as teachers and they discover that the MSC curriculum does most of the work for them. We often tell beginning teachers, "Trust the curriculum . . . and love 'em up!" Indeed, most problems resolve themselves as the course proceeds, and most students leave the program happy and satisfied.

Encouraging Attendance and Participation

One purpose of the first MSC session is to have a second session, and participants are more likely to return for a second session when they feel they belong in the group and can see how the program will meet their needs.

When students register for the program, they agree to attend every session. However, due to unforeseen circumstances, this may not always be possible. If students wish to receive credit for completing the MSC course (i.e., as a prerequisite for teacher training), they need to attend seven of the nine meetings (the eight regular sessions plus the retreat). Students who miss either Session 1 or Session 2, and possibly Session 3, should probably drop out of the course and take it later on. This is because Session 1 begins the process of connecting as a group, establishes group norms, and anchors the program in key concepts and practices. Session 2 provides key information about mindfulness, resistance, and backdraft—knowledge and skills required to safely negotiate the rest of the program. Session 3 is where participants begin to open up to one another and develop trust; those who miss Session 3 will take longer to bond with the group. Most students who attend the first three sessions are likely to finish the course and benefit from it. Each session, however, is scaffolding for the next session, so attendance at every session should be encouraged. Teachers may sometimes be willing to offer reading material and recorded meditations to students who miss a session, or work with them on the corresponding material in *The Mindful Self-Compassion Workbook* (Neff & Germer, 2018).

When students feel as if they are failing at self-compassion, they are likely to disengage from the program, miss sessions, or quit. Teachers should normalize the sense of failure, pointing out that self-compassion is actually surprisingly rare and that *most* students struggle in the learning process. The first half of Session 4 is designed to address these concerns, especially by reframing self-doubt as a sign of progress, and by giving students a chance to share their concerns with each other. Another common reason why participants drift away from the program is that they feel they don't belong in the group, perhaps due to a mismatch between the students' expectations and the reality of the course, cultural differences with other group members, or perhaps a personal conflict between group members. Finally, unexpected backdraft can make the program challenging for some participants. Most of these issues can be resolved when they are acknowledged and openly discussed.

The group learning experience is enriched when all members participate and share their experience. However, some group members are less talkative than others. Teachers should respect a student's wish to remain silent. For some shy participants, simply being in the group is a monumental challenge. Quiet people are more likely to speak in pairs and small groups. When a teacher senses that a participant is having difficulty connecting with others in the group, the teacher can serve as a lifeline to the group by connecting individually with the participant.

Talkative members are usually appreciated at the beginning of a course, but they may need to be reined in as the program progresses. Teachers can restrain excessively talkative members by reminding them to keep their comments practice-based. Sometimes it's necessary to speak privately with a talkative participant and ask the person to make room for others to speak.

The best way to encourage group participation is to validate each individual's experience as a valued member of the group. When students recognize this group norm, they become more confident and willing to share. Sometimes a participant will unintentionally invalidate the experience of another person in the room. When this happens, teachers can name something of value in what the first person shared, remind students that there are no "right" or "wrong" experiences, and reinforce the norm of inclusion. As trust builds, the depth and vulnerability of personal sharing also increases.

Managing Challenging Participants

Most MSC courses include one or two challenging participants. A challenging participant is one who can move a teacher out of a caring frame of mind and into a threat state. Examples of challenging students are those who:

- Complain about how the course is being conducted.
- Dismiss the feelings of other group members.
- Intellectualize rather than share direct experience.
- Consider themselves more expert than their teachers.
- Idealize or sexualize a teacher.
- Often arrive late or leave early.
- Talk excessively.
- Talk too little.
- Do not want to do home practice.

Such participants provide opportunities for you, the MSC teacher, to augment your compassion with wisdom—to discover how best to handle the situation. What follows are some general suggestions for working with challenging participants.

Practicing Compassion for Yourself

It helps to take a Self-Compassion Break (Session 1) when you feel challenged by a student: "This is a moment of suffering," "Suffering is also part of teaching," "May I be kind to myself." If there isn't enough time for a Self-Compassion Break, you can practice Giving and Receiving Compassion (Session 7) when challenged by a student—taking a nice, deep in-breath for yourself, and breathing out compassion for the challenging student.

Looking for the Pain

A moment of self-compassion often creates room for insight to arise about a student's motivation. *Why* might the student be talking so much? Or complaining so much? Or acting in an overbearing manner? Perhaps the student is feeling lonely, frustrated, or ashamed? When you understand what lies beneath the difficult behavior, the sense of threat is more likely to turn to care.

Seeing the Goodness

There is often an admirable quality hidden behind challenging behavior, even though it is expressed in a difficult manner. For example, a group member who dismisses the feelings of others may be courageous in the face of adversity; an excessively conceptual person may have a powerful intellect; and a person who does not do home practice may be finally asking herself, "What do I *really* need?" When students feel understood and appreciated, they are more likely to examine their behavior and make necessary changes.

Shifting to Caregiving

Most difficult behaviors are an unfortunate expression of the wish to be loved. Everyone, including MSC teachers, want to be loved, and we feel threatened when our students make it difficult to teach. We think we're failing, which makes us feel less lovable. Remembering that a challenging student *also* wants to be loved, just like you, can move you out of a threat state and into a care state.

Responding to Challenges

Some participants who challenge their teachers are earnestly trying to understand what self-compassion means, or they are not yet convinced that self-compassion is worth their time and effort. When challenges are met with openness, willingness, and kindness, these participants receive a direct dose of compassion that allows them to begin their own practice. Participants have their own way of responding to stress or confusion (e.g., intellectualizing, monopolizing, criticizing, withdrawing, disrupting, and grandstanding). A compassionate response can become a turning point that allows participants to drop the posturing and engage meaningfully with the group.

Protecting the Group

As a teacher, you have a responsibility to protect the group as a whole. When a particular group member monopolizes the discussions, consistently arrives late to class, disturbs other participants, or repeatedly challenges your authority, the behavior must be stopped to ensure the well-being of the group. If gentle efforts do not produce the desired result, you can meet for a private conversation with the challenging participant. The intention is not to shame the participant, but rather to enlist his cooperation in supporting the learning experience of the whole group.

Using Your Co-Teacher

Co-teachers are not necessarily challenged by the same students. For example, you may be upset by a participant who acts like an outside observer, whereas your co-teacher may see courage and perseverance in the same student who manages to show up each week despite feeling isolated and alone. It helps for you and your co-teacher to discuss your different perspectives and to put corrective measures in the hands of whomever feels less challenged by the participant. When *both* of you are bothered by a student's behavior, you can explore together what might be happening beneath the surface and address the problem together.

Knowing Your Limits

Sometimes a private conversation with a participant is required to set limits or manage expectations. For example, if a student shows sexual interest in you or a group member that interferes with the learning process, you may need to gently confront and redirect the student to finding other ways of meeting those needs. On rare occasions, a participant will not adjust to limits or respond to efforts to improve cooperation. In that case, the challenging participant should be asked to leave the program. This can be a painful conversation, but ideally it occurs with as much mutual understanding as possible, and with backup from your co-teacher.

POINTS TO REMEMBER

* MSC training is most effective within a culture of kindness. When students experience compassion outside themselves, they are more likely to find it inside.

* Compassion training depends on a sense of safety. Students take responsibility for their own safety, and teachers support their efforts.

* Students will become emotionally overwhelmed if they strive too hard to become self-compassionate. Teachers should encourage students to learn slowly, and to close emotionally when they need to.

* Focusing on the resource-building function of MSC, rather than the therapeutic aspect, helps participants to modulate how much emotional pain they experience during MSC.

* Backdraft, or the opening of wounds in the context of compassion, can cause distress for students until they understand the process and know how to respond. Backdraft is an intrinsic part of emotional transformation through self-compassion.

* Special effort may be needed to help trauma survivors access and implement safety strategies.

* The mood of a group needs to be generally positive to facilitate new learning. Teachers can regulate the mood of the group by adjusting their own moods, as well as by varying the types of experiences that students engage in.

* Ideally, students will attend every session and share their practice experiences with the group. The main reasons why students leave the program are that they don't feel they belong in the group, they think they are failing at self-compassion, or they experience unexpected backdraft.

* Challenging participants are those who make teachers feel anxious or who disrupt the group. Co-teachers should work together to understand and resolve these problems.

Chapter 9

Engaging in Inquiry

The art of teaching is the art of assisting discovery.
—MARK VAN DOREN (1961)

The sixth and final domain of competence for MSC teachers is *engaging in inquiry*. Inquiry is a powerful teaching tool. It is a particular way of joining in conversation with individual students about their experience of a practice, typically immediately after the practice is completed. The purpose of inquiry is to strengthen the resources of mindfulness and self-compassion. Inquiry is a self-to-other dialogue that ideally mirrors the self-to-self relationship that teachers wish their students to cultivate, namely, loving, connected presence. Since inquiry is both a personal and a public encounter, everyone gets the chance to learn from the exchange.

Inquiry is the component of teaching that intrigues and confounds most teachers. We can become adept at teaching topics, leading meditations, informal practices, exercises, and reading poetry, but inquiry will always be an unpredictable and unrepeatable experience. Inquiry is as complex as any authentic human relationship, and it's as simple as showing up. Inquiry is a *real* encounter between *real* human beings about *real* experiences and is guided by curiosity, respect, and humility.

Inquiry is also an art that we can develop as long as we are engaged in teaching. The best way to learn inquiry is through lots of practice, and by observing and experiencing inquiry under the guidance of seasoned teachers. Fully one-half of the practice time in the MSC teacher training program is dedicated to the art of inquiry. Readers who wish to teach mindfulness and self-compassion in other settings, such as psychotherapy or business, are encouraged to integrate elements of the inquiry process into their familiar style of teaching. To illustrate the inquiry process further, Part III of this book offers an example of inquiry after each formal or informal practice and exercise.

What Inquiry Is *Not*

To understand what inquiry is, it helps to consider what it is *not*:

- *Discussion.* A discussion is an exchange of ideas *about* an experience, whereas inquiry is a collaborative touching of moment-to-moment experience itself, including thoughts, sensations, and emotions.
- *Elaboration.* Inquiry is a distillation, not an elaboration. Inquiry is the opposite of telling stories about our experience.
- *Interpretation.* Interpretation refers to what our experience *means.* Meaning making depends on our current mood or past experience and is therefore more conditional than direct experience.
- *Asking why.* Inquiry asks *what,* not *why.* It is anchored in present experience rather than a retrospective evaluation or analysis.
- *Fixing.* Inquiry is opening to what is happening in the present moment. A priori attempts to fix how we feel or who we are is often an effort to avoid our experience.
- *Therapy.* The purpose of inquiry is to build the resources of mindfulness and self-compassion, rather than to heal old wounds.
- *Objective.* Since our experience is always subjective, no one has all the answers. However, the best experts on students' experiences are the students themselves.
- *You–me.* Inquiry arises out of *we,* a unique interpersonal field, complex and new.
- *Doing.* Inquiry is a way of being, not doing. It is *being with.*
- *Q&A.* Inquiry is a gentle unfolding, not digging for answers.
- *Formulaic.* Inquiry is a natural human encounter, and rules about inquiry can often get in the way.

Mindfulness and Self-Compassion

MSC, as its full name suggests, cultivates both *mindfulness* and *self-compassion.* A teacher might invite a class to inquiry by asking such questions as "What did you notice?", "What emotions arose for you?", or "How did you respond?" When inquiry is used for training mindfulness, it focuses primarily on the *content* of a student's experience—precisely what the participant noticed from moment to moment—and on whether the awareness was spacious and nonjudgmental. When inquiry is used for training self-compassion, it focuses more on the *quality* of awareness ("Is it warm and accepting?"), especially whether students were relating to *themselves* with kindness and understanding.

Mindfulness questions that may arise in the mind of a teacher during inquiry include "Is the student experiencing any emotional discomfort?", "Can the emotion be named?", "Can it be found in the body?", and "How might the student respond with greater ease?" Self-compassion questions might include "Can the student hold himself with more kindness?" and "Is there anything the student needs, or that the student might find helpful?" When a student shares emotional distress during inquiry, an MSC teacher can assume that the student is fighting, resisting, or avoiding something. The follow-up question "How did you work with that?" could be either a mindfulness or a self-compassion inquiry question. At the end of inquiry, a mindfulness question might be "How are you feeling right now?" and a self-compassion question could be "Is there anything you need?." Either question would help to gently close the inquiry.

It is generally a mindfulness question when the question refers to spacious awareness of *experience,* and a self-compassion question when the teacher is curious whether the student could bring warmth and acceptance to *herself.* The overall purpose of inquiry is to help students adopt a friendlier relationship both to their experience and to themselves. In actual practice, MSC inquiry appears like a single cloth with subtly woven threads of mindfulness and self-compassion.

The Three R's: Radical Acceptance, Resonance, and Resource-Building

Teachers can focus on three components of inquiry, which we refer to in MSC as the "three R's," as a guide for how to engage in inquiry. *Radical acceptance* is the overall attitude of the inquiry process; *resonance* is the primary mode of engagement; and *resource-building* is the desired outcome of inquiry.

Radical Acceptance

Radical acceptance means "fully entering into and embracing whatever is in the present moment" (Robins, Schmidt, & Linehan, 2004, p. 40). In MSC, radical acceptance refers not only to embracing our experience, but also to embracing ourselves. This does not mean that we are perfect and have no need to change. It refers to knowing and accepting ourselves, right now, as a *foundation* for meaningful change.

In inquiry, radical acceptance is the attitude of not judging and not fixing. It is letting our students (and ourselves as teachers!) off the hook, at least for the few minutes of inquiry, of needing anything to be other than it is. A teacher is simply curious about how a student experienced a practice or exercise and how the student responded. Then, if the teacher detects that the student is struggling (which usually means the student is resisting the experience or fighting with oneself), the teacher and student can collaboratively explore what is going on, still without needing anything to change during the inquiry process. Since all beings instinctively resist distress, both personal and empathic distress, radical acceptance is rather an ideal than a constant reality during inquiry.

Radical acceptance also refers to respecting students—honoring their needs, cultural circumstances, vulnerabilities, and wholeness. Since teachers know very little about students' lives, they need to proceed with care. Speaking up in class can make a participant feel vulnerable and exposed, especially if old wounds have surfaced during the preceding exercise or practice. Therefore, when a teacher senses that a student is feeling vulnerable but the student would nonetheless like to continue with the inquiry process, the teacher may ask, "May I ask you a question?" or "Would you be willing to go a little further into this?" Even those questions should be asked without expectation because some students are unable to say "no." When in doubt, it's best to err on the side of safety and back off.

In general, open-ended questions are experienced by students as safer and more respectful than specific questions or statements. Open-ended questions give room for students to choose what they are willing to share. For example, a teacher might ask, "How do you feel right now?" rather than "Are you upset right now?" Another example of an open-ended question is ending an inquiry with "Is there anything you need right now—anything that would be helpful?" rather than suggesting what a participant should do next.

Radical acceptance also refers to how teachers relate to their *own* learning process. Teachers should be patient with themselves as they develop competence with engaging in inquiry. Just as striving to learn self-compassion can be an obstacle on the path to self-compassion for students, striving to get inquiry "right" can interfere with the flow between two people. It is better to be a natural, friendly person and make lots of mistakes rather than self-consciously trying to conduct a perfect inquiry. In other words, the intention for teachers is to learn what their students experienced during a practice, not to act as if they are doing inquiry.

Resonance

The primary task of MSC teachers during inquiry is to *resonate* emotionally with their students. Resonance is 90% of inquiry. When resonance is happening, not much else needs to occur during inquiry.

While resonating, teachers listen not only with their ears, but also with their bodies. Resonance is *embodied* listening. Resonance occurs when students can say, "I know that you know how I feel." They *feel felt* (Siegel, 2010, p. 136). Another measure of resonance is that a teacher is in a state of loving, connected presence. In other words, a student senses the warmth of the teacher, perceives a sense of intimacy, and feels understood.

The intimacy of emotional resonance evokes a sense of deep connection. One student reported, "When my teacher and I were speaking, it felt not only like *she* was talking to me, but also like *I* was talking to me. No difference." In this way, inquiry can activate and strengthen the compassionate voice within each student. Moreover, since other participants are also likely to resonate with the student engaged in inquiry, the dyadic inquiry process can activate self-compassion in everyone in the room.

Resource-Building

The final key component of inquiry is *resource-building*. Resources are not cultivated through resonance alone, but also through validating how a student has used the resources of mindfulness and self-compassion in the preceding practice or by evoking mindfulness and self-compassion during the inquiry itself.

For example, when a student gets derailed during an exercise because of strong emotions, the teacher can return to the point in the exercise where the student got lost, bring mindfulness or self-compassion to the scene, and then escort the student through one or more remaining phases of the exercise. Here's an inquiry with a participant, Joan, after the Meeting Unmet Needs exercise in Session 7.

JOAN: I don't know about that exercise. I just checked out.

TEACHER: Can you remember when you checked out?

JOAN: Not really. Wait . . . it was when you asked us to let go of the person who hurt us and go deeper into what we were feeling. I didn't want to do that. I want an apology from the person.

TEACHER: I can understand that. Don't we all, when we feel hurt by someone? It's so natural.

JOAN: Yeah.

TEACHER: I'm curious. When we got to the part of the exercise that asked what unmet need was driving your feelings of hurt, were you able to identify anything?

JOAN: No, I was just stuck feeling sad and hurt.

TEACHER: Do you mind considering the question now? For example, did you want to be treated more respectfully, or be seen, or be valued?

JOAN: Yes, I really loved this person and needed to be loved back. I just wanted to be loved back (*eyes becoming moist*).

TEACHER: Of course you did. You needed to be loved back. (*Pause*) It hurts so much when we don't feel loved back. (*Pause*) I wonder, what would you say to a good friend who felt this longing, just like you?

JOAN: Oh, I'd say, "You are *so* lovable. You are *so* beautiful." I'm afraid he just couldn't see that.

TEACHER: Yes, you would say, "You are *so* lovable. You are *sooooo* beautiful." Is it okay if we do a little experiment together?

JOAN: Sure.

TEACHER: Let's just say those words together. Maybe even as a whole group, silently. If others are willing, let's close our eyes and just say those words silently to ourselves: "You are *so* lovable. You are *so* beautiful." (*Long pause*)

JOAN: (*Smiling*) I get it.

TEACHER: What do you get?

JOAN: It will take some time, but I get it. I can give it to myself. I actually feel much better right now.

In this short exchange, the teacher referred Joan back to the moment in the Meeting Unmet Needs exercise when she "checked out." That grounded the conversation in direct experience. Then the teacher escorted Joan through the next set of instructions in the exercise, which were about discovering unmet needs behind hurt feelings. When Joan was able to complete that activity, she was guided into the final part of the exercise—giving ourselves compassion in response to unmet needs, and meeting our needs directly. Joan was able to finish the exercise this time, with the help of the teacher and the rest of the group. The inquiry process also reminded the whole group about different elements in the exercise that they had just completed, especially how to meet our unmet needs from old relationships by using the resource of self-compassion.

Motivation for Sharing

At the start of inquiry, when a student raises a hand, the teacher begins to assess the student's motivation. The aim is to ascertain as quickly as possible if there is a problem that needs to be addressed, or if the student simply wishes to share an insight or observation.

No Problem

When there's no problem, or if the student *had* a problem that resolved itself, the student may be speaking in order to:

- Feel part of the group.
- Acknowledge a success.
- Strengthen an insight.
- Find words for a new discovery.
- Help others by sharing an interesting experience.

All these motivations are welcome. In general, when there is no problem, the teacher can simply resonate with the student and validate the resource that was evident during the sharing. For example:

- *The resource of mindfulness:* "It seems that you were able to make a lot of space for your anxiety. That takes some courage."
- *The resource of self-compassion:* "And then you put your hand over your heart and you felt reassured. That's wonderful. Is this something you might like to try again the next time you feel like that?"

Sometimes a simple "thank you," a warm smile, or a nod is all that's needed. This can also give group members confidence that they can share what they like, and that the teacher will not try to keep them talking. When a teacher acknowledges a few comments in succession without much discussion, it can create an atmosphere of quiet, mutual appreciation. Some students articulate their experience so beautifully, like a Rembrandt painting, that it is unnecessary to add any more to it.

Ongoing Problem

Sometimes there is an ongoing difficulty that a student would like to address, so the student may speak in order to:

- Alleviate discomfort left over from the practice.
- Find a solution to an ongoing life dilemma.
- Confirm whether he is practicing correctly.
- Connect with others and feel less alone in her struggle.
- Speak as a means to avoid discomfort.

This is when inquiry can be used to discover, activate, or strengthen the resources of mindfulness and self-compassion. For example:

- *The resource of mindfulness:* "When you say you feel hopeless, is there some place in your body where you feel the hopelessness right now?"
- *The resource of self-compassion:* "I'm wondering what you might say to a dear friend who was struggling in the same way as you are now."

Overcoming obstacles to practice is what makes inquiry most interesting for everyone in the room. In the first few weeks of MSC, participants have a tendency to share only positive experiences and insights. It's necessary to invite students early in the course to share challenging experiences as well, so they don't feel alone with their difficulties.

Moving from Resonance to Resource-Building

When it is time for teachers to speak, where do they start? What part of a student's experience should a teacher highlight in conversation? How does the teacher move from resonance to resource-building? The way to begin is to follow the *pings*. A ping in MSC is a little internal tap, or moment of salience or interest, that a listener experiences in his body while another person is talking. A ping is a launching pad for inquiry. A student's motivation for sharing plays a role in the kind of pings that a teacher may experience during inquiry.

No Problem

When a student does not have a problem and is simply sharing an insight or experience, then a teacher can listen in an embodied way for what is most vivid and alive for the student. The teacher can make a mental note of what is being said at the moment of a ping, and then reflect the ping back to the student in a validating manner when the student has finished. In other words, the teacher looks for moments of mindfulness or self-compassion and "underlines" them. For example, a teacher might note an insight by a student, and then reflect it back with the words "And then you realized that the feeling of helplessness was behind your muscle tension." Or if the teacher has noted how an experience of common humanity helped a student to relax, that observation could be articulated with these words: "You had the courage to face your fear, and when you realized you weren't isolated or alone in your fear, you were able to exhale." In this way, resonating with students while remaining alert to ping moments gives teachers the capacity to reinforce or build the resources of mindfulness and self-compassion.

Sometimes the resources of mindfulness and self-compassion themselves may not be the most apparent features of a sharing; rather, strengths that *support* mindfulness and self-compassion may be evident, such as courage, determination, curiosity, sense of humor, confidence, humility, or receptivity. Recognition of these qualities are pings of appreciation, and they can also be named by teachers during inquiry. Appreciation and admiration are more likely to arise when teachers genuinely like their students and want to see the good in them.

Ongoing Problem

When a student describes a difficulty, embodied awareness can be practiced by the teacher by noting empathic discomfort in her own body—for example, the feeling of sadness as a student refers to a death in the family, or shame as the student relates a failure to do an exercise properly. Making note of these pings and gently sharing them can validate elements of the student's experience and help to illuminate the practice under consideration.

We can trust our curiosity as teachers and ask questions, respectfully, if we are speaking from a ping. Students usually like to be asked a question when it deepens their experience. It is important, however, to check humbly whether our reactions are accurate or not—for instance, "When you talked about your uncle dying, it felt like there was still some grief there. Is that right?" The student can then correct a misperception, if needed: "Actually, I'm not feeling much grief; I'm mostly relieved that he isn't suffering any more." If we are unsure where to begin, we can also simply ask a student, "Was there anything in particular about the practice or the exercise that stood out for you?" or "Where did that come up in your practice?"

Sometimes a student wants to discuss an ongoing problem because the student feels unable to handle it alone. That's when a teacher's presence is especially helpful, serving as a container for the student's feelings. When a teacher is genuinely moved by a student's plight, and the student feels the teacher's compassion, the student begins to experience the problem differently right there in the midst of inquiry. This is how self-compassion is taught relationally.

Sometimes the teacher can feel what a student is going through *before* the student is aware of it. For example, a female student once described a traumatic miscarriage in matter-of-fact terms while the teacher, and a few others in the room, welled up with tears. The openhearted response of other people opened the student to her own grief, and in that moment, the student's relationship to her trauma began changing.

Teachers should avoid the trap of putting the resource-building aspect of inquiry, such as exploring what to *do* about a problem, ahead of emotional resonance. Students will resist teachers' well-intentioned efforts to build resources if they don't feel heard. Sometimes a teacher may indeed hear what a student is trying to say, empathically feeling the student's distress, but launch into resource-building as an unconscious attempt to make the teacher's own distress go away. For instance, when a student tears up and displays intense sadness, if a teacher immediately suggests, "Do you want to try putting your hands on your heart?", the student may feel that the sadness is unwelcome. The optimal scenario is for a teacher to resonate with the student, hold the pain in loving awareness, validate it together with the student, and then collaboratively explore what might be most helpful. Asking an open-ended question such as "Is there anything that you need right now?", rather than offering a specific suggestion, will help the student feel that the pain is accepted while also reminding him of resources for holding it.

Conversely, some teachers resonate too strongly with a student's pain and forget about resources. A teacher only needs to *touch* pain as an occasion for building resources. In inquiry, this may mean just labeling a difficult emotion or locating it in the body before considering a compassionate response, such as calming with the breath if the participant feels anxiety, or focusing on common humanity if the student is absorbed in shame.

Engaging in inquiry itself can be an act of self-compassion by a student. For example, a student may want to break through silence about something embarrassing, and speaking up in class may do just that. Or a student who feels isolated in the classroom may engage in inquiry just to feel part of the group. When responding to students during inquiry, teachers should remember that the here-and-now experience of engaging in inquiry is also resource-building.

Enhancing Participation

At least one or two participants are usually willing to engage in inquiry after a practice, but occasionally no one volunteers. This potentially awkward situation is more likely to occur in the first few MSC sessions, before everyone feels safe, or near the end of a session, when participants are especially tired. Participants are also less likely to speak in larger groups (20+ people), or in classes taking place in cultures that value personal privacy.

Participants usually require a period of settling and reflection to shift from being immersed in meditation to thinking about it, to finding words for their experience, and then to speaking up in class. If teachers are patient, they will be rewarded by thoughtful comments from students. It also helps to open inquiry with *specific* questions. For example, teachers can ask a question about a *part* of a practice, such as "Did you receive an interesting gift from your compassionate friend during that meditation?" Other specific questions could include "Did anyone experience any challenges during that practice?"; "Was there anything particular in that practice that you liked? And if so, what was it?"; "Please raise your hand if you could feel [name of feeling]. What was that like?"; "Would anyone be willing to share a single word that captures something of your experience of that exercise?"

Generally speaking, teachers should guard against feeling anxious or distressed when no one speaks. When teachers get into a threat mode, they put subtle pressure on their students to speak, which makes the inquiry period unnecessarily stressful for everyone. In that case, it's better just to skip inquiry and move on to the next part of the program.

Anchoring Inquiry

MSC participants are instructed in Session 1 of the MSC course to keep their comments during class as practice-focused as possible—in other words, to share their *direct experience* of a practice. However, staying practice-focused is not always easy, since self-compassion can be emotionally activating and propel students out of their bodies and into their heads. When a student feels compelled to intellectualize or tell personal stories during inquiry, and a teacher wants to bring the conversation back into the room, it is important to redirect the student without cutting her off or making her feel that she is doing something wrong. The following approaches may be helpful:

- Asking the student about body sensations during the *inquiry process* itself (e.g., "Can you feel your grief in your body right now?").
- Asking the student to reflect on the sensations or emotions experienced during the *practice* itself (e.g., "Did these sensations arise during the exercise as well?").
- Asking the student at *precisely what point* in the preceding practice the student became derailed (e.g., "Was that at the point when you started to breathe compassion out for the other?").
- Keeping the *intention* of the preceding exercise or practice in mind, narrowing the student's attention to that purpose (e.g., "Were you able to warm up your awareness when you thought about someone you love?").
- Refocusing the student on the *skill* taught in the exercise or practice (e.g., "Were you able to find a phrase that was meaningful to you?").

By anchoring inquiry in this way, teachers are able to maximize the learning potential of the program's experiential components.

Some MSC students have relatively little practice in tracking their moment-to-moment experience—either because they are not introspective by nature, or because they have a tendency to think *about* what is happening rather than directly experiencing it. Teachers may feel frustrated by these students during inquiry, worrying that the students are setting a bad example for other students. Teachers should nonetheless give their students some leeway to express themselves in their own way, and then gradually reorient them to their direct experience.

Ending Inquiry

A teacher can usually tell when inquiry is over by a sense of ease in the body or the impression that there is nothing left to say. A teacher who is unsure whether a student has finished can simply ask, "How do you feel now?" A typical inquiry takes 2–3 minutes, but many inquiries take less than 1 minute, especially when a participant is sharing an insight and doesn't have a problem. An inquiry as long as 5 minutes is rare and carries the risk of over-exposing the student and losing the interest of the group. If a participant appears to have personal issues that require more than 5 minutes of inquiry time, the teacher can offer to speak with the student during the break or after class, or a co-teacher might go outside the room with the student.

Teachers are sometimes responsible for extending inquiry too long. For example, a teacher may feel a student's distress and want to keep the conversation going until it's resolved. Another reason why teachers may extend inquiry is that they want to feel they are doing a good job. Some teachers think they *should* keep talking to conduct a proper inquiry when there is actually nothing left to say. When teachers find themselves talking too much, they can apply the acronym WAIT, for "Why Am I Talking?" Less is more.

Sometimes *students* try to extend inquiry beyond its natural endpoint. There are many reasons for this, such as when a student is enjoying the attention, struggling to feel better, or looking for deeper understanding. Teachers should not be afraid to interrupt students who speak too much, especially if it is done with the clear desire to understand more deeply what a student is saying, and if it represents an attitude of caring rather than a wish to silence the student. When a teacher interjects with a question in order to get to the emotional core of a student's comments (e.g., "Would you mind if I ask a question? Are you saying that you could actually *feel* that the anger was masking grief?"), the student usually appreciates being interrupted because it leads to greater understanding. The rest of the group is generally appreciative as well.

Co-Inquiring

Generally speaking, the teacher who leads the practice conducts the inquiry. After inquiry has ended, if the co-teacher senses that something important has been overlooked, the co-teacher may ask the inquirer for permission to speak and contribute. The co-teacher should balance the inclination to continue the inquiry with how important the issue is and how it may feel to the inquirer if the co-teacher takes over. Teachers also don't want students to feel overexposed by an excessively long inquiry and the attention of both teachers. Respecting boundaries during inquiry helps to establish a norm of respect in the classroom.

Reorienting the Heart

Needless to say, no teacher resonates with all students all the time. As teachers, we may be unable to resonate with our students for a variety of reasons (e.g., we really don't know much about our students; our students get confused and don't know what *they* are trying to say; or we feel emotionally threatened or exhausted). These situations are normal and occur because we are all human beings.

We may find it easier to return to resonance when we know our own emotional triggers. Triggers might include seeing a participant yawn, feeling intellectually intimidated, being dismissed by a group member, or being unable to alleviate a participant's distress.

Another trigger is the experience of shame. All of us who sincerely wish to be good teachers will experience shame when it appears that we are failing at the task. Do we know what shame feels like in our bodies; can we recognize it when it arises; and can we be kind to ourselves, knowing that this is part of the teaching experience? Recognizing shame when it arises creates inner space and protects us from shaming our students in return. It also removes a major obstacle to resonating with the experience of others.

No matter what the reason may be for losing connection with a student during inquiry, the first step back into connection is for us to recognize and admit to ourselves that we're lost. Our breathing can then help us back into connection—for example, by breathing in for ourselves, allowing our attention and compassion to go inside, and then breathing out for the student, allowing our attention and compassion to flow out to the student (see the discussion of compassionate listening in Chapter 14). We can do this a few times, and when connection is restored, we can return to embodied listening.

When we feel lost during inquiry, we can also reorient ourselves by asking ourselves a simple question: "What is most salient and alive for the student?" If it is clear that the student is struggling, then the question is "Where's the pain?" For example, maybe a student fell asleep during the practice and feels distraught about that. Then we may ask, "And how did you feel when you *noticed* you fell asleep? Were you okay with that, or was there some judgment?" In other words, sometimes the pain is experienced within the practice itself, and sometimes the pain comes from how the student is *approaching* the practice. No matter what the source, our task as teachers is primarily to recognize and hold the pain of our students with kindness and understanding, and then to teach the students how to do the same.

The safest way to do inquiry is to be humble and openhearted, learning together with our students. MSC participants are very forgiving of us as teachers when they know that we care and also want to learn. Just being human is the best example we can set for others who are on the path to self-compassion.

POINTS TO REMEMBER

* Inquiry is a self-to-other dialogue that mirrors the mindful and self-compassionate self-to-self dialogue that we are cultivating in MSC.

* The three R's of inquiry are radical acceptance, resonance, and resource-building.

* *Radical acceptance* is accepting the participant and the participant's experience just as they are. Radical acceptance also refers to respecting the needs and capacities of our students.

* *Resonance* is a state of loving, connected presence that enables students to "feel felt." Resonance is 90% of inquiry.

* *Resource-building* is using inquiry to affirm, activate, strengthen, and build the skills of mindfulness and compassion. This is a collaborative process of discovery, rather than an effort to fix or change a student.

* Students typically speak up during inquiry either to share an experience or to find a solution to a problem. In either case, teachers can listen in an embodied manner for what is most salient and alive to the students.

* When students stray from practice-based comments, they can be brought back into the room by focusing on body sensations or by referring to what happened during the exercise.

* Teachers should not feel shy about interrupting their students if they can bring the conversation to a deeper level of understanding. A typical inquiry lasts 2–3 minutes and ends when the teacher and student have a sense of closure.

* There are many times during inquiry when teachers cannot resonate with their students or understand their struggles. Maintaining a humble and collaborative attitude is the safest and most beneficial stance for a teacher during inquiry.

* The goal of inquiry is to model how to hold pain with compassion. Sometimes pain arises during the inner journey of a practice, and sometimes it arises from how a student *relates* to a practice itself (e.g., striving, sleeping). Both are valid topics for inquiry.

PART III

Session by Session

There is no teaching until the pupil is brought into the same state
or principle in which you are; a transfusion takes place; he is you,
and you are he; then is a teaching; and by no unfriendly chance
or bad company can he ever quite lose the benefit.

—RALPH WALDO EMERSON (1841/1883, p. 35)

The following chapters contain detailed descriptions of each of the eight
MSC sessions, plus the half-day retreat. This material can be used as a
resource for readers who want to integrate the principles and practices of
self-compassion into their professional activities (e.g., counseling, coaching, teaching, medicine, business), and as a reference for MSC teachers.
Many details are provided (e.g., research, quotations, poems, and videos).
Our purpose is not to overwhelm the MSC teacher, but rather to provide
a solid platform for teaching. As already mentioned, *connection* is as
important as the *content* when teaching self-compassion, and *how* we
teach is as essential as *how much* we teach. Ideally, students will experience the warmth and ease of self-compassion during every MSC class—
loving, connected presence—and will also hear about self-compassion in
the unique voices of their teachers.

Some material in Part III has already been presented in the previous
chapters and is mentioned again to show how those points can be woven
into the curriculum. In the following chapters, the components of each
MSC session are identified by the icons in the box on page 146.

Some readers may feel that they are ready to teach MSC after
reviewing the domains of competence (Part II) and reading the detailed
descriptions of each session in this part of the book (Part III). Seasoned
mindfulness teachers or experienced psychotherapists are especially likely
to feel that way. Indeed, MSC has so much in common with mindfulness
training and psychotherapy, but MSC also has its own unique characteristics that require in-person teacher training and often multiple rounds
of practice to adequately understand and communicate MSC to students.

Components of MSC

Meditation
Most sessions begin with a formal meditation, followed by inquiry.

Practice Discussion
Participants are invited to discuss their home practice.

Session Theme
Participants are oriented to what they will learn in the session.

Topic
Each topic provides a conceptual map for subsequent practices and exercises.

Informal Practice
An informal practice is a brief practice that can be integrated into everyday life.

Break
All sessions include a 15-minute refreshment break.

Soft Landing
A soft landing allows students to gently settle into the present moment after the break.

Exercise
An exercise is a classroom activity designed to illustrate a key concept or concepts.

Home Practice
Participants are reminded of the practices they have learned in the session and are encouraged to practice during the week.

Closing
Each session closes with a brief group activity.

Our hope is that the following chapters will convey the subtlety and complexity of teaching MSC, and that readers will be inspired to seek out formal teacher training if they wish to teach the MSC course.

At the formal teacher training, trainees receive helpful classroom materials (i.e., teacher handbook, session guide, handouts, forms) that augment this professional textbook and make the experience of teaching smoother and easier. Graduates of the teacher training program can also join the worldwide community of MSC teachers and further develop their teaching skills through online resources and continuing education.

Chapter 10

Session 1

DISCOVERING MINDFUL SELF-COMPASSION

Overview

Topic: Welcome

Exercise: Why Am I Here?

Topic: Practical Details

Topic: How to Approach MSC

Exercise: Guiding Principles

Break

Soft Landing

Exercise: How Would I Treat a Friend?

Topic: What Is Self-Compassion?

Exercise (Optional): Gestures of Self-Compassion

Topic: Misgivings about Self-Compassion

Topic (Optional): Research on Self-Compassion

Informal Practice: Soothing Touch

Informal Practice: Self-Compassion Break

Home Practice

Closing

Getting Started

- In this session, participants will:
  - Introduce themselves to one another and become oriented to the program.
  - Understand what self-compassion is and what it isn't.
  - Explore the link between self-compassion and well-being, scientifically and experientially.
- These subjects are introduced now to:
  - Establish a conceptual foundation for self-compassion before students embark on the path of practice.
- New practices taught this session:
  - Soothing Touch
  - Self-Compassion Break

On Teaching Sessions 1 and 2

Although the recommended length of time for each MSC session is 2 hours and 45 minutes, it may be necessary to schedule 3 hours for Session 1. Both Sessions 1 and 2 contain more didactic material than subsequent sessions because they provide participants with a conceptual foundation for the rest of the course.

Session 1 introduces the topic of *self-compassion,* and Session 2 lays the groundwork for *mindfulness.* The first half of Session 1 welcomes participants to the course and helps them get to know one another. This conversation is crucial to establish a sense of safety and connection in the classroom. The second half of Session 1 familiarizes participants with the meaning and practice of self-compassion.

Teachers should carefully prioritize what they would like to teach in Sessions 1 and 2. This is especially the case for Session 1, since there is a wealth of theoretical and scientific material to choose from. Generally speaking, the experiential components of a session (meditations, class exercises, and informal practices) are more important than the didactic material, so teachers should focus on teaching all the practices in a session. Many beginning teachers find it difficult to conduct Session 1 in a spacious, interactive manner. In that case, teachers may consider the following two options:

1. *Orientation session.* As mentioned in Chapter 5, a separate orientation session can be offered to prospective participants before the 8-week course begins. This is an opportunity to present some of the didactic material

in Session 1 (e.g., components of self-compassion, misgivings, research), so that those attendees who continue with the program will already have been exposed to this material and it doesn't have to be repeated.

2. *Outside reading.* Students can be offered relevant material before or after Session 1. For example, Neff's (2015) article "The 5 Myths of Self-Compassion," or an article in *Scientific American Mind,* "The Self-Compassion Solution" (Krakovsky, 2017), can be distributed to students before Session 1; this may enable teachers to focus more on the experience of self-compassion during the class. Additional materials can be found in *The Mindful Self-Compassion Workbook* (Neff & Germer, 2018), chapters from our books (Appendix B), and other written or online materials (Appendix C).

Welcome
(15 minutes)

The course begins with a few minutes of casual, welcoming conversation, and then teachers guide participants in a brief meditation that gives them a taste of mindfulness and self-compassion. Teachers can improvise how they offer this introduction. Here are some examples:

- "Now that everyone is *physically* present, we would like to bring our *hearts* and *minds* into the room as well."
- "Please sit in a comfortable position, any way you like, and let your eyes close partially or fully."
- "Let's begin by simply listening to the sounds in the room, just sitting in the midst of sounds, letting them come to you."
- "Now, in your mind's eye, finding your own body in the room. Perhaps welcoming yourself into the room, greeting yourself with an inner smile."
- "Inclining your awareness toward yourself as you might toward a dear friend."
- "Now dropping your awareness into the body and noticing the physical sensations in the body as they come and go—pleasant (*pause*), unpleasant (*pause*), and neutral (*pause*)."
- "Are there any *pleasant* sensations? (*Pause*) If so, can you take a moment to *appreciate* and *savor* them?"
- "Are there any *un*pleasant sensations? (*Pause*) If so, can you make some *space* for them, allowing them to be there, if only for this one moment?"

- "Remembering that you are *not alone*—that uneasiness and discomfort is part of the human condition."
- "And if there is discomfort, can you let your heart *soften* a little, be a little tender, simply *because* this is so."
- "Or maybe offer yourself some *words of encouragement,* like 'It's okay. You can handle this.'"
- "And finally, appreciating the effort and the good intentions that brought you here—already an act of compassion and self-compassion."
- "Gently opening your eyes."

Afterward, teachers can mention that all three components of self-compassion were contained in this brief meditation: *mindfulness* (paying spacious attention to what we are experiencing), *common humanity* (remembering that we are not alone), and *self-kindness* (offering ourselves some warmth or encouragement). The MSC course that the participants are about to embark upon is designed to move mindfulness and self-compassion from a *concept* to a *felt experience* in each person's life, to let the experience *sink in,* and to *provide tools* for evoking mindfulness and self-compassion in everyday life.

To begin the process of building connections between group members, teachers can conduct a general survey of the group, asking questions such as these:

- "Is there anyone in the room who is *new* to meditation?"
- "How many people have *some* experience with meditation?"
- "How many people meditate as a *regular* practice?"
- "How many people *aspire* to have a regular practice?"
- "Please raise your hand if you have a *loving-kindness* or *compassion* meditation practice."
- "Is there anyone with a devotional practice, such as prayer?"
- "Does anyone hope to integrate self-compassion into their *work*? If so, what type of work?"
- If professionals indicate that they are taking the course primarily for the sake of their work, gently suggest that they approach the course as an opportunity to experience mindful self-compassion in their own lives first, as a foundation for teaching self-compassion to others.

Thereafter, teachers can invite all participants to say their names, indicate where they live, and (depending on the size of the group) briefly share why they are interested in taking this course.

Why Am I Here?
(25 minutes)

To help participants focus on their goals and intentions for taking the course, they are invited to close their eyes and reflect upon two questions:

- " 'Why am I here?' " (*Pause*)
- " 'Why am I *really* here?' (*Pause*) See if you can peel back the onion a little and discover something deeper: 'Why now, at this particular stage in my life, at this particular time . . . why am I *really* here?' " (*Pause*)

There are usually a few chuckles in the room when the second question is asked.

To reinforce each participant's intention and to begin the process of connecting the members of the group, participants are invited to form small groups of three persons, introducing themselves to one another and sharing *why* they are taking the class, but only sharing what feels safe and comfortable. Some responses to the first question ("Why am I here?") may be "To learn self-compassion," "Because my wife/husband/partner asked me to come," or "Because my life is a mess." In response to the second question of why a person is *really* at the workshop, we hear comments like "Because I'm so self-critical," "I'm hoping self-compassion will make me a happier person," and "I get angry too easily, and I think this could help me." We ring a bell after 6–8 minutes, letting participants know that they will have many more opportunities to interact with one another, and adding that we as the teachers also hope to connect personally with each group member during the course.

Then the teacher or teachers share what brought them to self-compassion, especially sharing a few personal details that illustrate why they are passionate about practicing and teaching self-compassion. Teachers should not feel shy about stating their professional credentials or teaching experience if doing this would help create a sense of trust in the participants.

Practical Details
(5 minutes)

Participants will want to know the following practical details about the course that make it run smoothly.

- *Schedule.* The course schedule is reviewed with participants. Participants are told that there will be a break at the midpoint of each session, but that they should feel free to use the restroom at any time.

- *Nametags.* Knowing names makes it easier to connect with one another. In larger classes, participants are asked to wear their nametags throughout the course.

- *Seating.* Participants are invited to occasionally change where they are sitting as the course proceeds, if that feels right. Shifting seats gives participants new neighbors and sometimes different perspectives.

- *Workbook.* Students can follow the topics and practices of the MSC course, using *The Mindful Self-Compassion Workbook* (Neff & Germer, 2018). Teachers usually purchase copies of the workbook for their students as companion reading for the course.

- *Recordings.* Ideally, MSC teachers make audio recordings of MSC meditations in their own voices and share the recordings with participants. Alternatively, recordings of the three core meditations and selected other MSC practices can be streamed or downloaded from this book's companion website (see the box at the end of the table of contents). *The Mindful Self-Compassion Workbook* also has a companion website featuring the audio recordings.

- *Research.* Participants can find a comprehensive reference list of research on self-compassion on Kristin Neff's website (*https://self-compassion.org*).

- *Weekly feedback.* Participants are invited to provide weekly feedback about their daily practice and bring it to each session. Providing this feedback is an opportunity to reflect on this practice and to communicate with the teachers.

- *Teacher availability.* Participants are informed about how to contact their teacher(s) when they need to do so. If there are co-teachers, they are also reminded that what they share with one teacher may be shared with the other teacher unless a participant specifically asks for privacy.

- *Notes.* Paper-and-pencil exercises are included in most sessions, so participants are asked to come prepared with writing materials. Some students also like to keep a diary of their experiences during the program.

- *Recording.* To create a safe, confidential learning environment, participants are discouraged from recording the sessions. In special cases, a participant may be allowed to record the spoken words of the teachers only.

- *Email.* Most teachers communicate with their students via email between classes (e.g., summarizing what was taught, encouraging home practice, sending a poem, or sharing a personal anecdote). Students should inform the teacher(s) after class if they do *not* wish to be included in the email list.

How to Approach MSC
(25 minutes)

We have found that the following orientation to MSC helps make the program safe, effective, and enjoyable. As much as possible, the following material should be presented interactively, with leading questions and discussion.

MSC Is an Adventure

Teachers can open with the question: "MSC is a journey, and it is an adventure. What is the difference between a journey and an adventure?" An adventure takes us into uncharted territory where we are likely to encounter unexpected obstacles. The process of discovering and mastering those obstacles makes MSC more like an adventure than a journey—an *inner* adventure.

Participants should also be invited to take a curious, investigative approach to everything that transpires during MSC. Many different elements will be introduced into the laboratory of their own experience—new attitudes, thoughts, words, images, and sensations—and each participant is encouraged to be a good scientist and explore what happens. Teachers can ask, "What are some qualities of a good scientist?" A good scientist is open-minded, curious, honest, and flexible—willing to follow the evidence wherever it leads, without too many preconceptions about what should happen or what it means.

Students are told that during the course they will learn 7 meditations and 20 informal practices designed to evoke mindfulness and self-compassion in their daily lives. The rationale behind the practices will also be explained, so participants can understand and tailor the practices to meet their own individual needs—in other words, to become their own best teachers. As they go along, students are encouraged to ask themselves, "What works for me?", and to record their experience of the practices in the weekly feedback they provide.

Difficult Emotions

Compassion is a positive emotion associated with happiness and well-being. Therefore, learning self-compassion is mostly a positive experience. However, there is a saying: "Love reveals everything unlike itself." This means that difficult emotions will show up for almost everyone who participates in MSC. Teachers can ask, "What kinds of difficult emotions do you think could arise during self-compassion training?" Common responses are grief, loneliness, longing, anger, fear, and self-doubt. Self-compassion opens old wounds, but it also allows people to meet these old wounds in a new way and transform them for the better. MSC is a *resource-building* program; it is designed to build the emotional skill and capacity to meet challenges from a position of strength.

Lest students worry that the course will be hard work, they should be advised that a moment of self-compassion is actually a *relief*—not hard and not work. Work is what we do when we struggle to improve our lives. Mindfulness and self-compassion involve letting go of that struggle without compromising our goals.

A moment of *mindfulness* has the sound of a delicious exhale—"Ahhh." A moment of *compassion* has a tender sound—for example, "Awww" when we feel moved by someone's struggle, "Ohhh" when we lean forward with empathic understanding, or "Ahhh" as we lean back having finally understood the fullness of what's happening. In contrast, the sounds of struggle are more like "Grrr" and "Aargh." Voice is a powerful vehicle for communicating emotion and attitude (Kraus, 2017). Teachers can make these sounds with the class and encourage their students to experiment with the sounds of mindfulness and self-compassion whenever they find themselves struggling in the course. Although self-compassion training can be challenging, teachers aspire to make it as easy and pleasant as possible.

The MSC program itself is a training ground for self-compassion. If MSC increases a participant's stress, the student is probably trying too hard. The *path* and the *goal* of self-compassion should be the same—taking a kinder approach to ourselves and our experience. Participants should allow themselves to be "slow learners" in the MSC course. Too much zeal on the path to self-compassion can lead to emotional overwhelm. As MSC teachers like to say: "Walk slowly, go further."

Opening and Closing

There will be sessions when participants find it impossible to pay attention—when the mind is closed. Opening and closing are natural, like the expansion and contraction of the lungs. Students should be encouraged to let themselves close when needed and to open up when the time comes. Forcing the mind to open when it needs to close is not self-compassionate.

How do we know when we're opening? We are opening when we feel alive and when our thoughts, feelings, and sensations are particularly vivid. A sense of ease or relief may accompany opening, including tears for no apparent reason. Tears often signify the end of a struggle. For example, beauty pageant contestants cry when they win and when they lose, but in either case the contest is over. Ironically, most of our struggles occur unconsciously, such as our perpetual struggle to be loved or connected, and tears may come when we feel love and connection during a moment of compassion.

What are some signs of closing? We are closing when we feel distracted, fatigued, angry, or critical—when we need to shut down or push away our experience. At those times, students can explore the quintessential self-compassion question "What do I need?" For example, a participant who feels tired or overwhelmed can choose not to participate in a particular class exercise, or even take a brief nap. Afterward, the student can explore for herself: "Do I feel ashamed about taking a nap? Am I worrying that I missed a critical lesson? Or was taking a nap necessary in order for me to care for myself in the moment?" In other words, was taking a nap a self-compassionate act or not, and was the student's *reaction* to the nap self-compassionate? Every moment of class time can be an experiment in self-compassion. Again, self-compassion means letting ourselves open when we're opening and letting ourselves close when we need to close, even during the MSC course itself. As long as closing is done consciously, in the service of responding to oneself with kindness, it still develops the habit of self-compassion.

Safety

MSC participants need to take responsibility for their own well-being. Teachers can put three concentric circles on the flipchart or whiteboard as shown in Figure 6.2 (Chapter 6)—*safe, challenged,* and *overwhelmed*—to help students make decisions that ensure safety and enhance learning. Learning and growth happen best in the challenged circle. For example, if students find that they are in the safe circle and not practicing (which could be avoidance), they can remind themselves that the benefits of self-compassion are dose-dependent, and then nudge themselves into the challenge circle by experimenting with more practice. On the other hand, if students are practicing in the overwhelmed circle and it isn't going well for them, they might ask themselves what they can let go of to make their practice easier, perhaps by cutting back on formal meditation and focusing more on informal exercises in daily life. If and when students find themselves emotionally overwhelmed, they should close and move back toward safety—the inner circle. Instructions for closing are given throughout the program.

Meditation

MSC is not designed to turn every participant into a meditator. The purpose of MSC is twofold: to help participants (1) *know* when they're suffering and (2) *respond* with kindness and understanding. Sometimes the most skillful response to suffering is compassionate *behavior*—drinking a cup of tea, taking a warm bath—rather than meditation or mind training.

Many participants are convinced that they can't meditate. This is usually because they have mistaken notions about what to expect in meditation. Meditation is really quite simple; for example, if you can feel your breath in your body, you can meditate. We humans are hardwired for wandering attention, however. Therefore, a good measure of progress in self-compassion meditation is not how *often* the mind wanders, but how *tenderly* we bring the mind back to the object of our attention.

Another struggle for aspiring meditators is lack of time. This is really only a problem when we think meditation means sitting down and practicing for an extended period, perhaps 20–45 minutes daily. We can also sit in meditation for 5 minutes. Stopping to sit down is the toughest hurdle for aspiring meditators to overcome.

We can also practice *informally* throughout the day, taking even *less* than 5 minutes to practice. Everyone can find time to practice informally. Practicing self-compassion informally in daily life makes special sense because we need a bit of suffering to evoke compassion, and suffering is more likely to occur in everyday situations. Evidence also shows that informal practice is no less effective than formal meditation (Elwafi et al., 2013; Neff & Germer, 2013). A combination of formal meditation and informal practice is probably the best way to cultivate mindfulness and self-compassion. People also discover that their desire to meditate increases when they experience the relief of bringing warmth and kindness to their everyday experience.

Levels of Experience

Some MSC participants have been practicing meditation for decades, and others are trying it out for the first time. Very experienced practitioners are encouraged to practice in a way that is familiar to them, perhaps by adding a little loving-kindness or compassion to their existing practice. Beginning meditators can be encouraged to start where they are, perhaps appreciating the benefits of a *beginner's mind*—a mind with fewer preconceptions and more possibilities. There are also many different ways to practice self-compassion in meditation, including prayer (Knabb, 2018), and course participants are invited to apply self-compassion in a manner that feels just right for them.

Practice-Focused Comments

Participants are often asked during class to comment on their direct experience of a practice or class exercise that just transpired ("What did you notice?", "What did you feel?", "How did you respond?"), or to describe how their practice is unfolding over time ("Any insights, challenges, or successes?"). Practice-focused comments help everyone learn from the experience of others. A useful question that participants can ask themselves before speaking is "Is this comment useful to me *and* to others in the group?"

Another strategy for reducing conceptual discussion is to create a special page on a flipchart called the "Parking Lot." Conceptual questions or comments can be written down on the Parking Lot page for later consideration in the group. Parking Lot questions should also be relevant to others, whereas more personal questions can be addressed individually with a teacher.

Introverts and Extroverts

Some MSC participants are introverts, and others are extroverts. *Introverts* are encouraged to say as little or as much as feels comfortable, but also to nudge themselves to speak when they get the urge. *Extroverts* are encouraged to make room for introverts, who might be hesitant to take "air time" from others. The goal is for all participants to be themselves, and to be heard, but also to work the edge of their habitual ways of relating to others. MSC also includes small-group conversations (in dyads and triads), which make it easier for introverts to speak and connect with others. The purpose of all group discussions is to foster a sense of common humanity in class.

Personal Needs

The body is the physical platform of mental and emotional work so participants are encouraged to take good care of their bodies by getting enough rest, eating well, and exercising regularly.

If any students have private concerns that interfere with their participation in the program, they are encouraged to speak with one of the teachers. When participants need to skip a session, they are requested to inform one of the teachers beforehand. An understanding attitude by teachers toward their students' ways of coping helps students communicate their needs openly and honestly.

Guiding Principles
(15 minutes)

This class exercise is an opportunity for participants to reflect on group norms that create an atmosphere of safety and ease—a culture of kindness.

A sense of safety is necessary for compassion to arise. Teachers ask participants to write down their responses to these two questions:

- " 'How would I like to be treated so I feel safe and comfortable in this program?' " (*Pause for 2–3 minutes*)
- " 'How would I like to treat *others* so *they* feel comfortable and safe with me?' (*Pause*)
- In other words, what *guiding principles* should we keep in mind as we go through the program together?" (*Pause*)

Then the entire group engages in a general conversation about how the members would like to treat and be treated by others. Comments and reflections can be written on the flipchart or whiteboard. If any of the following guidelines are not mentioned, teachers can add them to the discussion.

- *Protecting confidentiality.* "We don't discuss outside the group what individuals share in session."
- *Letting go of fixing.* "Imagine that nobody in the room needs fixing, including yourself."
- *Avoiding advice giving.* "Advice is usually experienced as interference."
- *Practicing nonjudgment.* "We're all doing the best we can."
- *Respecting differences.* "Allow others to be different from you."
- *Honoring diversity.* "Be open to what you do *not* know about a person."
- *Supporting inclusion.* "Remember we all wish to belong."
- *Giving space.* "Some people need more privacy than others."
- *Respecting physical boundaries.* "Not everyone likes or wants to be touched."
- *Being mindful of romantic attraction.* "Focus on the purpose of this training and avoid causing pain to others outside the class."
- *Protecting your own safety and comfort.* "Nobody knows you, or can protect you, better than yourself."

Group members usually get a sense of what teachers are aiming for, and they clarify their personal aspirations during the conversation as well, so a summary or wrap-up is usually not necessary at the end of this discussion. Teachers may note at the end of the discussion, however: "Most of us will probably break our own rules by unwittingly hurting someone or not living up to our own expectations. That is perfectly human and provides a golden opportunity to practice self-compassion."

Diversity and Inclusion

Teachers are encouraged to expand on the concept of *respect*—respect for *individual differences*. There are differences we can see and those that are less visible, which inevitably have an impact on our life experience and our identity. The purpose of discussing diversity is to encourage an attitude of inclusion (see Chapter 7). The following is an example of how to introduce diversity and inclusion:

- "One of the guidelines that was just mentioned is 'respect.' Respect often means 'respect for *differences*.' In MSC, we want to honor our differences as well as our commonalities."
- "There are differences that we *may be able to see* and those that are perhaps *less visible*. What are some examples of differences that *we may be able to see*?" Here are some examples:
  o Age
  o Gender
  o Race
  o Ethnicity
  o Body type
- "And what are some differences that may be *less visible*?" Here are a few examples:
  o Sexual orientation
  o Gender identity
  o Socioeconomic status
  o Religion
  o Politics
  o National origin
  o Early childhood experiences
  o Chronic illness
  o Educational level
  o Physical and mental ability
- "And what are some of our *commonalities*?" Here are some examples:
  o We are all breathing.
  o We all struggle in life.
  o We all have emotions, such as joy and sadness, fear and anger.
  o We all wish to be happy and free from suffering.
  o We all wish to be loved.
- "It is important to honor our differences and commonalities since certain cultural identities can be a source of pain due to societal oppression, discrimination, and biases. This is *cultural identity pain*."

- "Some groups suffer *disproportionately* from cultural identity pain, due to longstanding legacies of oppression brought against them. Suffering is universal, but not equal across individuals and groups."
- "It is also important to remember that some people develop remarkable strength and resilience in the face of cultural oppression and adversity.
- "Self-compassion can open cultural wounds. Although the external world is often not just or kind, we can at least learn to treat *ourselves* in a more just and kind manner, providing the stable emotional platform we need for the work of cultural change."
- "We want to create a "brave space" (Arao & Clemens, 2013) in the MSC course where everyone can feel safe and welcome just as we are. Toward that end, it's worth reminding ourselves that:
  - 'We are all different.'
  - 'We are all human.'
  - 'Everyone has a voice.'
  - 'Everyone belongs.' "

For teachers, cultivating an attitude of "not knowing" the unique experience of each participant creates space for open, honest communication. Teachers are also encouraged to stay engaged, both personally and professionally, in the cultural conversation about diversity and inclusiveness.

Forgiveness

Since teachers and students know very little about one another, and because we all have unconscious biases, there is a possibility that participants will unintentionally hurt one another during the course. A teacher may also unwittingly hurt a student as the course proceeds. Therefore, teachers can offer the following "intention to forgive" on behalf of themselves and all of the participants:

- "Please forgive *me*, in advance, for any hurt that I may unconsciously cause you during this course." (*Asking for forgiveness*)
- "May we all forgive *ourselves* for any hurt that we may unconsciously cause to others in this course." (*Forgiving others*)
- "And, by the end of the program, may we forgive *others* for any hurt that they may have caused us, probably entirely unconsciously and because they didn't know enough about us." (*Giving forgiveness*)

Teachers can repeat these forgiveness phrases at the end of the program as well.

Poetry

Poetry is an optional component of MSC, and teachers are encouraged to read poems that they particularly enjoy. Suggested poems are given for each session. At this point in Session 1, many teachers like to read the poem "Start Close In" by David Whyte (2012, p. 262–263), which emphasizes the importance of honoring our own experience and beginning where we are. This poet also has a CD titled *The Poetry of Self-Compassion* (Whyte, 1992).

Break
(15 minutes)

Each MSC session includes a break of 15 minutes so that participants can use the restroom, have a snack, or connect informally with one another. The physical and emotional well-being of participants is paramount in MSC. Teachers can follow the energy and mood of the group to determine the best time to take a break, but every session should include a break.

Soft Landing
(2 minutes)

Soft landings are very brief practices that gently guide participants into the present moment (see the discussion of soft landings in Chapter 5). Being present can be difficult when the present moment includes physical or emotional pain; it can feel like an airplane landing hard in stormy weather. A soft landing is touching down softly with the support of loving-kindness and compassion. The present moment may be easier to bear, for example, when we let ourselves be rocked by the rhythm of the breath, offer ourselves words of comfort and kindness, or give ourselves a warm, inner smile.

Soft landings are also an opportunity to remind students of what they have already learned, especially practices they can use on the spot throughout the day. Soft landings should be simple, brief, and easy to follow. Here is an example:

- "Let's take a couple of minutes to settle back into the present moment and into our bodies, making it a soft landing by including the component of compassion."
- "Let's just give ourselves a few deep breaths, letting out an audible 'Ahhh' with each exhalation." (*Pause*)
- "Now closing your eyes, turning your attention inward, and noticing

if there is tension or stress in any part of your body. If so, offering yourself a silent, inner compassionate 'Awww,' allowing your heart to melt a bit with each 'Awww.' " (*Pause*)

Soft landing instructions can be concluded by ringing a bell or by simply saying "thank you" and pausing before continuing with the rest of the session.

How Would I Treat a Friend?
(15 minutes)

After the break, the session changes its focus to the meaning of self-compassion, misconceptions about self-compassion, research, and simple ways to practice self-compassion in daily life. Since self-compassion involves being a good friend to oneself, teachers can begin by asking participants to reflect on how they treat themselves when they are struggling compared to how they treat dear friends in similar situations.

Instructions

- Ask participants to take out a sheet of paper, close their eyes, and reflect for a moment on the following question:

    "Think of a time, or various times, when you've had a *close friend* who was suffering in some way. Not a partner or family member—they are sometimes *too* close—but a friend you really cared about who was struggling. For example, maybe your friend had a misfortune, failed, or felt inadequate. How do you typically respond to your friends in such situations? What do you *say*? What *tone* do you use? How is your *posture*? What *nonverbal* gestures do you use?" (*Pause*)

    Ask participants to write down what they have discovered.

- Then invite the group members to close their eyes again for the next question:

    "Now think about various times when *you* were suffering in some way—had a misfortune, failed, or felt inadequate. How do *you* typically respond to yourself in these situations? What do you *say*? What *tone* do you use? How is your *posture*? Which *nonverbal* gestures do you use?" (*Pause*)

    Again, invite participants to write down what they learned.

- Then ask, "Do you notice any *patterns of difference* in how you respond to yourself and others?"

- Ask the class to form groups of three and take a total of 5 minutes to share what they have discovered. Participants should be reminded to share only what they feel comfortable sharing, and to avoid the tendency to advise one another or try to fix any problems.

Inquiry

When laughter can be heard in the small groups, this is usually a sign that the groups have completed their task. Teachers can take another few minutes with the whole group to inquire what participants noticed in this exercise. Participants usually report that they are tougher on themselves than on others (e.g., are more impatient, are less understanding, use harsher words or a more strident tone, and argue with themselves more than they would with a good friend). Some people will notice that when we have perspective on our own suffering or the suffering of others—when we can see ourselves or others from a little distance—compassion is more likely to arise. A sample inquiry follows.

> CARINA: (*Shyly*) I noticed that I reach out to others when they're struggling, but I close others off from others when I'm feeling bad.
>
> TEACHER: Does it feel different to reach out and to close off?
>
> CARINA: Sure does.
>
> TEACHER: May I ask how?
>
> CARINA: Well, I feel all tight and contracted inside myself when things go wrong for me, and I feel soft, like I can feel my heart beating, when others feel bad about themselves.
>
> TEACHER: That seems like an important discovery. What does it suggest to you?
>
> CARINA: I'd really like to feel like that with *myself*! (*Giggling*)
>
> TEACHER: Do you think you can?
>
> CARINA: That's why I'm here, I guess.
>
> TEACHER: (*Laughing*) Yes, I guess we all are! Let's see how it goes.

To normalize the difference between how we treat others versus ourselves, teachers can cite the preliminary evidence gathered in Neff's research lab (Knox et al., 2016) suggesting that the vast majority of the general population in the United States (78%) are more compassionate toward others than themselves, 16% are about equal in their compassion for themselves and others, and only 6% are more compassionate to themselves than to others.

Teachers can close the exercise by offering two informal definitions of self-compassion:

- "Self-compassion is treating ourselves with the same kindness and understanding as we would treat a friend when things go wrong. (It's the reverse of the Golden Rule: Do unto *yourself* as you would do unto others.)"
- "Self-compassion is treating ourselves as we would like *others*— family and friends—to treat us."

What Is Self-Compassion?
(10 minutes)

Now that participants have had a chance to reflect on how they instinctively react when things go wrong in their lives, and are beginning to get a sense of how they *could* treat themselves more compassionately, the scientific construct of self-compassion is introduced. As before, teachers are encouraged to present this topic (and all topics in MSC) as interactively as possible. They can offer leading questions to the group, elicit responses, and then identify common themes that illuminate the topic.

For example, the concept of self-compassion can be introduced by first asking students to consider what ingredients are necessary to feel compassion for *others*: "Imagine that there is a homeless person asking for change at a busy street corner. What does it take to have compassion for that person?" Participants usually mention that first they need to *notice* the person is there, especially the fact that the person is struggling; then they need to feel a sense of humanity and connectedness ("There but for fortune go I"); and they also need to feel kindness or understanding rather than judgment at the sight of this unfortunate person. The themes of mindfulness (noticing suffering), common humanity (recognizing that we all struggle), and kindness (responding with warmth or tenderness) are all needed for compassion to arise. Then a teacher can make the bridge to *self*-compassion, pointing out that for self-compassion to arise, first we also need to know when *we're* suffering, frame our suffering as part of the human experience, and respond to ourselves with kindness rather than self-criticism.

The three components of self-compassion (Neff, 2003b) should be clearly understood by all participants because they form the conceptual foundation for most of the exercises in the MSC program (see Chapter 2). A summary of the three components is given on the next page. Teachers can embellish this discussion by soliciting participants' comments, by sharing examples from their own lives, and/or by including research on self-compassion.

Self-Kindness versus Self-Judgment

- "Treating ourselves with kindness, care, understanding, and support, just as we would treat a good friend. Most people treat themselves more harshly, saying cruel things to themselves that they would never say to others."

- "Compassion includes the wish and effort to alleviate suffering. There is an action component to self-compassion. It involves actively comforting, protecting, and supporting ourselves when we're in pain."

Common Humanity versus Isolation

- "Seeing our imperfections as part of the larger human experience. Also recognizing that everyone suffers."

- "When we struggle or fail, we often feel that something has gone wrong—that this shouldn't be happening. This creates a feeling of abnormality ('*I am wrong!*'), leading to shame and isolation."

Mindfulness versus Over-Identification

- "Knowing that we *are* suffering, while we suffer. This is a prerequisite for compassion to arise. Mindfulness allows us to turn toward painful feelings and 'be with' them as they are."

- "Mindfulness is a balanced state of awareness. We don't suppress or avoid what we're feeling; nor are we carried away by the dramatic storyline of what's happening. This process can be referred to as *over-identification.*"

The three components of self-compassion may be lyrically rephrased as *loving* (self-kindness), *connected* (common humanity), *presence* (mindfulness). This helps students understand what the state of self-compassion feels like.

The Yin and Yang of Self-Compassion

Most people assume that self-compassion is primarily soft and receptive because compassion is associated with nurturing relationships. However, compassion and self-compassion can be strong, even fierce. For example, soldiers in the military endanger their own lives to protect the lives of others, and parents may struggle to put food on the table, even working multiple jobs. Both of these are also examples of compassion. People can have fierce compassion for *themselves* as well, such as refusing to use an addictive substance despite severe withdrawal symptoms or performing acts of courage (e.g., standing up to an abusive boss, speaking out against social injustice). Being fully self-compassionate requires both the yin and yang of self-compassion (see also Chapters 2 and 6). Teachers can explain this as follows:

- "The yin of self-compassion contains the attributes of 'being' with our pain in a compassionate way—*comforting, soothing,* and *validating* ourselves."
- "The yang of self-compassion is associated with 'acting' in the world—*protecting, providing,* and *motivating* ourselves."

These two aspects of self-compassion are different but equally essential ways of *caring.* MSC includes both yin and yang aspects. As meditation teacher Joan Halifax says, "strong back, soft front" (Halifax, 2012a).

Gestures of Self-Compassion (Optional)
(5 minutes)

The optional Gestures of Self-Compassion exercise is as an opportunity for participants to feel the three components of self-compassion in their own bodies and also to experience the yang side of self-compassion. Students can be invited to stand up for this exercise, if they wish, and to stretch their legs.

Instructions

- The teacher asks participants, "Please hold your hands out and squeeze your fists" (while both teachers, if there are co-teachers, demonstrate the same). After about 20 seconds, so that group members start feeling some discomfort, participants are invited to tune into their bodies and explore what emotions might be arising while maintaining this hand gesture. Then participants are asked to say out loud, randomly (we call this "popcorn-style" responding), how they feel. We typically hear words like "Tense," "Angry," "Strong," or "Afraid." This hand gesture is then described as a metaphor for *struggling with ourselves or our experience*—something most of us do unconsciously much of the time.
- Now the teacher giving the instructions asks, "Please open your palms, turned upward," while both teachers demonstrate the gesture. Class participants are invited to drop inside their bodies again and discover what feelings arise with open palms, also noting how different this gesture feels from the last one. "What do you feel? Please say out loud what emotions arise for you." Typical comments include "Peaceful," "Release,"

"Acceptance," "Ease," or "Openness." Teachers can then suggest that this is what *mindfulness* feels like when we accept what's happening with open, spacious awareness.

- "Now extend your arms forward, perhaps imagining that you are holding a person or the whole world in your arms." Teachers demonstrate outstretched arms with hands very slightly turned toward each other. "What emotions does this gesture evoke inside you?"

- Participants usually say things like "Embracing," "Connecting," "Reaching out," or "Inclusive." Teachers can suggest that this gesture gives a sense of *common humanity*—what it feels like when we go beyond our separate selves and include others.

- "Now place one palm in the other, and slowly bring them both to the center of your chest. Feel the warmth and gentle pressure of your hands on your chest. Breathe gently." Teachers demonstrate, pause a little while, and then elicit responses—which typically include "Safe," "Calm," "Refuge," "Loved," "Soft," or "Peaceful." Teachers can then share that this gesture arouses *self-kindness*—comforting ourselves when we need it.

- Teachers note that the *combination* of these three gestures captures a sense of what it is like to be in a state of self-compassion, especially yin self-compassion. Teachers should note that the gesture of self-kindness—putting one or two hands over the heart—does *not* feel safe or comforting for some people (it can cause anxiety), so later on in the session alternative gestures will be explored that may feel more soothing.

- Participants are now led into an experience of the yang side of self-compassion: "While you are still standing, or if you are willing and able to stand up, please find your way into a 'horse stance.' This is a posture from martial arts, such as tai chi or karate. A horse stance is a wide, stable stance with a low center of gravity." A teacher demonstrates, and then asks, "How does it feel to be in this posture?" Students typically say things like "Strong," "Stable," or "Flexible." Teachers can then explain that when we feel centered and anchored, we are in a strong position to take action.

- "We can *protect* ourselves (a teacher can demonstrate stretching out their arm with palm raised while firmly saying 'no'; do this two more times). Notice how you feel when you do this, the energy that rises up within you. We can also *provide* for ourselves as well as others (a teacher can demonstrate sweeping their arms out in a gathering motion and bringing them back inward while saying 'yes' and then sweep them outward in a motion of giving to others and once again saying 'yes'). Take a moment to feel that in your body, the balance between oneself and others. Finally, we can *motivate* ourselves to do difficult things (a teacher can demonstrate giving a thumbs-up while saying, 'You can do this!'). And if you succeed, you can celebrate (teacher turns to co-teacher and gives a 'high five' and invites students to do the same) and if you fail you can give yourself some yin self-compassion (teacher puts both hands on heart again and makes a tender 'aww' sound). Both yin and yang are always available when we need them."

Misgivings about Self-Compassion
(10 minutes)

Many people have misgivings about self-compassion that prevent them from engaging wholeheartedly in practice. A *misgiving* is a worry that self-compassion could have unintended negative consequences (Robinson et al., 2016). Even if class participants feel generally positive and optimistic about self-compassion, underlying uneasiness may express itself when they are discussing self-compassion with friends and colleagues.

Misgivings are typically based on *misconceptions* about what self-compassion really is. Teachers can begin dispelling misconceptions by gathering a list of concerns from the group and then addressing them one by one in light of the scientific evidence, or by further clarifying the meaning of self-compassion (see below). The following misgivings are typically mentioned (see also Chapters 2 and 3).

Self-Compassion Is a Form of Self-Pity

- Self-compassion reminds us that everyone suffers (common humanity) and doesn't exaggerate the extent of suffering (mindfulness). It is not a "Woe is me" attitude.
- Research shows that self-compassionate people are more likely to engage in perspective taking than to focus on their own distress (Neff & Pommier, 2013). They are also less likely to ruminate on how bad things are (Raes, 2010).

Self-Compassion Is Weak

- Self-compassion is strong; it offers resilience when people are faced with difficulty.
- Research shows that self-compassionate people are better able to cope with tough situations like divorce (Sbarra et al., 2012), trauma (Hiraoka et al., 2015), or chronic pain (Wren et al., 2012).

Self-Compassion Is Selfish

- By *including* ourselves in the circle of compassion (a humble agenda!), we lessen our sense of separation from others.

- Research shows that self-compassionate people tend to be more caring and supportive in romantic relationships (Neff & Beretvas, 2013), are more likely to compromise in relationship conflicts (Yarnell & Neff, 2013), and are more compassionate toward others (Neff & Pommier, 2013).

Self-Compassion Is Self-Indulgent

- Compassion emphasizes long-term well-being over short-term pleasure (just as a compassionate mother doesn't let her child eat all the ice cream the child wants, but says, "Eat your vegetables").
- Research shows that self-compassionate people engage in healthier behaviors like exercise (Magnus et al., 2010), eating well (Schoenefeld & Webb, 2013), drinking less (Brooks et al., 2012), and going to the doctor more regularly (Terry, Leary, Mehta, & Henderson, 2013).

Self-Compassion Is a Form of Making Excuses

- Self-compassion provides the safety people need to admit mistakes, rather than creating a need to blame someone else for them.
- Research shows that self-compassionate people take greater personal responsibility for their actions (Leary et al., 2007), and are more likely to apologize if they've offended someone (Breines & Chen, 2012).

Self-Compassion Will Undermine Motivation

- Motivation with self-compassion comes from the desire for health and well-being. Self-compassionate people are actually *more* motivated to change because they motivate themselves with encouragement (as a supportive coach does), rather than with harsh self-criticism.
- Research shows that self-compassionate people have high personal standards; they just don't beat themselves up when they fail (Neff, 2003b). This means that they are less afraid of failure (Neff et al., 2005) and are more likely to try again and to persist in their efforts after failing (Breines & Chen, 2012).

The key message is that the scientific evidence points in the opposite direction of the misgivings. Many of these misgivings, as well as misgivings about *practice* (e.g., self-compassion is a lot of work, or too emotionally activating), will resurface as the course goes on and will need to be addressed again.

What Gets in the Way?

If there is time remaining, teachers can lead a "repeated questions" exercise that helps uncover *personal* obstacles to self-compassion rather than misconceptions. This exercise also helps participants to open up and feel connected to one another. It taps into what Gilbert and colleagues' (2011) call "fears of compassion," such as "I fear that if I am too compassionate with myself bad things will happen," "If I am too compassionate with myself, others will reject me," and "I have never felt compassion for myself, so I would not know where to begin to develop these feelings."

The group breaks into pairs; for 3 minutes, one person in each pair asks the same question while the other person answers, and then they switch roles. Again, participants should be reminded to only share what they feel comfortable sharing. A lighthearted way to start the exercise is for a teacher to say, "Please get into pairs and decide who will be the first questioner—the one with the longer last name." Then the questioner asks, "What gets in the way of your being more self-compassionate?" After an answer is given, the questioner says, "Thank you. And *what else* gets in the way of your being more self-compassionate?" A bell is rung after 3 minutes, and participants then switch roles. After everyone has spoken, teachers can ask the whole group, "What did you discover?" Participants are likely to encounter these obstacles in their self-compassion practice as the course unfolds.

 ## Research on Self-Compassion (Optional)
(15 minutes)

Teachers can add their own research talk to Session 1, depending on the needs and interests of the group. This topic will extend the session beyond 2¾ hours, but it is usually worth the effort. A comprehensive summary of the science of self-compassion can be found in Chapter 3, and an up-to-date bibliography is available at *https://self-compassion.org.*

The main message of the research is that self-compassion is consistently linked to well-being. Self-compassion is associated with lessened negative states like depression, anxiety, stress, shame (Johnson & O'Brien, 2013; Zessin et al., 2015), and body dissatisfaction (Albertson et al., 2015), and with increased positive states like happiness, life satisfaction, and optimism (Neff, Rude, & Kirkpatrick, 2007). It's also linked to better physical health (Friis et al., 2015; Hall et al., 2013). When pain is wrapped in the warm embrace of self-compassion, negative states are alleviated, while positive states are generated.

Other areas of interest are the relationship of self-compassion to self-esteem, and the physiology of self-compassion and self-criticism (both of these areas are covered in Chapter 3). Finally, teachers may want to summarize the research on self-compassion *training*, especially the MSC program itself (see Chapter 4). Understanding the research gives participants confidence to proceed with training.

Soothing Touch
(5 minutes)

MSC provides multiple pathways for evoking self-compassion in daily life. One approach is somatic, with soothing or supportive touch. Evidence shows that touch is a reliable way of expressing kindness and compassion to others (Hertenstein, Keltner, App, Bulleit, & Jaskolka, 2006; Keltner, 2009); that it triggers physiological changes (Maratos et al., 2017); and that even *watching* a simple gesture like putting a hand over the heart can influence how people think and feel (Parzuchowski, Szymkow, Baryla, & Wojciszke, 2014). Anecdotal evidence suggests that giving soothing touch to *oneself* can have similar effects. However, a small percentage of participants find that placing a hand over the heart can provoke anxiety, perhaps because they feel embarrassed about self-care or because the gesture makes them feel vulnerable. Therefore, we invite participants to explore alternative ways of supporting themselves with touch, especially since touch is such an important communicator of yin self-compassion.

Instructions

Teachers lead group members through the following gestures to help them discover for themselves which form of touch might be most soothing or supportive:

- Two hands over the heart.
- Cupping one hand over a fist over the heart, symbolizing strength with kindness.
- One hand on the belly and one over the heart.
- Two hands on the belly.
- One hand on a cheek.
- Cradling one's face in the hands.
- Gently stroking one's arms.
- Crossing one's arms and giving a gentle squeeze.
- Gently stroking one's chest, either back and forth or in small circles.
- Cupping the hands in one's lap.

Then teachers give participants another minute to explore these or other options on their own.

Usually there is no inquiry after Soothing Touch, and teachers move right on to the next informal practice, the Self-Compassion Break. If teachers notice that students are having difficulty with Soothing Touch, they can expand the practice and ask, "Is there any *other* way you can physically soothe or support yourself, such as petting your dog or taking a warm bath?" Inquiry may also be useful if it appears that one or two students are still struggling with the exercise.

Inquiry

Here is an example of inquiry following Soothing Touch.

> TEACHER: I'm wondering whether anyone found a place on the body that is soothing or supportive?
>
> GEORGE: I found a bunch of places that were definitely *not* like that!
>
> TEACHER: For example?
>
> GEORGE: Well, when I put my hands on my belly, I was reminded how fat I am, and when I put my arms on my shoulders, I felt ridiculous . . . pathetic, really, like "Why am I hugging myself?!"
>
> TEACHER: So you discovered self-judgment as you were searching for places of comfort? Is that fair to say?
>
> GEORGE: Yes, I guess it is.
>
> TEACHER: (*To the group*) Did self-judgment come up in anyone else's mind during this exercise? (*Half of the group members raise their hands.*) You see, George, you're not alone in that. That's human. But was there anywhere on your body that touch actually felt good?
>
> GEORGE: Yes, it was weird . . . resting my head in one hand. I have a photograph of my dad doing that at the dinner table, smiling at the camera, after a long day at work.
>
> TEACHER: So that gesture brought up good memories. Did it also feel *physically* good to rest your head in your hand?
>
> GEORGE: (*Repeating the gesture*) Yes, I suppose it does.
>
> TEACHER: Great! And please feel free to use the same gesture at home, if you like. Maybe you already found the right soothing touch, or maybe it's somewhere else.
>
> GEORGE: Got it, thanks.

This inquiry allowed the whole group to explore the topic of self-soothing, and to see how self-judgment can be an obstacle to self-soothing. Students should be reminded to continue the exploration at home, and should also be told that the *wish* to be soothed and supported is already an act of self-compassion. Soothing touch may not feel good every time, but the goodwill behind the gesture is the real point of the practice.

Self-Compassion Break
(15 minutes)

The Self-Compassion Break is an informal practice that participants can apply whenever they find themselves in a stressful situation. It is taught in class as a meditative reflection to unpack the different elements of the practice, but with sufficient training, it only takes a minute to apply in daily life. The Self-Compassion Break is usually taught immediately following Soothing Touch (without a break for inquiry when class time is limited).

Instructions

- "Think of a situation in your life that is difficult, that is causing you stress right now, such as a health problem, a problem in an important relationship, a work problem, or perhaps someone crossed your boundaries or disrespected you. Please choose a problem in the mild to moderate range, not a big problem. We don't want to overwhelm ourselves as we're first learning the skill of self-compassion."

- "Allow yourself to see, hear, and feel your way into the problem, to the extent that you experience some uneasiness in your body. Where do you feel it the most? Make contact with the discomfort that you feel in your body."

- "Then say to yourself, slowly and clearly, 'This is a moment of suffering.' That's mindfulness. Other options include 'This hurts,' 'Ouch!', or 'This does not feel good.'"

- "Next, say to yourself, again slowly and clearly, 'Suffering is a part of living.' That's common humanity. Other options include 'Others would feel just like me,' 'I'm not alone,' or 'Me too.'"

- "Now put your hands over your heart, or wherever it feels supportive, feeling the warmth of your hands. Say to yourself, 'May I be kind to myself.' 'May I give myself what I need.' That's self-kindness. Perhaps asking yourself what quality of self-compassion you need right now, yin or yang? Yin language might be "May I accept myself just as I am" or "May I care for myself tenderly in this moment." Yang language might be 'No, I will not allow myself to be harmed in this way" or "May I have the courage and strength to make a change."

- "If you're having difficulty finding the right words, imagine that a dear friend or loved one is having the same problem as you. What would you say to this person, heart to heart, without giving advice? If your friend were to hold just a few of your words in her mind, what would you like them to be? What message would you like to deliver? (*Pause*) Now, can you offer the same message to yourself?"

Settling and Reflection

Students are usually given a minute to let the practice settle inside and to reflect on what just transpired, even taking notes if they wish. During the reflection period, teachers may prime their students for inquiry by asking, "What did you notice?" or "What did you feel?" More specific questions related to the theme of this particular practice can also be asked, such as, "Did you notice an internal shift when you said, 'This is a moment of suffering?'", "What happened when you reminded yourself that all living beings suffer?", or "Were there any words of kindness that spoke to you in your situation? Did you need yin or yang self-compassion?"

Inquiry

The Self-Compassion Break is the first exercise that uses language to evoke self-compassion. Since the meaning of words is so context-dependent, the suggested phrases are unlikely to appeal to everyone. Finding authentic phrases that evoke self-compassion is a personal, inner journey that is explored further in Session 3 (Chapter 12). Here is a sample inquiry about the Self-Compassion Break.

> TEACHER: Did anyone notice an internal shift when you said, "This is a moment of suffering"?
>
> TIANA: Yes, I felt like I wasn't so engulfed with my struggle any more, like the struggle was there and I was here. There was a bit of distance from it. I even sighed with relief. (*Smiles and sighs again*)
>
> TEACHER: Sounds like your body got the message. How about the second phrase, "Suffering is part of life," if I may ask?
>
> TIANA: That one just made me depressed. I don't like to think about how much everyone struggles.
>
> TEACHER: You probably have a lot of empathy for the pain of others.
>
> TIANA: Not really. When I think about how much others suffer, I say to myself, "So who are you to complain?"

TEACHER: Oh, I see. That part of the exercise actually made you feel *more* alone, not less.

TIANA: I guess that wasn't the point, was it? (*Smiling wryly*)

TEACHER: I wonder if there are different words that would work better for you.

TIANA: (*Pause*) I'm trying to remember everything that you said, but I can't. I got stuck on "Everyone has problems." It reminded me of my mother telling me to stop complaining.

TEACHER: So you've been told that the sufferings of others matter more than your own?

TIANA: (*Tears welling up*) Yes, that's probably true. (*Longer pause*)

TEACHER: It takes some courage to see that. (*Waiting*) Would you still like to know what those other words were?

TIANA: Yes, I would.

TEACHER: They were "I'm not alone" and "Others are just like me."

TIANA: That makes sense. I guess I got a bit swept up in the earlier ones.

TEACHER: Happens all the time. How do you feel now?

TIANA: I'm okay. I just don't want to take any more time from others.

TEACHER: I understand. Thanks for speaking up, though.

In this inquiry, the teacher took Tiana through different parts of the practice, both to assist her and to deepen the whole group's understanding of the Self-Compassion Break. Tiana had an important personal insight: that opening to the sufferings of others meant to her that she had to invalidate her own problems. This mental habit also made her feel alone. The inquiry closed when Tiana felt uneasy receiving the attention of the class, but only after she recognized the value of common humanity, after she noticed how she tended to separate herself from others when she struggled, and after she found language to connect with others during difficult moments in the future ("I'm not alone").

The Self-Compassion Break is one of the most popular informal practices in MSC. Students can apply any of the three components singly or together, using the practice to comfort oneself (yin) or to move bravely into the world (yang). Over time, a simple gesture (such as soothing or supportive touch) might be able to evoke the experience of the entire Self-Compassion Break without needing to practice each component. Teachers can also remind students to practice the Self-Compassion Break during the MSC course itself, whenever they need it.

Home Practice
(5 minutes)

Every session concludes with a review of the practices that participants are encouraged to try at home. Since this is the first session, participants should be told that the amount of positive change from self-compassion training depends, in part, on how often the student practices. The benefits of self-compassion practice are dose-dependent.

Starting to Practice

The new practices from this session are:

- Soothing Touch.
- Self-Compassion Break.

When participants register for the MSC program, they commit to practicing mindfulness and self-compassion for at least 30 minutes each day in any combination of formal and informal practices. However, since the practices taught in Session 1 are all short informal ones, participants are not expected to practice as long during the following week. Instead, they should be encouraged to recognize stressful moments in their daily lives, and to explore what happens when they respond with Soothing Touch or the Self-Compassion Break.

Weekly Feedback

The purpose of weekly feedback is briefly mentioned, to facilitate the learning process for students through self-reflection and to communicate with the teachers. Students are invited to bring written feedback to the next class. Feedback may include (1) the student's general experience of self-compassion during the week, (2) which specific practices were tried out and how they went, and (3) how the MSC course itself is going. Participant feedback is kept strictly confidential by the teachers.

Emails

Participants are told that they will receive group emails from the course instructors. Any students who prefer not to receive emails, or who do not want their email addresses shared with other group members, are requested to inform one of the teachers.

Closing
(3 minutes)

Teachers have individual preferences for how to close an MSC session. Sometimes they offer a word of thanks or encouragement; they may invite participants to listen mindfully to the sound of a bell; or perhaps a teacher reads a poem. The following poem, which beautifully captures the humility, tenderness, and common humanity of self-compassion, was written by an MSC participant shortly before completing the program.

JUST FOR ME
by Ana Villalobos
What if a poem were just for me?
What if I were audience enough because I *am,*
Because this person here is alive, is flesh,
Is conscious, has feelings, counts?
What if this one person mattered not just for what
She can do in the world
But because she is *part* of the world
And has a soft and tender heart?
What if that heart mattered,
if kindness to this one mattered?
What if she were *not* distinct from all others,
But instead connected to others in her sense of being distinct, of being
    alone,
Of being uniquely isolated, the one piece removed from the picture—
All the while vulnerable under, deep under, the layers of sedimentary
    defense.

Oh, let me hide
Let me be ultimately great,
Ultimately shy,
Remove me, then I don't have to . . . be.

But I am.
Through all the antics of distinctness from others,
or not-really-there-ness,
I remain
No matter what my disguise—
Genius, idiot, glorious, scum—
Underneath, it's still just me, still here,
Still warm and breathing and human
With another chance simply to say hi,
and recognize my tenderness
And be just a little bit kind to *this* one as well,
Because she counts, too.

Chapter 11

Session 2

PRACTICING MINDFULNESS

Overview

Opening (Core) Meditation: Affectionate Breathing

Practice Discussion

Session Theme: Practicing Mindfulness

Topic: Wandering Mind

Topic: What Is Mindfulness?

Informal Practice: Soles of the Feet

Break

Soft Landing

Topic: Resistance

Exercise: How We Cause Ourselves Unnecessary Suffering

Topic: Backdraft

Informal Practice: Mindfulness in Daily Life

Informal Practice: Self-Compassion in Daily Life

Informal Practice (Optional): Here-and-Now Stone

Topic: Mindfulness and Self-Compassion

Home Practice

Closing

Getting Started

- In this session, participants will:
  - Bring mindful awareness to present-moment experience.
  - Warm up awareness by combining breath meditation with savoring and appreciation.
  - Understand how resistance causes suffering.
  - Recognize and work with backdraft.
  - Anchor awareness with mindfulness and self-compassion in daily life.
  - Explore the meaning of mindfulness and self-compassion.
- These subjects are introduced now to:
  - Help students become mindfully aware of suffering and make room for a compassionate response.
  - Stabilize their awareness when difficult emotions are activated.
- New practices taught this session:
  - Affectionate Breathing
  - Soles of the Feet
  - Mindfulness in Daily Life
  - Self-Compassion in Daily Life
  - Here-and-Now Stone (Optional)

Affectionate Breathing
(30 minutes)

Affectionate Breathing is the first of the three core meditations taught in MSC. The sensation of breathing is a handy object for meditation because it is relatively easy to notice and is available everywhere we go.

Allowing ourselves to be comforted and soothed by the rhythm of our breathing adds important elements to traditional breath meditation—a sense of being supported by the breath, pleasure in breathing, and gratitude for how the breath nourishes the body. Focusing on the soothing rhythm of the breath was inspired by Paul Gilbert (2009). Affectionate Breathing differs from Gilbert's method in its emphasis on savoring the natural rhythm of the breath, rather than intentionally breathing in a rhythmic manner to calm the body.

One reason for savoring the breath in meditation is to make it easier to practice. If we approach meditation as work (e.g., training the mind, learning to concentrate, becoming a better person), we subtly introduce an attitude of striving. However, when we experience the breath as something positive, perhaps noticing how it soothes, calms, and nourishes us all by itself, then our attention will naturally incline in that direction. Furthermore, the experience of being rocked or cradled by our breathing can be deeply soothing—an important source of yin self-compassion. Finally, when we feel safe and held by our breathing, we may even be willing to surrender to it—even allowing ourselves to *become* the breath for brief periods of time. This selfless state is usually accompanied by a deep sense of well-being.

Teachers should be aware that some novice meditators or trauma survivors may experience anxiety when they are invited to surrender to their breathing. Those participants should simply be invited to feel the rhythm of their breath, rather than to experience the internal caress of the breath or let go and "become" their breathing.

Some meditation practitioners struggle with breath meditation because their breath becomes constricted by the effort to focus. Others do not like feeling embodied, perhaps due to illness or trauma. Anecdotal evidence suggests that these adverse reactions are less likely to occur when a practitioner focuses on the rhythm of the breath, especially the whole body being gently rocked by the breath, rather than the more specific sensations of breathing in and breathing out. A student who continues to struggle with breath meditation can choose a different object of focus, such as the experience of soothing touch (see Soothing Touch, Session 1) or repetition of phrases (see Finding Loving-Kindness Phrases, Session 3).

Some people are distractible by nature and want to become more focused. Teachers should be careful not to subtly reinforce an adversarial relationship to a wandering mind. However, when it appears that participants have a friendly attitude toward their minds and just want to gather their attention a little more, one helpful strategy is to give their minds more to do. For example, these practitioners can combine the breath with repetition of loving-kindness phrases. Or they can count their breaths from 1 to 10, over and over, or say "in" and "out" with each inhalation and exhalation. However, the main purpose of breath meditation in MSC is not to enhance concentration, but rather to warm up awareness by tenderly returning attention to the breath and by experiencing the breath as a source of nourishment and support.

At the beginning of Session 2, the class members are told that they will be guided for 20 minutes through the first core meditation of MSC. (Tips for guiding meditation have been given in Chapter 6.) Students are encouraged to take a relaxed, almost playful attitude toward meditation, letting their experience be just as it is—no better and no worse.

Instructions

* "Please find a posture in which your body is comfortable and will feel supported for the duration of the meditation. Then let your eyes gently close, partially or fully. Take a few slow, easy breaths, releasing any unnecessary tension in your body."

- "If you like, placing a hand over your heart or another soothing place as a reminder that you're bringing not only awareness, but *affectionate* awareness, to your breathing and to yourself. You can leave your hand there or let it rest at any time."
- "Now beginning to notice your breathing in your body, feeling your body breathe in and feeling your body breathe out."
- "Perhaps noticing how your body is nourished on the in-breath and relaxes with the out-breath."
- "Just letting your body *breathe you*. There is nothing you need to do."
- "Now noticing the *rhythm* of your breathing, flowing in and flowing out. (*Pause*) Taking some time to *feel* the rhythm of your breathing."
- "Perhaps inclining your attention toward your breathing as you might toward a beloved child or a dear friend."
- "Feeling your *whole body* subtly moving with the breath, like the movement of the sea."
- "Your mind will naturally wander like a curious child or a little puppy. When that happens, just gently returning to the rhythm of your breathing."
- "If you notice there's a sense of *watching* your breath, see if you can let that go and just *be* with your breath, *feeling* it."
- "Allowing your whole body to be gently rocked and caressed—*internally caressed*—by your breathing."
- "If you like, even *giving yourself over* to your breathing."
- "Just breathing. *Being* breathing." (*Long pause*)
- "And now, gently releasing your attention to your breathing, sitting quietly in your own experience, and allowing yourself to feel whatever you're feeling and to be just as you are."
- "When you are ready, slowly and gently opening your eyes."

Settling and Reflection

After the meditation has ended, teachers can introduce the settling and reflection period:

> "Now please take a minute and let your mind settle, to soak in what you just experienced. (*Pause*) Also, please give yourself a chance to reflect on what you just experienced: 'What did I notice?', 'What did I feel?', 'How do I feel now?' Did you find anything particularly enjoyable, or challenging, in this meditation? If you wish, please feel free to take notes on what you experienced."

Inquiry

Teachers can open inquiry in a general way, as given above, or they can ask more specific questions about the practice to facilitate sharing, such as these:

- "If you were familiar with breath meditation, how was it to bring *affection* and *appreciation* into the practice—allowing yourself to be soothed by your breathing?"
- "Did you notice that your attention naturally gravitated to your breath when you *enjoyed* it?"
- "Did you encounter any *obstacles* or *challenges* during this meditation?"

The following is a sample of inquiry following Affectionate Breathing.

MAURA: I've been practicing breath meditation for many years now, and this variation was new to me. I found I was able to really drop into my breathing this time.

TEACHER: Could you describe how it felt in your body to really drop into your breathing?

MAURA: Well, yes, I felt really relaxed . . . soft and relaxed.

TEACHER: And your breathing?

MAURA: It was like that was all there was. Just breathing.

TEACHER: Were you able to connect to the *nurturing* quality of the breath?

MAURA: Yeah, it felt really good and comforting. I think that's why it was easier than usual for me to stay focused. I need to remember that . . . to just let myself be rocked and caressed by my breathing. Heck, it's doing that all the time anyway; I just didn't realize it!

TEACHER: Sounds good, Maura. Thanks for sharing your experience.

In this inquiry, Maura just wanted to share an insight and she didn't have a problem, so the teacher simply validated her discovery. Now let's consider a problem that arose for Carlos during Affectionate Breathing.

CARLOS: I'm not a very good meditator, I'm afraid. I just can't seem to concentrate. No sooner do I feel my breath than I'm off to the races.

TEACHER: How long does it take before you're off to the races, Carlos?

CARLOS: Oh, maybe 3 seconds!

TEACHER: (*To the whole group*) May I see by a show of hands how many people noticed that their attention usually wandered away from their breathing within 3 seconds? (*Half of the group members raise their hands.*)

CARLOS: Well, I guess I'm not alone (*laughing*), but I wish I could do this better.

TEACHER: Don't we all! Did you happen to hear the instruction to bring your mind back to the sensation of breathing like redirecting a puppy or a child who has wandered off?

CARLOS: Yeah.

TEACHER: What was that like?

CARLOS: Truth be told, I didn't actually follow the instruction because I started thinking about my son, Bryan. He's a toddler, and I'm chasing him around all day long. He's really cute.

TEACHER: I wonder what would happen if you treated your wandering mind like you treat Bryan, maybe with the same feeling. When your mind wanders off, it's like "Theeeere he goes . . . !" You could then bring your attention back the same way you might take Bryan's hand and lead him back to where he needs to be.

CARLOS: I get what you're saying. I'll try that. Thanks.

TEACHER: Sure thing.

During this inquiry, the teacher identified self-judgment as an impediment to meditation practice and connected Carlos's natural loving-kindness toward his son as a new model for how to relate to his own mind. The inquiry process was geared toward enhancing a sense of friendliness and warmth in the meditation.

The inquiry period usually takes about 10 minutes when a new meditation is taught. There are often more questions or comments than teachers can address in the available time, so they have to decide eventually when to close the inquiry period—perhaps by saying, "Okay, we have time for one more comment," and selecting a final speaker. However, it takes courage to speak up in a group, so teachers should try to let each participant speak the first time the person raises a hand.

Inquiry into Affectionate Breathing can be concluded by reading a poem such as "This Constant Lover," by John Astin (2013). This poem speaks to the integration of love and awareness. Another poem that can be read after Affectionate Breathing is Jane Pujji/O'Shea's (2007) "My Balm," which beautifully captures the sense of being held and caressed by one's own breathing. Sometimes teachers like to read poetry when a meditation is completed but before participants open their eyes because poems can be heard more deeply when received in a state of meditative awareness.

Practice Discussion
(15 minutes)

Participants now have a chance to share their experience of self-compassion practice during the previous week. An inclusive way to begin the practice discussion is for each participant to say one word—we call these "one-word shares"—that capture something about their practice. One-word shares are a way of helping each person contribute to the group experience. One-word shares also give teachers a chance to assess the needs of their group members from week to week.

The discussion usually focuses on the practices that were learned in the previous session. In this case, they were these two:

- Soothing Touch
- Self-Compassion Break

Speaking with students about home practice can be a delicate topic because students may feel guilty or ashamed when they didn't practice much. Furthermore, teachers often believe that *they* are failing if their students don't practice. Therefore, it's important for everyone to remember that the main purpose of MSC is to cultivate self-compassion, not to become conscientious meditators. It's even possible to make progress and *never* practice (Germer & Neff, 2013).

Teachers can ask, "Did anyone feel the *need* to practice Soothing Touch or the Self-Compassion Break last week?" Students are more likely to answer that question than "Did anyone practice last week?" Even when students think they didn't practice much, they may still recall a time during the previous week when they spoke in a kinder way to themselves or put a hand over the heart. Sharing even minor successes encourages practice.

The practice discussion is conducted by teachers via the inquiry method because it discourages participants from engaging in cross-talk or giving each other advice. Here is a sample of inquiry during the practice discussion.

> JOHN: Truth be told, I didn't practice at all last week. I just didn't have the time, with all the changes going on at work right now.
>
> TEACHER: Thanks for being so candid, John. It takes some courage to say that.
>
> JOHN: I wonder if my timing is off and I shouldn't be taking this course right now.
>
> TEACHER: Could be, but do you think, realistically, that you'd have more time in the future?
>
> JOHN: (*Laughing*) Not really. My life is just too crazy.

TEACHER: Can you feel how crazy it gets in your body?

JOHN: Yeah, I get jaw pain. I clench my teeth so much that I need to take Advil.

TEACHER: (*Smiling*) Would you like to add some self-compassion to your Advil regimen?

JOHN: Well, yes. The jaw pain is the slap in the face that brought me here in the first place. (*Laughing again, appreciating the irony of slapping himself into compassion*)

TEACHER: What could you do that doesn't take too much of your precious time, John?

JOHN: I'm embarrassed to say this, but I think putting a hand on my chest—like we did last week—and saying, "Love ya, man," might do the trick. It calms me down. It's like remembering that I matter.

TEACHER: That sounds like a great practice. Maybe "Love ya, man" is enough for now?

JOHN: Maybe so. Thanks.

The main aims during the practice discussion are to celebrate successes and remove obstacles to practice. In this case, John didn't practice at all, and he felt embarrassed about it. Rather than judging him, the teacher explored the consequences of his hectic lifestyle and helped him consider what might be a realistic way to practice. Especially when participants are learning self-compassion, practice doesn't have to be formal. Just taking a kinder, gentler approach toward oneself still counts. Shame tends to undermine the formation of new habits, so a conversation about *not* practicing needs to be radically accepting of a participant's needs and circumstances.

While sharing their experiences, group members should be reminded to keep their comments as practice-based as possible. When a participant tells a story that is only vaguely related to practice, it helps for a teacher to identify the emotional core of what's being said and to explore whether the student responded to it with self-compassion. For instance, Mariana came to class distraught by news of a hit-and-run car accident in her neighborhood.

MARIANA: What kind of world do we live in when people do these kinds of things? It makes me sick! I can only imagine the pain that the family must be feeling right now. It's awful. Sometimes I think human beings are a lost cause.

TEACHER: Yes, there is so much sadness in this world, so much pain.

MARIANA: I find it just unbearable. It breaks my heart.

TEACHER: How do you respond when your heart breaks like this?

MARIANA: I just cry. It's just so painful.

TEACHER: Did you consider taking a Self-Compassion Break when you got the news about the car accident?

MARIANA: No, I didn't. I thought that was only for when I was going through a hard time myself, not when others are in pain.

TEACHER: But weren't you also in pain—feeling the pain of the grieving family?

MARIANA: I guess in a way, the pain of others *is* my pain.

TEACHER: Yes, it is. It's all of ours, even just listening to your story. Why don't we all put our hands on our hearts for a moment and breathe together? (*Whole group does this.*)

MARIANA: (*Smiling now*) You know, maybe there's hope for us humans after all.

In this case, Mariana originally wanted to speak about how upset she was about an event outside class, and not about any of the exercises taught the previous week. The teacher took the opportunity to identify Mariana's empathic pain and link it to the practice of Soothing Touch and the experience of common humanity; this made the inquiry a learning opportunity for everyone.

As stated earlier, *how* we practice is more important than *how much* we practice. Most MSC students discover during MSC that a moment of self-compassion practice is actually a relief rather than a chore, which makes self-compassion practice self-rewarding. A participant's life may not radically change during the 8-week program, but each moment of self-compassion is planting a seed of transformation.

Practicing Mindfulness
(1 minute)

After the practice discussion, participants are introduced to the topic of the day, Practicing Mindfulness. They are given a very brief overview of what will be included in the class and offered an explanation for why this material is presented now.

Students can be told, for example, that they have already established a foundation for self-compassion training in Session 1 by exploring the meaning of self-compassion, addressing misgivings about self-compassion, and learning two simple strategies for evoking a felt sense of self-compassion—Soothing Touch and the Self-Compassion Break. Session 2 focuses specifically on mindfulness. Mindfulness is a prerequisite for self-compassion because we need to be *aware* when we're suffering in order to have a compassionate response. Usually we're too swept up in our thoughts to know what's going on within us. The price we pay for our inattention is that suffering may persist for a long time. Mindfulness, in contrast, is a skill that enables us to turn toward emotional discomfort in a healthy new way—with spacious, tender awareness.

Session 2 is the only session dedicated *primarily* to the theory and practice of mindfulness, but mindfulness continues to be taught throughout the course in practices such as the Compassionate Body Scan, the Sense and Savor Walk, Compassionate Movement, and Working with Difficult Emotions, and indirectly through the inquiry process after each practice.

Session 2, like the first session, contains more didactic teaching than the other sessions because participants need to build a conceptual foundation for both self-compassion and mindfulness before practicing those skills throughout the course. Students who came to the program hoping for more experiential training can be reassured that subsequent sessions will have more practice and less didactic teaching.

Wandering Mind
(5 minutes)

Below is some background information that can be condensed into a 10-minute presentation on the wandering mind. Understanding that human attention has been hardwired to wander helps students to be more compassionate with themselves when this happens during meditation.

Teachers can lead the discussion with a teasing question: "Did any of you notice that your mind wandered during the Affectionate Breathing meditation?" One of the first insights gleaned by mindfulness meditation students is that the mind wanders much more frequently than they ever imagined. This can be particularly distressing for students who want to "get it right." Even those who have practiced meditation for decades may be embarrassed to admit that their attention wanders from the breath (or another object of awareness) every few seconds. Concentration tends to improve during silent meditation retreats, but participants' attention always tends to wander.

Mind wandering is normal. Teachers can summarize a research study published by Matthew Killingsworth and Daniel Gilbert (2010) in *Science*. These authors found that mind wandering occurred 46.9% of the time, and rarely less than 30% with any activity (except for making love, when minds wandered only 10% of the time). In their study, participants were contacted though an iPhone application at random intervals and asked three questions: "How happy do you feel right now?", "What are you doing right now?" (e.g., working, reading, shopping, talking), and "Are you thinking about something other than what you're currently doing?" Killingsworth and Gilbert discovered that people were less happy when their minds wandered, *regardless of their activity*. Hence, mind wandering comes with a price.

Default Mode Network

Why does the mind wander so much? Teachers can explain that we're hardwired for mind wandering. A distinct network of structures, called the *default mode network* (DMN), is active in the brain when the mind wanders (Gusnard & Raichle, 2001; Hasenkamp & Barsalou, 2012). The DMN was identified from brain scans, and it appears that most of the brain structures in the DMN are located down the midline of the brain from the front to the back. The DMN is primarily engaged when we're left alone to think—remembering the past, envisioning the future, and taking the perspective of others (Buckner, Andrews-Hanna, & Schacter, 2008).

DMN activity also consists of self-referential thinking: "What happened to *me* in the past? What will happen to *me* in the future? How am *I* doing?" We might say that a key function of the DMN is to create a separate self and protect it from danger. Unfortunately, looking for threats to our well-being in every spare moment is not a prescription for happiness. It seems that we humans are hardwired for survival, not for happiness.

Ample research suggests that when we are left alone with our thoughts, we start to ruminate and focus on our faults (Nolen-Hoeksema, Wisco, & Lyubomirsky, 2008). As Anne Lamott (1997) wrote, "My mind is a bad neighborhood I try not to go into alone."

Luckily, we don't need to be left unprotected with our thoughts. Mindfulness is a tool for inhabiting the mind more safely and happily. Brewer, Garrison, and Whitfield-Gabrieli (2013) found that key structures in the DMN, especially the posterior cingulate cortex (PCC), were relatively *inactive* in experienced practitioners during meditation. The PCC may represent the process of "getting caught up in" one's experience rather being mindful of it. Taylor and colleagues (2013) found that reduced DMN activity persisted *beyond* the state of meditation in experienced meditators. When experienced meditators (with over 1,000 hours of practice) and beginners were placed in an fMRI scanner and told simply to rest, their DMNs were less tightly organized than those of beginners—an indication that experienced meditators were less caught up in the wandering mind.

What Is Mindfulness?
(10 minutes)

MSC students come to MSC with varying levels of understanding and practice of mindfulness. The following information can be adapted to accommodate the individual needs of group members.

The most common definition of *mindfulness* is "the awareness that emerges through paying attention, on purpose, in the present moment, and non-judgmentally to the unfolding of experience moment by moment" (Kabat-Zinn, 2003, p. 145). It may also be defined as "awareness of present experience, with acceptance" (Germer, 2013, p. 7). Teachers can solicit various definitions of mindfulness from students. Ultimately, however, mindfulness cannot be captured in words because it's a nonconceptual, nonverbal moment of awareness. Thoughts and words are representations—symbols that stand for reality, not reality itself. For example, we can't smell, taste, or eat the word *apple*. Mindfulness allows us to contact the world directly, not just through the lens of thought.

A practical definition of mindfulness is "knowing what you are experiencing *while* you're experiencing it." As an example, teachers can ask their students to raise their hands and wiggle their fingers. If they can feel their fingers wiggling, that's mindfulness. Mindfulness itself is not unusual, but *continuity* of mindfulness is rare indeed. This is where practice comes in. Mindfulness practice is a conscious attempt to return with warmhearted awareness to present moment experience, again and again.

Teachers can invite their students to experience mindfulness through using each of their senses:

- *Hearing.* "Please close your eyes and take a moment to listen to the sounds in the environment. Letting the sounds come to you. Noting what you hear, one sound after another, with an inner nod of recognition. There is no need to name what you hear."
- *Seeing.* "Now please open your eyes and allow your eyes to have a soft, wide-angle gaze. Again, note whatever you see, one visual impression after the other."
- *Touching.* "Gently rub your hands, noticing how your hands feel as you move them."
- *Smelling.* "See if you can notice any smells on your hands, staying aware that you are smelling."
- *Tasting.* "Are there any flavors or tastes left in your mouth, perhaps from your last meal?"

Afterward, teachers can solicit a few comments from students about their experience, and then inquire, "What would it be like to be mindful all the time?" Students are likely to say that it could be overwhelming. To illustrate how intense, as well as poignant, our lives might be if we were mindful all the time, teachers can show a short video, *Moments* (which can be found online by using the search terms *Moments* and *Radiolab*).

Soles of the Feet
(10 minutes)

Soles of the Feet (based on Singh, Wahler, Adkins, Myers, & Mindfulness Research Group, 2003) is a simple and effective mindfulness practice that students can use to calm the mind when they feel emotionally over-whelmed. It is an anchoring practice: It uses a single mental object (i.e., sen-sations in the feet) to which attention can return, again and again. Teachers can lead Soles of the Feet to illustrate present-moment awareness, or they can also introduce it after the discussion of backdraft later in this session as a grounding and stabilizing practice for times when backdraft arises.

People who have difficulty balancing or walking can practice Soles of the Feet while sitting in a chair and disregard the walking instructions; if they use wheelchairs, they can focus on the sensations in their hands, mov-ing their wheelchairs instead of the soles of their feet. It is respectful to have this conversation with participants who have disabilities *before* beginning this informal practice, and to adjust the instructions accordingly.

Instructions

- "Begin by noticing the sensations—the sense of touch—in the soles of your feet on the floor."
- "To better feel sensation in the soles of your feet, try gently rocking for-ward and backward on your feet, and side to side. If you are standing, perhaps making little circles with your knees, feeling the changing sensa-tions in the soles of your feet."
- "Feel how the floor supports your whole body."
- "When the mind has wandered, just return to feeling the soles of your feet."
- "Now beginning to walk, slowly, noticing the changing sensations in the soles of your feet. Noticing the sensation of lifting a foot, stepping for-ward, and then placing the foot on the floor. Now doing the same with the other foot. And then one foot after another."
- "As you walk, perhaps appreciating how small the surface area of your feet is, and how your feet support your entire body. If you wish, allowing a moment of gratitude for the hard work that your feet are doing, which we usually take for granted."
- "If you like, leaving an *imprint* of kindness or peace on the floor with each step—whatever you may wish your life to stand for."
- "Or you can imagine the ground rising up to support you with each step."
- "Continuing to walk, slowly, feeling the soles of your feet."
- "Now returning to standing again, and expanding your awareness to your entire body—letting yourself feel whatever you're feeling, and let-ting yourself be just as you are."

Inquiry

After participants have returned to their seats, teachers can ask, "What did you notice when you anchored your attention in your feet?" or "Did your mind calm down or rev up when you focused on your feet?" Inquiry can help to clarify the *purpose* of an exercise through the students' direct experience, as in this example.

TANYA: I may be the only one, but I noticed how wobbly I was as I walked. I felt like a klutz.

TEACHER: (*Smiling*) I suspect you were not the only wobbly person in the group. Anyone else notice that? (*Many hands go up in the room.*) And you also felt like a klutz?

TANYA: Yeah, I felt kind of embarrassed that I wobbled so much, and I found myself focusing on stabilizing myself rather than feeling the soles of my feet.

TEACHER: So you didn't want to *look* wobbly.

TANYA: Yes, I'd rather have the balance of a ballet dancer (*smiling cynically*).

TEACHER: Who wouldn't? Did you notice *during* the practice that you were paying more attention to stabilizing yourself than feeling the soles of your feet, or did that occur to you afterward?

TANYA: Only after we started talking about it. It's funny how easily self-consciousness crept in there, though. Self-*judgment*, really. I think that happens a lot in my life.

TEACHER: Join the club! Self-judgment and paying attention to what we're doing can be opposite ways of thinking. Thanks for pointing that out. I think that *noticing* this difference is already a step forward.

TANYA: Glad to hear I'm not just hopelessly wobbly (*smiling*).

Inquiry helped Tanya to strengthen her mindfulness muscle. During the practice itself, Tanya noticed that she wobbled while she walked; she felt embarrassed and became self-critical ("You're a klutz"), and then spent the remainder of the practice trying to walk in a smoother way. Using gentle questions, the teacher reminded Tanya (and the class) about the purpose of the exercise—mindfulness of sensation—and noted how easily self-consciousness and self-judgment can compete for our attention. To avoid overexposing Tanya, especially in this early session in the MSC program, the teacher focused on the universality of self-judgment rather than Tanya's personal tendency to judge herself.

Break
(15 minutes)

Teachers can suggest a break at any time during a session. They will know it is time for a break if their students seem restless or distracted, or if they themselves are tired. A 15-minute break should always be taken in every 2¾-hour session, regardless of how much time pressure a teacher may feel.

Soft Landing
(2 minutes)

MSC includes new practices each week from which to customize a 2-minute soft landing. Teachers should keep soft landings simple—few words, few elements—giving students a chance to settle easily into their experience. The practices learned so far include listening to sounds; feeling the soles of the feet; soothing touch; gentle vocalizations ("Ahhh" or "Awww"); an inner smile; the three components of the Self-Compassion Break (validating distress, recognizing common humanity, and offering ourselves words of self-kindness); and letting oneself be soothed by the gentle rhythm of the breath. Here is an example of a soft landing that could be used in Session 2:

- "Let's take 2 minutes to practice what we have learned as a way of settling into the present moment."
- "Please close your eyes, partially or fully, and begin to notice how your body breathes itself, feeling the chest expand and contract with each breath."
- "Now focusing on the *rhythm* of your breathing, rising and falling, just like the sea, and letting yourself be gently held and rocked by your breathing." (*Pause for 1 minute.*)
- "And then gently opening your eyes. Thank you."

Resistance
(10 minutes)

Mindfulness has two key aspects: *awareness* and *acceptance* of present-moment experience. *Resistance* is the opposite of acceptance. Resistance refers to the struggle that occurs when we believe that our moment-to-moment experience should be other than it is. Teachers should help students understand the concept of resistance, and also notice when it arises in their daily lives. Recognizing and letting go of unnecessary resistance reduce suffering and are at the heart of mindfulness and self-compassion practice.

Teachers can construct a concise talk about resistance, using points from the following paragraphs.

After offering a definition of resistance, teachers can engage students by asking, "How do you *know* when you're resisting? What are the signs and symptoms of resistance?" Here are some examples of resistance: when our attention bounces off unpleasant events, when we incessantly worry, when our muscles tense up (as if to create a shield against physical injury), when we distract ourselves with meaningless entertainment, or when we drink or eat too much to avoid what we're feeling.

Without resistance, we would be easily overwhelmed by the intensity of ordinary life. The poet Emily Dickinson (1872) wrote, "To live is so startling, it leaves but little room for other occupations." Resistance helps us to function, but resistance also has a cost. There is a saying that "What we resist, persists." Pain is inevitable in life—loss of loved ones, physical injury or illness, financial hardship—but we often prolong and amplify our pain by resisting it. For example, what happens when we find ourselves awake in the middle of the night and struggle to fall asleep? The struggle is likely to keep us awake even longer, isn't it? Over time, a simple episode of sleeplessness can develop into a case of insomnia. Similarly, when we fight grief, it can develop into depression; when we try to avoid anxiety, it can become a case of panic disorder. One MSC participant joked, "What happens when you fight your daughter's lousy boyfriend? You get a lousy son-in-law!"

Meditation teacher Shinzen Young (2017) has created a clever formula to describe the power of resistance: *suffering = pain × resistance*. Pain is inevitable; suffering is optional. Without resistance, our suffering is reduced to zero. Unfortunately, most of our resistance is unconscious—the myriad ways we fight or avoid our experience, wishing it were other than it is. Sigmund Freud's defense mechanisms (e.g., denial, projection, dissociation) are examples of unconscious resistance. Resistance is hardwired into the human mind.

The opposite of resistance is expressed in another saying: "What we can feel, we can heal." When we *accept* our moment-to-moment discomfort, we increase the possibility that it will change on its own.

For a dramatic illustration of resistance, teachers can show a short video, *The Fly*, by Hanjin Song (the video can be found online by using the search terms *The Fly* and *mindfulness*). In this film, a martial artist is bothered by a fly while he's meditating. He attempts to kill the fly by cutting it in half with his sword, but the bisected fly quickly morphs into two flies. The process continues as more and more flies appear. Finally, the martial artist collapses, exhausted by the struggle, and meditates in the midst of a swarm of flies. In the final scene, he opens his clenched fist, and a lone fly spreads its wings and flies away.

How much of our lives do we endure like this—with clenched fists rather than open palms? That's resistance. Fortunately, we can let go of the fight and live more amicably with our moment-to-moment experience.

That's *mindfulness*. We can also let go of the battle we wage against ourselves—the constant struggle to be better persons—and learn to befriend ourselves just as we are. That's *self-compassion*. Together, mindfulness and self-compassion are powerful antidotes to resistance.

How We Cause Ourselves Unnecessary Suffering
(20 minutes)

After the concepts of mindfulness and resistance have been introduced, group members participate in a reflection exercise that demonstrates how resistance directly affects the quality of their lives, and they explore how mindfulness and self-compassion can help to reduce unnecessary resistance. This class exercise requires paper and a pen.

Instructions

- "Think of a current situation in your life in which you may be resisting the reality of an unwanted experience, and you suspect the resistance is causing you unnecessary suffering and may actually be making things worse. We are not referring here to resisting unjust situations in our lives, but rather how we *feel*, moment-to-moment, when we resist something unpleasant. Also, for the sake of this preliminary exercise, please choose a relatively benign situation such as harboring resentment toward a loud neighbor, avoiding your taxes, or ignoring a talkative friend's phone calls. [Teachers can give illustrations from their own lives.] We'll be sharing this in small groups, so please choose an example that you feel comfortable telling others, and then write it down."

- "How do you know that you are resisting? Is there any discomfort in the body or the mind? Can you describe it?"

- "How might resistance be *benefiting* you in some way? Perhaps resistance is helping you to cope temporarily? If difficult feelings arise, please be kind to yourself. Honor your resistance, knowing that it allows you to function in the world."

- "How might resistance *not* be serving you? For example, how might your life be easier if you stopped resisting, or resisted a little less?"

- "Now please consider how *mindfulness* or *self-compassion* might help lessen your resistance in this situation? For example, perhaps using the components of the Self-Compassion Break—validating the pain ('This is tough'), seeing common humanity ('This is how people feel in these situations'), or offering yourself kindness ('It's not your fault,' 'I'm here to support you')."

Discussion

Group members now form pairs, and the partners each take 5 minutes to discuss their situation and how mindfulness and self-compassion might make it easier. Teachers can acknowledge that sharing an ongoing personal difficulty with unfamiliar people can make anyone feel vulnerable, so participants should only discuss what feels comfortable. The partners should also be reminded to respect each other's privacy, listen with an open heart, and avoid giving advice.

Inquiry

After small-group conversations, the entire group reconvenes for a brief inquiry period. Here's one dialogue in which a participant focused mainly on how mindfulness could help overcome unnecessary resistance.

TEACHER: What did you discover?

MICHAEL: I am a cyclist, and I like to ride every day. Sometimes I ride with a friend who is a really good athlete, and he always tells me to "love the hills." That always aggravates me because it just reminds me how much better an athlete he is than I am. Anyhow, I think I get it now because when we're riding together and a steep hill is coming up, I brace myself for the pain and exhaustion—and when it happens, I think how awful I feel and I look ahead to see how much longer I will have to endure it. Sometimes I even feel exhausted *before* I leave home when I think about the hills.

TEACHER: And did you discover anything new in this exercise?

MICHAEL: The crazy thing is that I love to exercise, and I feel great afterwards *because* of the hills. I need to stop making my life miserable over them.

TEACHER: I wonder if your resistance to the hills has been *serving* you in some way?

MICHAEL: I thought about that. I think part of me just wants to enjoy myself and not be so disciplined all the time.

TEACHER: That makes sense. I know this is another crazy question, but might there be a way for you to *enjoy* the hills?

MICHAEL: That's a tall order! I guess I could focus on the burn in my thighs and see that as a good thing. It *is* a good thing—it just doesn't feel good. I have to think about that.

TEACHER: (*With a teasing smile*) Anyhow, we might not want your friend to be right about the hills.

In this exercise, Michael was able to recognize resistance and how resistance reduced his enjoyment of cycling. The inquiry brought the conversation closer to a mindful embrace of the pain of physical exertion, but stopped short of advice giving, leaving Michael with an open-ended challenge.

Below is an inquiry example with another group member who found the exercise more challenging. It's important to ask the class about challenges, so struggling participants don't feel isolated and so working through difficulties in inquiry will provide a learning opportunity for everyone.

HOLLY: I heard you say that we should open to what's causing us suffering, but I'm afraid that if I do that, I simply couldn't function. My father has Alzheimer's disease, and I recently quit my job to care for him. It's a tough situation, and when I think about it, I get pretty overwhelmed.

TEACHER: I see, that sounds really hard, Holly. There are probably one or two people in this room right now who have an idea what you're talking about.

HOLLY: I know I'm not alone—my whole generation is doing this—and I need to take it one day at a time to cope.

TEACHER: That's probably a good idea. May I ask where in your body you feel stress the most, even now as you speak?

HOLLY: It's in the center of my heart, the core of my being.

TEACHER: Would you be willing to put your hand over your heart for a moment and just give yourself a little kindness? (*Everyone is quiet for 5 seconds.*)

HOLLY: It does calm me, but it doesn't change my situation.

TEACHER: I know. I also wish you didn't have to go through this.

HOLLY: (*Pause*) Yeah.

TEACHER: (*Pause*) Is there anything you could do to support yourself while you're in this situation?

HOLLY: It's just awful. It's not fair. (*Starts to sob.*)

TEACHER: (*More quiet*) Sometimes there's nothing we can do. Do you think we can all just be together with this for a little while?

HOLLY: (*Still sobbing as one participant offers a tissue and another puts an arm around her*) Thank you.

TEACHER: (*To the group*) This is real opening, the kind where words fail.

HOLLY: (*To the people who are comforting her*) Thank you so much. I'll be all right.

TEACHER: I'm sure you will. It may take a while, though. Thank you for sharing your situation with us.

Holly was already feeling overwhelmed by caring for her dying father and believed that "opening" to it meant being further overwhelmed by her plight. Holly resented that she was in this unfair situation (a form of resistance), a natural consequence of grieving for the loss of her career as well as her father. When she located the resistance in her body and experienced the kindness and support of the group, she began to let go a little and experienced the relief of tears. This inquiry demonstrates how resistance can be released during inquiry itself.

Backdraft
(15 minutes)

Backdraft refers to distress that arises when we give ourselves compassion. This topic is introduced now as an explanation for why uncomfortable sensations, thoughts, and emotions may arise during self-compassion training. It comes after the discussion of resistance because our students will inevitably resist backdraft during the course. Backdraft is an important part of emotional transformation through self-compassion, and identifying backdraft helps students to work more effectively with it. An example of how this topic may be presented follows.

A teacher can begin by saying, "Please raise your hand if, sometime when you practiced self-compassion, you felt good? Bad? Nothing at all?" Pleasant feelings make sense because compassion is a positive emotion. We may feel nothing when we're distracted or emotionally closed. But why would unpleasant thoughts, sensations, or emotions arise when we practice self-compassion?

One reason we may feel worse is that we require *contrast* to know anything—light–dark, high–low, hot–cold. Self-compassion works by creating contrast in the relational matrix of our lives. When we give ourselves unconditional love, we discover the conditions under which we were unloved. If we say to ourselves, "May I love myself just as I am," we may remember old messages telling us the opposite: "Don't be so full of yourself!" or "Listen, stupid, why can't you . . . " or "There you go again; you're always getting it wrong."

A metaphor for this phenomenon is *backdraft* (Germer, 2009, pp. 150–152). Backdraft is a term that firefighters use to describe what happens when a fire has used all available oxygen, and then fresh oxygen is introduced through an open door or window: The fire dramatically intensifies. A similar effect occurs when the doors of our hearts open with self-compassion. Our hearts hold a lot of pain, often old wounds that we have pushed aside in order to function in our daily lives. When we feel loved and the doors of our hearts open, the love goes in and the pain comes out. As mentioned last session, there is a saying: "Love reveals everything unlike itself." Those difficult feelings are not *created* by self-compassion; we're simply reexperiencing them because we feel safe and secure enough to do so.

Another metaphor, perhaps less dramatic, is what happens when our hands become numb in very cold weather and then hurt when they begin to warm up. The pain is actually a good sign because it means our hands are warming up. Similarly, we may have become numb to the pain in our lives, and when we warm up with self-compassion, hidden pain reveals itself as well.

Backdraft can be experienced mentally, emotionally, or physically. Here are some examples of backdraft:

- *Mental.* "I'm all alone," "I'm a failure," "I'm unworthy."
- *Emotional.* Shame, fear, grief.
- *Physical.* Body memories, aches, and pains.

Teachers can ask the class for examples of backdraft that they may already have experienced during the training.

Backdraft is part of the healing process. We transform old wounds by first *activating* them with mindfulness and self-compassion, and then *meeting* them with mindfulness and self-compassion. In this way, we have an opportunity to "re-parent" ourselves—to give ourselves the kindness and understanding we may have missed earlier in our lives (Shonin & Van Gordon, 2016).

Backdraft is not inherently problematic; it's our innate *resistance* to backdraft that causes so much suffering. Examples of resistance to backdraft are muscle tension, social isolation, overintellectualizing, criticism of ourselves or others, and spacing out/dissociation. Mindfulness and self-compassion help us to meet backdraft with less resistance, and hence with less suffering. When we do that, "ka-boom" may become "ka-*bloom*."

Backdraft is actually a good sign; it means that self-compassion training is starting to work. To extend the firefighting metaphor, when firefighters know there is a fire behind a door, they poke holes in the wall or break windows, letting oxygen in slowly. Similarly, practitioners of self-compassion should practice slowly and carefully. As we develop the capacity to hold ourselves and our experience in loving awareness, backdraft subsides. The 4th-century Christian saint Amma Syncletica used another fire-based metaphor for this: "It is just like building a fire: at first it's smoky and your eyes water, but later you get the desired result" (quoted in Chittister, 2000, p. 40).

Backdraft is often associated with "fears of compassion" (Gilbert et al., 2011; Kelly et al., 2013). In this case, we are not afraid of self-compassion per se; we are afraid of the discomfort that we may experience when we give ourselves compassion. We may also have fear of backdraft when the practice of self-compassion goes against our personal or cultural values (Robinson et al., 2016).

MSC teachers who are also psychotherapists may be tempted to explore the emotional histories of group members who are experiencing backdraft. Although this impulse is well intentioned, teachers will not be able to give participants the individual attention they need to do this kind of work. Students who want to go more deeply into the content of their backdraft should seek out individual counseling (see Part IV of this book).

Working with Backdraft

MSC students are taught to work with backdraft in a variety of ways. First, participants can *make space* and *allow* backdraft to percolate in the background of their awareness, and see whether it dissipates on its own. Second, participants can *reduce* whatever practices they were doing when backdraft occurred. Finally, if backdraft remains an issue, participants can (1) regulate emotions by regulating attention and/or (2) practice mindfulness and self-compassion in daily life.

Regulating Attention

Where and how we place our attention (mindfulness) have an impact on our emotions. For example, distraction is a key aspect of emotion regulation (Denkova, Dolcos, & Dolcos, 2014). The following mindfulness practices can be applied in response to backdraft:

* Label the experience as backdraft: "Oh, this is *backdraft*!."
* Name the strongest emotion and validate it with a kind voice ("Ahhh, that's *grief*").
* Explore where the emotion physically resides in the body, perhaps as tension in the stomach or hollowness in the heart region, and offer the self soothing touch. (We explore this further when we describe Session 6 in Chapter 16.)
* Redirect attention to a neutral focus inside the body (e.g., the breath), or a sensation at the boundary of the body (e.g., soles of the feet), or a sense object in the outside world (e.g., ambient sounds)—whatever is easiest.

Mindfulness and Self-Compassion in Daily Life

If backdraft continues to cause emotional distress, participants should discontinue whatever *mental* practices they were doing and focus instead on *behavioral* practices. Doing this keeps MSC safe. Behavioral practices are ordinary ways of living that we already enjoy, but done as a means of caring for ourselves. The behavioral practices described below and on the next page are Mindfulness in Daily Life and Self-Compassion in Daily Life.

Mindfulness in Daily Life
(5 minutes)

Mindfulness is more than a strategy or a technique; it is a way of life. Mindfulness can be practiced at any time, day or night. For example, we can feel the water on our backs while we shower, savor the flavors of our food, or listen to the sound of crickets in the evening. Mindfulness brings us "home" to the present moment. However, in the midst of our hectic lives, we usually need to make a conscious choice to be mindful. The following steps can be taken to experience ordinary life more mindfully.

Instructions

- "Pick an ordinary activity. You might choose drinking a hot beverage in the morning, brushing your teeth, or taking a shower. It may help to select an activity that occurs early in the day, before your attention is pulled in many directions."
- "Choose *one* sensory experience to explore in the activity, such as the sensation of taste as you drink a cup of tea, or the sensation of water touching your body while you are showering."
- "Immerse yourself in the experience, savoring it to the fullest. Return your attention to the sensations again and again when you notice it has wandered away."
- "Bring friendly awareness to the activity until it has been completed."

    After reviewing this exercise with the class, teachers can ask participants to choose one activity they might wish to engage in mindfully during the coming week. Teachers can also ask for examples from the class, to inspire other participants to think creatively about the possibilities for mindfulness in daily life.

Self-Compassion in Daily Life
(5 minutes)

The goal of MSC is to be self-compassionate in daily life. This might seem like a distant dream for many people, but most of us are closer to it than we realize because we've been caring for ourselves our entire lives. Self-care becomes self-compassion when it is done with the conscious intention to alleviate suffering. It's also an important form of yang self-compassion— *providing* for ourselves in the world.

Teachers can introduce this practice with the question "How do you care for yourself already?" and ask participants to write down three self-care activities. Then teachers can invite volunteers to share, "popcorn-style" (see Chapter 10), what they do for themselves. To cover the full range of activities, teachers can keep in mind the following self-care categories:

- *Physical.* Exercise, get a massage, take a warm bath, sip a cup of tea.
- *Mental.* Meditate, watch a funny movie, read an inspiring book.
- *Emotional.* Have a good cry, pet the dog or cat, listen to music.
- *Relational.* Meet with friends, send a birthday card, play a game.
- *Spiritual.* Pray, walk in the woods, help others.

The challenge, of course, is to *remember* to do these self-care activities when we struggle in daily life.

 # Here-and-Now Stone (Optional)
(5 minutes)

Another practice for anchoring attention in the present moment, especially in the midst of emotional distress, is the Here-and-Now Stone. It is an adaptation of *suiseki,* the Japanese art of stone appreciation (Covello & Yoshimura, 2009). The practice requires fairly large (1.5- to 2-inch) polished stones; teachers can ask participants to bring such stones to class, or teachers can buy them online for their group members. The sensation of rubbing the stone is used to bring the practitioner into the present moment. It is also a savoring practice when participants allow themselves to *enjoy* their stones.

When teachers bring stones to class for their students, they can put them on a plate and ask participants to each choose one that they find most attractive. This task should probably be started earlier in the session, after the break, so that students will be ready with their stones when the exercise is introduced.

Instructions

- "Let's start by carefully examining our stones. Noticing the colors, the angles, and the way the light plays on the curves of your stone."
- "Allowing yourself to *enjoy* the sight of the stone."

- "Now, closing your eyes and exploring the stone with your sense of touch. First, closing your hand around the stone and squeezing it, feeling its hardness. Then noticing its texture. Is it smooth or rough? What is its temperature?"
- "Opening your eyes again and letting your gaze become absorbed in your stone, and the experience of handling this beautiful stone."
- "Noticing that when you are focused on your stone, with appreciation, there is little room for regret or worry—you are home in the present moment."
- "Feel free to take your here-and-now stone home with you. You can keep it in your pocket, and whenever you're under stress, you can feel your stone, enjoy the sensation of rubbing it, and come into the present moment."

Mindfulness and Self-Compassion
(10 minutes)

This topic helps participants to make sense of this session as a whole, especially the conceptual relationship of mindfulness to self-compassion. Seasoned mindfulness meditators are often particularly curious about this relationship. Since the topic comes at the end of the session, teachers should try to deliver it as concisely and interactively as possible.

Mindfulness practitioners may want to know how mindfulness is integrated into MSC training. Mindfulness has four important roles:

1. Knowing that we're suffering while we're suffering. We need to be aware of suffering to have a compassionate response.
2. Anchoring and stabilizing awareness in present-moment experience when we are emotionally overwhelmed.
3. Managing difficult emotions by finding them in the body and relating to them with mindful awareness.
4. Balancing compassion with equanimity, or calm, spacious awareness. We need a stable mind to choose compassionate action.

How do mindfulness and self-compassion relate to one another? Self-compassion is the heart of mindfulness when we meet suffering (see also Germer & Barnhofer, 2017). Warmth creates space, and space creates warmth. Without self-compassion, we cannot tolerate difficult emotions. Conversely, we need mindfulness to be self-compassionate. When either mindfulness or compassion is in full bloom, both are present. However, our mindfulness or self-compassion is often partial or incomplete—tinged with desire, aversion, or confusion—so it helps us to understand the differences between mindfulness and self-compassion in order to practice skillfully. In our modern understanding, these are some key differences:

- Mindfulness is loving awareness of *experience,* whereas self-compassion is loving awareness of the *experiencer.*
- Mindfulness asks, "What am I *experiencing* right now?", and self-compassion asks, "What do I *need* right now?"
- Mindfulness says, "*Feel* your suffering with spacious awareness," while self-compassion says, "*Be kind* to yourself when you suffer."
- Mindfulness regulates emotions through *attention.* Self-compassion regulates emotions through *affiliation.*
- Mindfulness is *calming,* and self-compassion is *warming.*

People may argue about the relative merits of mindfulness and self-compassion, but mindfulness and self-compassion don't argue. They are best friends.

Together, mindfulness and self-compassion constitute a powerful formula for alleviating suffering. When we feel emotionally overwhelmed and cannot make space for our experience, we can still give compassion to *ourselves*—focus on ourselves and validate our pain as we might for a dear friend. Both mindfulness and self-compassion alleviate suffering by allowing us to live with less resistance.

Self-compassion may seem more *intentional* than mindfulness because we are adding warmth and kindness to our awareness, but it is not more *effortful.* Self-compassion is allowing our hearts to melt in the heat of suffering—letting go of resistance—not pushing suffering away. The central paradox of self-compassion is this: When we struggle, we give ourselves compassion not to feel better, but *because* we feel bad. One metaphor for this is a child with the flu. We are naturally kind to a child with the flu, not to make the illness go away, but simply because the child is sick. Can we offer ourselves the same kindness when we feel bad? This paradox is very important for students to understand because if they start using self-compassion to make the pain go away it becomes a form of resistance. When we give ourselves compassion just because it hurts, however, then we provide ourselves the warmth and safety needed to hold our pain in mindful awareness without resisting it.

Some mindfulness practitioners worry that self-compassion will strengthen the sense of a rigid, separate "self" and thereby increase suffering. However, both mindfulness and self-compassion reduce and soften the sense of self. Mindfulness *dismantles* the self into moment-to-moment experience. Self-compassion *melts* the sense of a separate self by generating warmth and connection.

Home Practice
(5 minutes)

Teachers should remind their participants of the new practices learned in this session:

- Affectionate Breathing
- Soles of the Feet
- Mindfulness in Daily Life
- Self-Compassion in Daily Life
- Here-and-Now Stone (Optional)

Students can now practice up to 30 minutes each day, formal and informal practice combined, since they have learned a core meditation this session— Affectionate Breathing. For beginners in meditation, it may help to listen to guided meditations. Participants who already have a meditation practice are encouraged to continue in their own way, perhaps adding elements from Affectionate Breathing and other MSC practices that they find interesting or appealing.

It is not easy to establish a regular meditation practice. In general, home practice needs to be pleasant and easy, and it is best to start with short meditations, perhaps only 10–15 minutes long. Informal practice is also as valuable as formal practice, and many participants find informal practice easier to integrate into their daily lives.

Closing
(2 minutes)

Session 2 can be closed in a variety of ways—for instance, by engaging in another circle of one-word shares, having a moment of silence, ringing a bell, or reading a poem. A recommended poem that captures key themes from this session, especially mindfulness and overcoming resistance, is "Unconditional" by Jennifer Welwood (1998/2019).

Chapter 12

Session 3

PRACTICING LOVING-KINDNESS

Overview

Opening (Core) Meditation: Affectionate Breathing

Practice Discussion

Session Theme: Practicing Loving-Kindness

Topic: Loving-Kindness and Compassion

Exercise: Awakening Our Hearts

Break

Soft Landing

Topic: Loving-Kindness Meditation

Meditation: Loving-Kindness for a Loved One

Informal Practice (Optional): Compassionate Movement

Topic: Practicing with Phrases

Informal Practice: Finding Loving-Kindness Phrases

Home Practice

Closing

Getting Started

- In this session, participants will:
  - Understand the difference between loving-kindness and compassion.
  - Learn to evoke a felt sense of loving-kindness and compassion.
  - Discover and learn how to use phrases in loving-kindness meditation.
- These subjects are introduced now to:
  - Help participants bring loving awareness to *themselves*, after learning in Session 2 to bring loving awareness to *moment-to-moment experience*.
- New practices taught this session:
  - Loving-Kindness for a Loved One
  - Compassionate Movement (Optional)
  - Finding Loving-Kindness Phrases

Affectionate Breathing
(20 minutes)

The session begins with a guided, brief Affectionate Breathing meditation. Affectionate Breathing is practiced three times in MSC (twice in the regular sessions, once during the retreat) because it is a core meditation that participants can practice throughout the course. Please refer to Session 2 (Chapter 11) for instructions on guiding this meditation. An inquiry period follows the meditation.

Practice Discussion
(15 minutes)

Teachers can start the practice discussion with a one-word sharing circle or can inquire right away about the participants' experience of home practice, especially the new practices. The new practices from Session 2 were these:

- Affectionate Breathing
- Soles of the Feet
- Mindfulness in Daily Life
- Self-Compassion in Daily Life
- Here-and-Now Stone (Optional)

To stimulate discussion, teachers can ask, "Did anyone encounter any obstacles to practice last week?" and then conduct inquiry. Here is an example.

WILMA: I wanted to practice Affectionate Breathing at home, since I really enjoyed that meditation when we did it together in class last time, but my in-laws were in town for the holidays. I just didn't get to it.

TEACHER: Sounds like you were pulled in two directions—you wanted to take care of your in-laws, and you also wanted to take care of yourself.

WILMA: Yeah, and the in-laws won out. No surprise there! (*Laughing*)

TEACHER: Were you aware of your struggle at the time?

WILMA: Yes, I was. I was really frustrated because they needed me to make breakfast in the morning when I wanted to meditate. I also didn't want to come to this class and admit that I didn't meditate.

TEACHER: So what did you do when you felt frustrated?

WILMA: I tried to ground myself, and silently repeated, "Soles of the feet . . . soles of the feet." Actually, that calmed me down, but it wasn't what I really wanted to do.

TEACHER: So you still practiced mindfulness, just in a different way?

WILMA: Yes, I guess I did! Okay, perhaps I'm not as delinquent as I thought. (*Smiling*)

TEACHER: No, I guess you're not. (*Also smiling*)

This short inquiry illustrates how participants can use any life situation to practice, including the experience of *not* practicing. Obstacles are ideal opportunities for all of us to practice, if we only *remember* to practice. Wilma remembered and used her frustration as an occasion to anchor her awareness in her feet (mindfulness practice).

The home practice discussion is a good opportunity to teach participants how to motivate themselves with self-compassion (see also Session 4). Self-compassion occupies the middle ground between the extremes of *self-indulgence* ("I don't feel like practicing") and *excessive striving* ("Because it's good for me, damn it!"). For students on the side of excessive striving, teachers can help them discover how to motivate themselves with encouragement rather than self-criticism. The following questions may help:

- "How can I make my practice *easier*—less like work?"
- "How can I make my practice *more enjoyable*?"
- "What *voice* am I listening to: critical or encouraging?"
- "What do I really *need* in this moment?"

For students on the self-indulgence side, teachers should bear in mind that self-indulgence can be an important first step—not practicing at all.

However, teachers should be careful not to establish a group norm of not doing home practice for the sake of one or two participants.

To develop a habit of self-compassion, students need to discover for themselves that moments of self-compassion provide genuine relief. This is the insight teachers are angling for in practice discussions when they focus on small, informal acts of self-compassion, such as a kind word or a hand on the heart, in response to stressful situations in daily life. Teachers can also focus on little shifts during formal meditation that may make practice more pleasant, such as sitting more comfortably or keeping meditation as simple as breathing, without further expectations. In general, practice becomes self-reinforcing when it is easy, pleasant, or meaningful.

Practicing Loving-Kindness
(1 minute)

Teachers can explain that this session, Practicing Loving-Kindness, builds upon the previous session on mindfulness: "Last week we learned to warm up our awareness and now we will find ways to direct loving-kindness toward ourselves. When our loving-kindness is directed toward ourselves *in the midst of struggle*, it becomes self-compassion." In this session, participants will explore the conceptual differences between loving-kindness and compassion, have a direct experience of loving-kindness and compassion in dyads, learn to practice meditation using phrases (loving-kindness meditation), and then do an exercise in which they discover phrases that are authentically their own.

Loving-Kindness and Compassion
(2 minutes)

This short topic serves as a segue to the next exercise, rather than as an opportunity for conceptual discussion. Teachers can invite participants to write down their questions on the Parking Lot page of the flipchart (see Session 1, Chapter 10) for later consideration.

Compassion and Self-Compassion

Teachers can start by offering an operational definition of *compassion*, such as "the feeling that arises when witnessing another's suffering and that motivates a subsequent desire to help" (Goetz et al., 2010, p. 351). This definition contains the aspects of *recognizing* and *empathizing* with the pain of another person, along with the *wish to help*. There is often a behavioral aspect to compassion as well—*doing* something to alleviate suffering.

Together, compassion involves *seeing, feeling, wishing,* and *doing. Self*-compassion is simply compassion directed toward oneself—*inner* compassion.

Loving-Kindness and Compassion

What is the difference between loving-kindness and compassion? The Dalai Lama (2003) describes it this way:

- *Loving-kindness* is "the wish that all sentient beings may be happy."
- *Compassion* is "the wish that all sentient beings may be free from suffering." (p. 67)

When loving-kindness bumps into suffering and stays loving, that's compassion. There is a saying from Myanmar: "When the sunshine of loving-kindness meets the tears of suffering, the rainbow of compassion arises." Compassion training helps us sustain the attitude of loving-kindness in the face of suffering. Both loving-kindness and compassion are the practice of *goodwill.*

Loving-kindness meditation (LKM) is a form of meditation that uses phrases to cultivate either loving-kindness or compassion. Phrases that point toward *happiness* may be considered loving-kindness phrases ("May I be happy," "May I live with ease") and phrases that address the experience of *suffering* in a loving way are considered compassion phrases ("May I be free from fear," "May I be kind to myself"). In MSC, we consider any meditation that uses phrases, regardless of whether they are loving-kindness or compassion phrases, to be LKM. This type of meditation derives from the ancient *metta* (Pali: loving-kindness, friendliness) meditation (Germer, 2009, pp. 130–131). Depending on the context, teachers should feel free to use words like *warmth, friendliness, goodwill, benevolence, kindness,* or *love* interchangeably with *loving-kindness.*

Awakening Our Hearts
(40 minutes)

The purpose of the Awakening Our Hearts exercise is to provide a direct experience of four different facets of goodwill—loving-kindness, self-kindness, compassion, and self-compassion—and to distinguish one from the other. It is also an opportunity to notice whether it feels similar or different when we are kind and compassionate toward others versus ourselves. This exercise also builds connection between members of the group and creates a safe space for emotional vulnerability. Teachers may want to offer their students a brief stretch break before introducing this exercise.

Awakening Our Hearts is based on a similar exercise adapted by Jack Kornfield (2008) from Joanna Macy (2007).

This exercise is the first of the class exercises that can be emotionally challenging for students (see Chapter 6). Teachers need to know this exercise very well before leading it. As with any challenging exercise, teachers should only lead the practice if they feel comfortable doing so and are capable of managing difficult emotions as they arise. Teachers should also have had previous training in leading exercises such as Awakening Our Hearts, and should be willing to access consultation from other MSC teacher trainers as needed.

Participants form pairs and face each other during the Awakening Our Hearts exercise. One person has eyes open and the other has eyes closed, alternately, with short periods (5 seconds) of looking into each other's eyes. This arrangement may be challenging or inappropriate for members of some cultural groups, and may make some participants feel unsafe, such as trauma survivors who are sensitive to being observed. Therefore, the exercise can be omitted from the class, depending on the participants, and vulnerable individuals can be given the option not to participate. Teachers can also control the intensity of this exercise by varying their tone and pacing. A lighter tone and faster pace (20 minutes vs. 25 minutes for this exercise) can reduce the intensity of the exercise. Many participants shed tears during this exercise, so tissues should be available.

Safety Suggestions

If participants hear the following safety caveats before they begin engaging in this exercise, most of them are likely to engage in the exercise and will find it meaningful. Teachers can offer the following safety suggestions, ideally conveyed in an easygoing manner so that participants are not scared off:

- "In the exercise we are about to do, we will first pair off, with the partners in each pair facing one another. During the exercise, one person will have eyes open, and the other person will have eyes closed. The partners in each pair will alternate back and forth four times, opening and closing eyes. There will also be very brief periods in which both partners have eyes open."
- "This exercise can be emotionally activating, mostly because it can be quite moving. You might want to have tissues on hand if you are a person who tears up easily—a 'leaky' person."
- "Please notice if you are emotionally opening or closing right now, and feel free to take a break and skip this exercise if you are closing. That, in itself, is good self-compassion practice."

- "You can also choose to sit alone in the room during this exercise and simply listen to the instructions, rather than being part of a pair. However, if you aren't sure, you will probably get more out of it by participating in a pair."
- "If you do the exercise and any discomfort arises, please take good care of yourself. This may include:
  - "Mindfulness practice—feeling your breath, naming the emotion you are feeling, making space for what you feel."
  - "Self-compassion practice—soothing touch, encouraging self-talk."
  - "Opening or closing your eyes as needed."
  - "Distraction, like drafting your next shopping list."
  - "Leaving the room."
- "This exercise also has sections where we imagine ourselves and others as children. If you think that doing this might be distressing for you, please feel free to ignore the instruction and just think about your adult self."
- "Any questions?"

Instructions

- "Now, please turn toward someone near you and sit face to face in a comfortable position that you can maintain for about 20 minutes. Then immediately close your eyes."
- "To begin, please place your hands over your heart or another soothing place on your body, as a reminder that we are not only paying attention to our experience, but paying *loving* attention. You can leave your hands on the soothing place during this exercise or let them rest in your lap."
- "We would like to offer you a direct experience of *loving-kindness* for self and other, and then *compassion* for self and other."
- "When I speak to the person with open eyes, the task is to mentally direct the words to your partner who has closed eyes. You can look directly at your partner or just glance at this person occasionally, depending on what feels most comfortable. At the same time, the person with closed eyes should mentally direct the words toward the self."
- "If some strong feelings arise in your partner, and you have a natural wish to touch or comfort your partner, please resist the impulse and let your partner have the fullness of her own experience."
- "Now please open your eyes and decide who will have eyes open first— perhaps the person with the longer first name—and then the other person should please close his eyes."

Loving-Kindness I

- "If your eyes are open, this is an opportunity to imagine the unique gifts and strengths that lie within your partner (or, if your eyes are closed, yourself). (*Pause*) Knowing there are gifts and strengths that are already realized, and those that are still seeds of potential. As in every human life, there are wonderful moments of strength, courage, humor, creativity, generosity, and tenderness. Your heart and the heart of this person, like all human hearts, are capable of more love and kindness than you ever dreamed possible." (*Pause*)

- "As you look, if your eyes are open, imagine your partner as a child. If your eyes are closed, you can imagine yourself as a child, if that feels right, or just keep imagining your adult self. (*Pause*) Recognizing that there is still a child that lies within all of us." (*Allow a longer pause to let participants form this image.*)

- "Letting yourself feel how much you want this child to be nurtured, to be able to grow into full adult potential. (*Pause*) How much you wish that this child would stay well, safe from harm, peaceful, and happy. How much you naturally want to bring forth and celebrate what is beautiful in this child."

- "If you are seeing this person's potential, and a wish is arising to cherish and honor this person, know that you are experiencing your innate capacity for *loving-kindness* (or, if you were directing the words toward yourself, that would be *self*-kindness). (*Pause*) And this capacity is there in you, always."

- "Both partners, please open your eyes and take a moment to silently acknowledge your partner with a soft gaze. (*Pause for about 5 seconds*) Then both partners, please close your eyes, taking a few moments to notice how you're feeling, letting yourself feel what you are feeling and be who you are. (*Pause*) Some people will be feeling loving-kindness; others will not. See if you can bring an accepting attitude to whatever your experience is."

- "Again, if it's the self-compassionate thing for you to do, please feel free to close—to tune out the instructions and just tune into your heart or your breath. You could even ask your partner for permission to take a break if you need to."

Loving-Kindness II

- "If your eyes were open before, please keep them closed now, and if your eyes were closed before, please open them now. If you like, offering yourself soothing touch as a reminder to be kind to yourself. Again, when I speak to the person with the open eyes, the task is to direct the words to your partner in a heartfelt way. At the same time, if you are the person with closed eyes, please direct the words to yourself."

- "If your eyes are open, this is an opportunity to imagine the unique gifts and strengths that lie within your partner (or, if your eyes are closed, yourself). (*Pause*) Knowing there are gifts and strengths that are already realized and those that are still seeds of potential. As in every human life, there are wonderful moments of strength, courage, humor, creativity, generosity, and tenderness. The heart of this person, like all human hearts, is capable of more love and kindness than you ever dreamed possible." (*Pause*)

- "As you look, if your eyes are open, imagine your partner as a child. If your eyes are closed, you can imagine yourself as a child, if that feels right, or just keep imagining your adult self. (*Pause*) Recognizing that there is still a child that lies within all of us." (*Pause to let participants form this image.*)

- "Letting yourself feel how you might want this child to be nurtured, to be able to grow into full adult potential. (*Pause*) How you may wish that this child would stay well, safe from harm, peaceful, and happy. How much you may want to bring forth and celebrate what is beautiful in this child."

- "If you are seeing this person's potential, and the wish is arising to cherish and honor this person, know that you are experiencing your innate capacity for *loving-kindness* (or, if you were directing the words toward yourself, that would be *self*-kindness). (*Pause*) And this capacity is there in you, always."

- "Both partners, please open your eyes and take a moment to silently acknowledge your partner with a soft gaze. (*Pause for about 5 seconds*) Then both partners, please close your eyes, taking a few moments to notice how you're feeling, letting yourself feel what you are feeling and be who you are. Now, taking a few slow, deep breaths and releasing these feelings of loving-kindness."

Compassion I

- "If your eyes were open before, please keep them closed now, and if your eyes were closed before, please open them now."

- "Once more, offering yourself a soothing or supportive gesture as you look at your partner or look within, letting yourself reflect on a measure of sorrow that lies within this person right now. The burdens that are carried, the suffering and pain accumulated over a lifetime, as in every human life." (*Pause*)

- "There are disappointments, failures, loneliness, loss, and hurts—things that may have seemed impossible to bear at the time, yet somehow were borne. Letting yourself open to this pain, turning toward it, acknowledging it. (*Pause*) You can't fix the pain or make it go away, but you can be with it, with a spirit of courage, and an open heart." (*Pause*)

- "Now, imagining your partner as a child (or, if your eyes are closed, imagining yourself as a child if that feels okay). Recognizing that there is still a child that lives within this person, sometimes frightened, hurt, confused, struggling." (*Pause*)

- "Letting yourself feel how you might naturally want to reach out, to soothe, to reassure. How much you may want that child to know that it's okay to lean on you for support, for understanding, for love and acceptance." (*Pause*)

- "If you are seeing this human vulnerability, and a wish is arising to help, to protect, and comfort this person in the midst of this suffering, know that what you are experiencing is *compassion*. (*Pause*) And if you were directing the words toward yourself, that would be *self-compassion*. And this capacity is there in you, always."

- "Both partners, please open your eyes now and take a moment to silently acknowledge your partner with your eyes. (*Pause for about 5 seconds*) Then both partners, please close your eyes, taking a few moments to notice how you're feeling, letting yourself feel what you are feeling and be who you are. Again, some people will be experiencing compassion; others will not. Can we give space for whatever arises?"

Compassion II

- "If your eyes were open before, please keep them closed now, and if your eyes were closed before, please open them now. If you like, offer yourself gentle, soothing touch."

- "Letting yourself become aware of a measure of sorrow that lies within this person right now—your partner if your eyes are open, yourself if your eyes are closed. The burdens that are carried, the suffering and pain accumulated over a lifetime, as in every human life." (*Pause*)

- "There are disappointments, failures, loneliness, loss, and hurts. Things that may have seemed impossible to bear at the time, yet somehow were borne. Letting yourself open to this pain, turning toward it, acknowledging it. (*Pause*) You can't fix the pain or make it go away, but you can be with it, with a spirit of courage, and an open heart."

- "Now, imagining your partner as a child (or, if your eyes are closed, imagining yourself as a child if that feels right). (*Pause*) Recognizing that there is still a child that lives within this person, sometimes frightened, hurt, confused, struggling." (*Pause*)

- "Letting yourself feel how you might naturally want to reach out, to soothe, to reassure. (*Pause*) How much you might want that child to know that it's okay to lean on you for support, for understanding, for love and acceptance." (*Pause*)

- "If you are seeing this human vulnerability, and a wish is arising to help, to protect, and comfort this person in the midst of this suffering, know that what you are experiencing is *compassion*. (*Pause*) And if you were directing the words toward yourself, that would be *self-compassion*. And this capacity is there in you, always."

- "Both partners, please open your eyes now and take a moment to silently acknowledge your partner with a soft gaze. (*Pause for about 5 seconds*) Then both partners, please close your eyes, taking a few moments to notice how you're feeling, letting yourself feel what you are feeling and be who you are." (*Pause*)

Discussion

Teachers can now invite participants to open their eyes slowly, thank their partners for what they have just shared, and take 10 minutes to discuss the experience with their partners. This is usually an animated conversation, so teachers may need to signal 2 minutes before the final bell so that participants can gracefully end their discussion.

Inquiry

The inquiry period could easily go beyond 10 minutes, but that isn't necessary because group members will have already processed their experience together in pairs. Before conducting this inquiry, teachers may wish to validate the courage it took to do this exercise and the natural anxiety that arises when people are thrown together in such an intimate way. Inquiry is helpful to remind participants of the purpose of the exercise. Teachers can explicitly ask:

- "Did loving-kindness feel different from compassion? If so, how? Was one easier to practice than the other?"
- "Was it easier to feel goodwill toward others or yourself?"
- "What were the obstacles you faced when giving or receiving loving-kindness or compassion?"

The inquiry period is also a good opportunity to remind students of the meaning of backdraft (explained in Session 2) when it arises in their direct experience. An example follows.

MEI: I've done an exercise like this before, with open eyes the whole time, and it was pretty intense. I was glad that we closed our eyes this time.

TEACHER: What did you prefer about keeping your eyes closed?

MEI: I could focus a little more on my own experience. For instance, at first I didn't think I could feel compassion for someone I don't know, but then I noticed that even though I don't know anything about my partner, I could connect with her losses, failures, and the like.

TEACHER: Sounds like you had an experience of common humanity?

MEI: Yeah, it was pretty cool.

TEACHER: I'm curious—did you find it easier to feel loving-kindness toward your partner, or compassion?

MEI: Definitely compassion. It felt deeper, like there was more traction. It was almost like my heart was ready to break because there was so much tenderness.

TEACHER: You could feel it in your body?

MEI: Yeah . . . right here (*pointing to her chest*). Like bursting.

TEACHER: May I ask whether the feeling of compassion was just as strong when you were directing the words toward yourself, when your eyes were closed?

MEI: Hmmm . . . let me think. (*Pause*) Not so much, to be honest. I got a bit lost in the feelings, especially a friend who died.

TEACHER: Oh, I'm sorry to hear that. Is that feeling still lingering around for you?

MEI: Only a little. I'm holding it tenderly. (*Shows by putting a hand over her heart.*)

TEACHER: Thank you for that. That feeling may be backdraft, as we discussed last session, and it seems like you are already meeting it with compassion. (*Pause*) And thanks for sharing so much about your experience of the exercise. This exercise is pretty rich, isn't it?

MEI: Sure is! I'm wondering if we can get a copy of this exercise to use with other people.

TEACHER: Well, we don't generally give out the instructions for this exercise because it can be a bit activating for people, and it's good to get some hands-on training in how to lead it. Does that make sense?

MEI: Yeah, that makes sense, thanks.

Mei had already been practicing mindfulness for a few years, so she and the teacher could quickly move through different aspects of the exercise—including differences in the felt sense of loving-kindness and compassion, and differences between directing attention toward ourselves and others. The challenging aspects of the exercise for some participants are being watched by another person, imagining themselves as children in pain, trying to imagine the inner life of someone they hardly know, and brief periods of eye contact. For most participants, however, the sense of vulnerability evoked by the exercise is matched by a sense of connection and mutual regard.

Teachers can bring closure to this exercise by reading a poem, such as the last two stanzas of Naomi Shihab Nye's (1995) poem "Kindness," in which she beautifully describes the intimate relationship of kindness and sorrow.

Break
(15 minutes)

Students usually need to stretch their legs and refresh themselves after Awakening Our Hearts. Some participants continue their discussion of the exercise into the break, but most prefer to walk around and chat informally. The break is also an opportunity for those students who sat out Awakening Our Hearts to reconnect with the group.

Soft Landing
(2 minutes)

The participants' repertoire of informal mindfulness and self-compassion practices continues to expand with each session, and teachers can improvise on those practices to create a soft landing. An anchoring practice is generally welcome after the preceding exercise, such as inviting participants to feel the rhythm of their breathing, followed by opening to any emotional echoes from Awakening Our Hearts, and then making room for all persons to *be* just as they are. Students can be reminded again to practice a soft landing during class when they feel the need, especially if they feel emotionally stuck or overwhelmed.

Loving-Kindness Meditation
(2 minutes)

The purposes of this short topic are to generate interest in the use of words or phrases as objects of meditation, and to describe the principles underlying LKM.

Using language in meditation can feel awkward for some practitioners, especially since the meaning of words depends heavily on the experience of each individual. LKM is also a complex meditation with a variety of different elements. Novice practitioners tend to be overly ambitious when they practice LKM, and they should keep it simple, focusing more at first on the sense of warmth than on mastering the technical details. Furthermore, one size does not fit all. Research even suggests that genes may have an impact on whether LKM will be a positive experience for a particular person (Isgett, Algoe, Boulton, Way, & Fredrickson, 2016).

LKM trains the mind to be more loving and compassionate by harnessing the power of words. To illustrate the power of words, teachers can ask, "Have any of you broken a bone in your lives? (*Pause*) Has it healed?" Then come these questions: "Has anyone been wounded by words? Is there anyone who is still hurting from words that may have been uttered many years ago?"

LKM harnesses the power of not only (1) *language*, but also (2) *imagery*, (3) *concentration*, (4) *connection*, and (5) *caring*. The concentration aspect (focused attention) is inherently calming, but LKM also calms through qualities of affiliation, including kind vocalizations, comforting images, a sense of being connected, and an attitude of caring.

As mentioned earlier, LKM is goodwill training; it cultivates good *intentions*. Intentions are the subtlest aspects of human psychology, and the ones from which other components—such as thoughts, emotions, and behaviors—emerge. Intentions drive our internal dialogue. In Session 4, the practice of good intentions (LKM) is expanded into a broader, internal compassionate conversation.

 ## Loving-Kindness for a Loved One
(20 minutes)

Traditionally, LKM starts with kindness toward oneself. The idea is that all living beings are trying to promote their own welfare, and if we recognize that, we will be kinder toward others. The problem is that in modern times, how we feel toward ourselves is no longer a reliable standard for how to treat others. Therefore, we begin LKM with how we feel toward a loved one and then sneak ourselves into the picture.

Instructions

- "Allow yourself to settle into a comfortable position, either sitting or lying down. If you like, putting a hand over your heart (or another location on your body that is comforting) as a reminder to bring not only awareness, but loving awareness, to your experience and to yourself."

A Living Being Who Makes You Smile

- "Now bring to mind a person or other living being who naturally makes you smile. Someone with whom you have an easy, uncomplicated relationship. This could be a child, your grandmother, your cat or dog—whoever naturally brings happiness to your heart. If many people or other living beings arise, just choose one."
- "Letting yourself feel what it's like to be in that being's presence. Allowing yourself to enjoy the good company. Create a vivid image of this being in your mind's eye." (*Pause*)

"May You . . ."

- "Now, recognize how this being wishes to be happy and free from suffering, and wishes to be loved, just like you and every other living being. Repeating softly and gently, feeling the importance of your words:
  - " 'May you be happy.'
  - 'May you be peaceful.'
  - 'May you be healthy.'
  - 'May you live with ease.' "
  (*Repeat twice, slowly, and then pause.*)
- "You can also use your own words to capture your deepest wishes for your loved one, or continue to repeat these phrases." (*Pause*)
- "When you notice that your mind has wandered, returning to the words and the image of the loved one you have in mind. Savoring any warm feelings that may arise. Taking your time."

"May You and I (We) . . ."

- "Now, adding *yourself* to your circle of good will. Creating an image of yourself in the presence of your loved one, visualizing you both together:
  - " 'May you and I—may *we*—be happy.'
  - 'May we be peaceful.'
  - 'May we be healthy.'
  - 'May we live with ease.' "
  (*Repeat twice, slowly, and then pause.*)
- "Now, letting go of the image of the other, perhaps thanking your loved one before moving on, and then letting the full focus of your attention rest directly on yourself."

"May I . . ."

- "Putting your hand over your heart, or elsewhere, and feeling the warmth and gentle pressure of your hand. Visualizing your whole body in your mind's eye, noticing any stress or uneasiness that may be lingering within you, and offering yourself the phrases:
  - 'May I be happy.'
  - 'May I be peaceful.'
  - 'May I be healthy.'
  - 'May I live with ease.' "

  (Repeat twice, slowly, and then pause.)
- "Finally, taking a few breaths and just resting quietly in your own body, accepting whatever your experience is, exactly as it is."
- *(Gently ring a bell.)*

Settling and Reflection

As usual, teachers should give some time for participants to let go of the practice and allow their awareness to linger in their bodies before reflecting on what they just experienced. Some people need more time than others to make the transition from inner contemplation to speaking in a group.

Inquiry

Inquiry can begin with general questions, such as "What did you notice?" or "What came up for you?" Or it can begin with a more specific question, such as "Did anyone find it easier to practice loving-kindness toward a loved one than yourself, or toward *both* yourself and a loved one?" or "Was there anything about this meditation that you found especially challenging?" Here is a sample inquiry.

> CAMILLE: It was kind of hard for me to find someone who makes me smile all the time. I started to realize how complicated all my relationships are! *(Laughs)*
>
> TEACHER: Did you eventually settle on one?
>
> CAMILLE: Not really. But I chose my teenage daughter because she's going through a tough time at college.
>
> TEACHER: Okay, so you took on a challenge in this meditation. It's true that most of our relationships with people have some ambivalence in them. That's why we include dogs and cats in the instructions. But how did it go from there?
>
> CAMILLE: Well, I think I spoke like a strict mother when I just focused

on her, but when it was her and me, it changed. By including myself in the mix—giving myself some attention, too—I could see how we've *both* been suffering in our relationship, and that we're both just trying to be happy.

TEACHER: That seems like an important insight. And what happened next?

CAMILLE: I followed along with the instructions, but I didn't like just being with myself, so I went back to my daughter and me.

TEACHER: What was wrong with just being with yourself?

CAMILLE: It felt so alone. I think I wanted to continue with the feeling of being connected with my daughter.

TEACHER: It sounds like that's where you needed to be. Can you let that be so?

CAMILLE: Happy to!

TEACHER: Please do. This is self-compassion training, and you're giving yourself what you need right now. Anyhow, the *recipient* of our loving-kindness is less important than our capacity to generate the *energy* of loving-kindness. You seem to have done that very effectively, even though you started out with a tough character—a teenage daughter!

CAMILLE: Thanks! (*Smiling*)

In this inquiry, Camille explored the nuances of loving-kindness for herself and others, and took the counsel of her own needs rather than dutifully following all the instructions. The teacher was able to point out to Camille and the rest of the class that the meditation is easier when it starts with a less ambivalent relationship. The teacher then validated a few of Camille's resources, such as the insight that we all wish to be happy, and her capacity to evoke compassion and stay with it despite instructions that would have pulled her elsewhere. In Camille's particular case, she needed a "we" rather than a "you" to activate the attitude of loving-kindness and compassion for herself.

For many participants, Loving-Kindness for a Loved One reveals the limitations of standard loving-kindness phrases and creates a wish among group members for personalized phrases, which they have a chance to discover later in the session. Nonetheless, LKM requires patience, and students should not feel that the practice is not working if they don't feel warm and fuzzy while practicing. There is a touching Hasidic tale that illustrates how LKM works:

A disciple asks the rebbe, "Why does Torah tell us to 'place these words upon your hearts'? Why does it not tell us to place these holy words in our hearts?" The rebbe answers, "It is because as we are, our hearts are closed, and we cannot place the holy words in our hearts. So we place them on top of our hearts. And there they stay until, one day, the heart breaks and the words fall in." (Moyers & Ketcham, 2006, p. 233)

 ## Compassionate Movement (Optional)
(5 minutes)

This practice can be offered to students any time they need a stretch break and are open to being guided again. Compassionate Movement asks and answers the question "What do I need . . . *physically?*" The main idea is to compassionately move the body *from the inside out,* rather than in prescribed ways. When done slowly and gently, the practice provides the yin of physical comfort and soothing to our bodies. However, teachers can mention that for students who need a bit more yang energy in the moment, they can move in a more energetic and vigorous manner, such as jumping, shaking, and so forth.

Instructions

Anchoring

- "Please stand up and feel the soles of your feet on the floor."
- "Then rock forward and backward a little, and side to side. Making little circles with your knees, feeling the changes of sensation in the soles of your feet. Anchoring your awareness in your feet."

Opening

- "Now opening your field of awareness and scanning your whole body for other sensations, noticing any areas of ease as well as areas of tension."

Responding Compassionately

- "Now focus for a moment on a place of *discomfort.* Gradually begin moving your body in a way that feels really good to you—giving yourself compassion. For example, letting yourself gently twist your shoulders, roll your head, turn at the waist, drop into a forward bend . . . whatever feels just right for you right now. (*Pause*) Giving your body the movement it needs."
- "Finally, coming to stillness, standing again and feeling your body, noting any changes since we began to move in this way."

Practicing with Phrases
(10 minutes)

This topic prepares students for the next practice of discovering personalized phrases that can be used in LKM. It describes what types of phrases are most useful in daily meditation, how to find them, and how to work with them in meditation. As usual, teachers can sort through the following points and develop a concise talk that reflects the interests of the teachers and the needs of the group.

The Language of Phrases

Finding loving-kindness phrases is like writing poetry—using words to express something that is beyond words. Good loving-kindness phrases have the power to evoke an attitude of loving-kindness and compassion in the practitioner, in the same way that good poetry can transmit a frame of mind to the listener with few words.

Loving-kindness phrases can be an object of attention in meditation, much as breathing is used in breath meditation. To tap into the power of concentration, however, it is helpful to find a few basic phrases that can be used over and over, perhaps for months or years. Other loving-kindness phrases can be created on the spot for informal practice during daily life.

Many MSC participants are already using traditional loving-kindness phrases in meditation that were given to them by their teachers, similar to the phrases used in Loving-Kindness for a Loved One. There is no need for anyone to switch to different phrases, but there is also no need to stick to phrases that do not feel resonant or authentic to the practitioner.

Ideally, phrases should be *simple, clear, authentic,* and *kind*. There should be no argument in the minds of practitioners when they are used. Instead, good phrases evoke a sense of gratitude when they are heard: "Oh, thank you! Thank you!" Good phrases allow the heart and mind to rest, as if practitioners have finally heard something that they have been waiting a very long time to hear. The phrases can be either yin (comforting, soothing, or validating) or yang (protecting, nourishing, or encouraging)—whatever we need to hear.

It is important to remember that loving-kindness phrases are wishes, not lofty positive affirmations (e.g., "I'm becoming stronger every day"). Research has shown that positive affirmations tend to make people with high self-esteem feel happier and people with low self-esteem feel worse (Wood, Perunovic, & Lee, 2009). If the contrast between the affirmation and living reality is too stark, practitioners will become disappointed. Loving-kindness phrases should be impossible to argue with; a *wish* can be true, no matter what our condition may be.

It also isn't necessary to use "May I . . ." in loving-kindness phrases if it feels awkward or too much like begging. The use of "May I . . ." is intended simply to incline the heart and mind in a positive direction—to cultivate goodwill. Any phrases can be used, as long as the inclination of heart is being practiced when they are repeated. "May I . . ." actually means "That it would be so . . ." or "If all the conditions would allow it to be so, then . . ." This type of phrasing is called the *subjunctive mood* in some languages. Loving-kindness phrases are like secular blessings or secular prayer.

We can address ourselves in different ways during LKM. Depending on what feels right, participants can say, "May *I* . . . ," "May *you* . . . ,"; use a proper name; or even use a term of endearment, such as "Sweetheart" or "Honey." For example, using "you" rather than "I" is more likely to motivate someone into action if that's the purpose of practice (Dolcos & Albarracin, 2014; Kross et al., 2014).

Another question is likely to arise: "Who is talking to whom?" In MSC, the person offering goodwill can be either a compassionate part of the individual self or a more universal Self that is inherently wise and compassionate. The *recipient* of loving-kindness and compassion is usually a general sense of oneself as a person, associated with the body, but it could also be a *part* of oneself, such as a childhood aspect or a wounded part.

The phrases should be kept general rather than specific. For example, it is better to say, "May I be healthy," than "May I be free from my diabetes." We cannot control the outcome of many situations in our lives, no matter how much we wish we could. The idea is to stick to the wishing side of the phrases rather than to get fixed on an outcome. Some beginning practitioners simply say, "May I," "May I," "May I" over and over again, without any object at all, to get a feeling for inclining the heart rather than going down the rabbit hole of expecting a specific outcome. Once the wishing attitude is deeply ingrained, it's even fine to use a single word such as "peace" or "love" rather than a phrase.

Finally, the tone in which the phrases are spoken matters a great deal. It's like talking to an infant or a beloved pet who responds to *how* we speak, not to *what* we say. We also feel the tone of our own internal dialogue, for better or worse. The phrases should be said slowly and warmly. There's no rush. The number of times we say a phrase matters less than the attitude that prevails during meditation.

"What Do I Need?"

One way to find authentic and meaningful phrases is to focus on the core question of self-compassion: "What do I need?" There is a difference between needs and wants. *Wants* are personal and arise from the neck up ("I want a better job," "I want to lose 10 pounds," "I want a new car").

Needs are universal and are discovered from the neck down. Wants are potentially unlimited and easily proliferate, whereas needs are fewer and easier to satisfy.

Examples of universal human needs are the need to be accepted, validated, seen, heard, protected, loved, known, cherished, connected, and respected. These are also *relational* needs. (A compelling way to discover a relational needs is to ask, "What do I need to hear from others?") Sometimes participants mention *material* needs such as food, clothing, and shelter, or *personal* needs such as wisdom, growth, and health, but mostly participants identify relational needs. If participants are having trouble identifying needs, teachers can say:

> "You may have difficulty discovering a wish for yourself because your need depends on others, such as the need for approval or the need for success. If that is the case, please ask yourself, 'How would that make me feel if I received all the approval in the world, or all the success in the world?' Perhaps then you could relax, you could smile, you would feel valued, or you would finally feel good about yourself? If so, you can wish *that* for yourself, such as 'May I live with ease,' 'May my heart smile,' 'May I know my own value,' 'May I be enough just as I am.' A good loving-kindness phrase allows the heart to finally rest."

The informal practice that follows, Finding Loving-Kindness Phrases, is designed to help participants discover what they *truly need* and what they need to *hear* from others. The question "What do I need to hear from others?" can activate old childhood longings, especially among participants who suffered childhood neglect or trauma, or remind participants about what they are missing in their present lives. Teachers should advise students about safety, especially the option not to do the practice if a student needs to close.

 ## Finding Loving-Kindness Phrases
(30 minutes)

The following instructions should be delivered slowly enough for students to reflect on the questions and allow answers to arise within.

Instructions

- "This is a pen-and-paper exercise. We will close our eyes and do some reflection, then open our eyes and write, and then close and open and close our eyes again."
- "Please wait until *after* the exercise if you have any questions."

- "The exercise is designed to help you discover loving-kindness and compassion phrases that are deeply meaningful to you. If you already have phrases and wish to continue using them, you can try this exercise as an experiment but please don't feel you need to find new phrases."
- "To start, please close your eyes, place a hand over your heart or elsewhere, and feel your body gently breathe."

"What Do I Need?"

- "Please take a moment and allow your heart to gently open—to become receptive –like a flower opens in the warm sun." (*Pause*)
- "Then ask yourself this question, allowing the answer to arise naturally within you:
  - 'What do I need?' (*Pause*) 'What do I *truly* need?' " (*Pause*)
  - "If this need has not been fulfilled in a given day, your day does not feel complete."
  - (*Pause*) "Letting the answer be a universal human need, such as the need to be connected, kind, healthy peaceful, or free." (*Pause*)
- "When you are ready, please open your eyes and write down what arose for you." (*Pause*)
- "The words you discovered can be used in meditation just as they are, or you can rewrite them as wishes for yourself, such as these:
  - " 'May I be kind to myself.'
  - 'May I *begin* to be kind to myself.'
  - 'May I know that I belong.'
  - 'May I connect with my basic goodness.'
  - 'May I know my own value.'
  - 'May I be free from fear.'
  - 'May I rest in love.' "

(*Longer pause*)

"What Do I Need to *Hear*?"

- "Now, please close your eyes again and consider a second question. This question may take you a little deeper, so feel free to only go as deep as you feel comfortable going. The question is this:
  - " 'What do I need to hear from others?' (*Pause*) 'What words do I need to hear because, as a person, I really need to hear words like this?' " (*Pause*)
  - "Some examples are: 'I love you,' 'I'm here for you,' 'I believe in you,' 'You're a good person.' "

- ○ "Opening the door of your heart and waiting for words to come." (*Pause*)
- ○ "If words are not coming for you yet, ask yourself: 'If I could, what words would I like to have whispered into my ear every day for the rest of my life—words that might make me say, "Oh, thank you, thank you!" every time I hear them?' " (*Pause*)
- ○ "Allowing yourself to be vulnerable and open to this possibility, with courage. Listening." (*Pause*)

- • "Now gently opening your eyes again and writing down what you heard. (*Pause*) If you heard a lot of words, seeing if you can make the words into a short phrase—a message to yourself." (*Pause*)

- • "The words you wrote down can be used in loving-kindness meditation just they are, or you can also rewrite them as wishes for yourself. Actually, words that we would like to hear from others again and again are words that we easily forget, or qualities we would like to realize in our own lives, or attitudes that we wish to implant firmly in our hearts. For example, needing to hear 'I love you' might mean that we wish to know we are truly lovable. That's why we need to hear it over and over again."

- • "What do you want to know for sure? If you like, you can reframe your words as wishes for yourself. For example:
  - ○ " 'I love you' can become the wish 'May I love myself just as I am,' or 'May I know that I am loved.' "
  - ○ " 'I'm here for you' can become the wish 'May I know that I belong.' "
  - ○ " 'You're a good person' can become the wish 'May I know my own goodness.' "

  (*Longer pause*)

- • "Now, please take a moment to review what you have written, and settle on one to three words or phrases you would like to use in meditation. (*Pause*) These words or phrases are gifts you will give to yourself. Please take a moment to memorize your words."

Practicing with Phrases

- • "Finally, let's close our eyes for a last time. We will repeat the words over and over to ourselves. See if you can let the process be as easy as possible, much like slipping into a warm bath. Nothing to accomplish. Just letting the words go where they need to go, and letting them do all the work."

- • "Beginning by saying your words or phrases, slowly and gently, perhaps *whispering* them into your own ear as if into the ear of a loved one." (*Pause for 3–4 minutes.*)

- • "Nothing to do, nowhere to go. Just surrounding yourself with kind words, letting them wash over you and through you—words that you need to hear."

- "And whenever your mind wanders, you can refresh your aim by offering yourself soothing touch or by just feeling the sensations in your body. And then offering yourself the phrases again."

- "And now, gently *releasing* the phrases and allowing yourself to rest in the experience, letting this practice be just what it was and letting yourself be just as you are." (*Pause*)

- "Please consider this exercise to be only the beginning of a search for phrases that are just right for you. Finding loving-kindness phrases is a soulful journey, a poetic journey. You will find yourself returning to this process ('What do I need?', 'What do I need to hear?') as you go forward."

- "And gently open your eyes."

Inquiry

Participants should be invited to share with the group the *process* of finding phrases, rather than their actual phrases, since the phrases are likely to reflect vulnerable needs that participants would rather keep to themselves. Here is a typical exchange after this practice.

> GINNY: I found some good phrases, I think, but I also got hung up in this practice. I was able to connect with what I *need*, but when I asked what I need to *hear from others*, I went straight back into my childhood and became flooded with feelings I don't like to feel.
>
> TEACHER: Are you still feeling those feelings, Ginny?
>
> GINNY: Yes.
>
> TEACHER: Would you be willing to *name* the emotion?
>
> GINNY: It's loneliness. Feelings of loneliness are just beneath the surface all the time for me.
>
> TEACHER: So connecting with what you need to hear from others brought up loneliness. That can happen in this exercise. That's backdraft. I especially appreciate that you have the courage to name it, since you're surely not the only person in the room who touched something like that.
>
> GINNY: Really? (*Looking around and seeing nodding heads*)
>
> TEACHER: Ginny, I'm wondering what you would say to a friend, heart to heart, who you discovered had also been living with loneliness for many years?

GINNY: (*Eyes misting*) I'd tell her, "I know, I understand."

TEACHER: And what do you think she would need to hear from you?

GINNY: Just that, really . . . knowing that she's not alone.

TEACHER: Would you be able to put that into a wish for her?

GINNY: Oh, I get it. Yes, I might say, "May you know that you are not alone."

TEACHER: Thank you, Ginny. And I also wish that for you . . . I think we *all* do.

GINNY: I think I can do this.

TEACHER: Yes, I believe so. But please don't try too hard . . . just say what feels right at the time, you know, not too much . . . what feels genuinely comforting to hear, okay?

GINNY: Okay. Got it. (*Smiling softly*)

In this case, Ginny was flooded with emotion when asked about her relational needs ("What do you need to hear from others?"), and she was unable to find a suitable phrase. The inquiry process brought Ginny back to the emotion that derailed her, and the teacher helped her find a loving-kindness phrase by connecting with how she might speak to a friend who felt the same way. Since Ginny seemed to be easily overwhelmed by past trauma, the teacher reminded her to go slowly and only use loving-kindness phrases that actually made her feel comforted and soothed. Toward that end, students can be advised to use qualifiers to titrate the intensity of an unmet need, such as "May I *begin* to . . ." or "May I *learn* to . . ."

Fortunately, most students have positive experiences while finding phrases and using them in meditation. Here's an example.

SIMON: Wow, that was deep! I've been using loving-kindness phrases for years, but didn't realize they could be so deep and moving.

TEACHER: I'm so glad you found phrases that touched you in a deep way. Could you describe what you felt?

SIMON: Well, the phrases spoke directly to me, in a personal way. It was like someone called my name and had all my attention. And each time I said the phrases, my whole body relaxed as if I were getting something I longed to receive for years—or hear what I longed to hear for years—and never knew what it was. It was physical, really, especially here in the center of my chest. I can still feel it.

TEACHER: I can feel it, too, as you speak, Simon. Thanks for letting us in, and for letting the words in.

In this inquiry, Simon simply wanted to share his surprise and wonderment, so the teacher allowed herself to resonate emotionally with Simon and thanked him for sharing. Inquiry can be quite short when there isn't a problem to address.

Home Practice
(5 minutes)

Participants should be reminded of the practices that were learned this session:

- Loving-Kindness for a Loved One
- Compassionate Movement (Optional)
- Finding Loving-Kindness Phrases

Teachers can invite participants to continue exploring what words or phrases are deeply meaningful to them. (This exercise is also downloadable from this book's companion website; see the box at the end of the table of contents.) The objective of Finding Loving-Kindness Phrases is for participants to settle eventually on a few phrases that can be used again and again in meditation. The same process can be used to discover what we may need at particular moments in our daily lives. For example, if we ask, "What do I need to have whispered into my ear *right now*?", new phrases may arise that can be applied on the spot as balm for a sore heart.

Students should be encouraged again at this point to provide weekly feedback and to bring it to each session. Again, the purpose of weekly feedback is not to embarrass those who don't practice 30 minutes per day, but to help participants reflect on the process of learning self-compassion and to communicate with the teachers. Teachers should also continue to send emails between sessions to remind and encourage students to practice, and to facilitate online sharing between students.

Closing
(3 minutes)

Teachers can close the session any way they like, perhaps with a moment of silence followed by ringing a bell, with another circle of one-word shares, or with a reading of one of these two poems by Irish poet John O'Donohue that reflect the power and universality of loving-kindness phrases: "Beannacht" (2011) and "For Belonging" (2008).

Chapter 13

Session 4

DISCOVERING YOUR COMPASSIONATE VOICE

Overview

Opening (Core) Meditation: Loving-Kindness for Ourselves

Session Theme: Discovering Your Compassionate Voice

Topic: Stages of Progress

Exercise: How Is MSC Going for Me?

Break

Soft Landing

Topic: Self-Criticism and Safety

Exercise: Motivating Ourselves with Compassion

Informal Practice: Compassionate Letter to Myself

Home Practice

Closing

Getting Started

- In this session, participants will:
  - Learn to practice loving-kindness in formal meditation.
  - Identify stages of progress on the path to self-compassion.
  - Begin motivating themselves with encouragement rather than criticism.
- These subjects are introduced now to:
  - Deepen the meditation practice of Loving-Kindness for Ourselves, using personalized phrases.
  - Review how participants are experiencing their progress in the MSC program, especially whether they are able to accept themselves more fully and where they are on the path to self-compassion.
  - Help participants cultivate a compassionate inner voice to motivate positive changes in their lives, based on the attitude of goodwill established in LKM.
- New practices taught this session:
  - Loving-Kindness for Ourselves
  - Compassionate Letter to Myself

Note to teachers: The home practice discussion is omitted in this session because a related exercise, How Is MSC Going for Me?, has been included.

Loving-Kindness for Ourselves
(30 minutes)

Loving-Kindness for Ourselves is the second core meditation of the MSC course. Participants have had a taste of this meditation at the end of Finding Loving-Kindness Phrases in Session 3, when they began offering their phrases to themselves. Some students may have already listened to recordings of Loving-Kindness for Ourselves during the previous week. This is the first chance to practice the full meditation as a group and engage in inquiry about it.

In this session, teachers should introduce the meditation by asking participants to review their phrases and decide in advance which ones they would like to use, so they do not use the following meditation for the purpose of finding new phases. New phrases may arise spontaneously, however, and that's fine when it happens. Additionally, since LKM can be rather complicated (compared to other meditations), teachers can invite students to let go of any unnecessary effort and expectations, and simply offer themselves the phrases in a relaxed manner without worrying whether they are doing it right—allowing the practice to be as easy as slipping into a warm bath.

Instructions

- "Please find a comfortable position, sitting or lying down. Letting your eyes close, fully or partially. Taking a few deep breaths to settle into your body and into the present moment."
- "Putting your hand over your heart, or wherever it is comforting and soothing, as a reminder to bring not only awareness, but *loving* awareness, to your experience and to yourself."
- "Now, feeling your breath move in your body wherever you notice it most easily. Feeling the gentle rhythm of your breathing (*pause*), and when your attention wanders, returning to the sensation of the gentle rhythm of breathing in your body."
- "Now, releasing the focus on your breathing—allowing the breath to slip into the background of your awareness—and beginning to offer yourself the words or phrases that are most meaningful to you. If you like, whispering them into your own ear." (*Long pause*)
- "Nothing to do, nowhere to go. Just bathing yourself with kind words, letting them wash over you and through you—words that you need to hear." (*Long pause*)
- "Or if it feels right, absorbing the words, letting them fill your being. Allowing the words to resonate in every cell of your body." (*Pause*)
- "And whenever you notice that your mind has wandered, you can refresh your aim by offering yourself soothing touch, or by just feeling the sensations in your body. Coming home to your own body. And then offering yourself the words. Coming home to kindness." (*Pause*)
- "Finally, releasing the phrases and resting quietly in your own body."
- "And then slowly opening your eyes."

Settling and Reflection

Students should be allowed 2–3 minutes to absorb what they have just experienced and to reflect on their experience of the meditation. Teachers can gently seed inquiry with questions like these: "What did you notice this time?", "Was any part of the meditation particularly important to you?", or "Was there anything challenging about the meditation?"

Inquiry

By Session 4, it becomes evident which participants are willing to speak up during inquiry and which participants prefer to listen. This is a good time to remind the group members that it is nice to hear from *everyone* because each sharing deepens the learning experience for the whole group. A sample inquiry after Loving-Kindness for Ourselves follows.

> GEOFF: I'm not sure about this meditation, to be honest. I like to keep meditation simple, and this one has a lot of moving parts. I used to do mantra meditation with a meaningless syllable, and now I do breath meditation, but the phrases just seem too long and awkward to me.

> TEACHER: This type of meditation isn't for everyone, that's for sure, and it sounds like you may have a good meditation practice already. I'm wondering, though, if we could back up a little. Can you tell me *when* the guided meditation began to feel awkward?

> GEOFF: I guess I didn't want to give up the breath and start in with the phrases.

> TEACHER: That makes sense. You actually don't need to give up the breath, but just let it move in the background of your awareness. But you especially didn't like *adding* phrases?

> GEOFF: That's right. I enjoyed the rhythm of my breathing and felt calm, and I didn't want to throw a wrench in the works.

> TEACHER: Of course, I get that. I'm wondering, though, whether the calmness of breath meditation ever disappears and you start having stressful thoughts or feelings?

> GEOFF: Yes, that can happen after a while.

> TEACHER: How do you think a few words of support and kindness would feel then?

> GEOFF: Probably not so bad.

> TEACHER: You have raised an important practice point for all of us, Geoff. It's really important to customize these practices for our own individual needs. Since you like breath meditation, you should stick with that and perhaps see if a few loving-kindness words might help you out when your mind goes to a dark corner. If not, why bother? Know what I mean?

> GEOFF: I do.

> TEACHER: Personally, I find that the phrases don't really land for me until my mind has settled after about 15–20 minutes of breath

meditation. Other people love the phrases from the start. We're all different.

GEOFF: I'm thinking that maybe I was just trying too hard, too.

TEACHER: Perhaps. We need to be relaxed with the phrases, saying them without any strings attached. They are like blessings.

GEOFF: I get it. Let's see.

TEACHER: Thanks, Geoff.

This inquiry could have taken several directions, and each direction would probably have been helpful. For example, the teacher could have focused on the particular phrases that Geoff was using that may not have suited him, or he could have resonated with Geoff's frustration and helped him bring compassion to his struggle, or he could have given Geoff permission to skip the use of phrases altogether. However, since Geoff spoke up, the teacher felt that Geoff still wanted to find some reason to try using phrases in meditation. He chose to connect with Geoff's frustration, using his own experience as a guide, and introduced to Geoff the idea that the *timing* of the phrases in meditation could be the reason the words seemed so cumbersome. The teacher was also thinking about the entire class when he discussed the importance of customizing one's practice and practicing LKM without expectations. It is fully acceptable for teachers to share bits of their own meditation experience, as long as it doesn't shift attention away from a student's experience or intrude on a student's reality.

 ## Discovering Your Compassionate Voice
(1 minute)

Teachers can orient participants to today's session, Discovering Your Compassionate Voice, by sharing the title of the session and a general outline, mentioning that we are now moving into the "muddy middle" of the course. The session begins with a review of the typical stages of progress in self-compassion training, followed by participants' reflections on their experience of MSC so far. Then teachers explore with participants how to motivate positive changes in their lives with kindness and understanding rather than criticism. The topic of compassionate motivation arrives after learning loving-kindness phrases because participants will use the good intentions generated in LKM to cultivate a compassionate inner dialogue. *Motivating* oneself to change also strengthens the yang-like, action element of self-compassion to balance the yin-like comforting and soothing practices already learned.

Stages of Progress
(15 minutes)

A review of the stages of progress in self-compassion training comes at this point in the course because many participants will have begun to doubt their capacity to be more self-compassionate. They are in the "disillusionment" phase that is actually a prelude to deeper practice (in the stages of progress adapted from Morgan, 1990). This topic—along with the group exercise that follows, How is MSC Going for Me?—helps participants feel less alone and overcome a sense of failure that could lead to abandoning their efforts.

The Stages of Progress topic should be presented in a lighthearted manner. After all, progress in self-compassion often means giving up the *idea* of progress. Teachers can open the discussion with questions like: "We are now in the 'muddy middle' of the program. Is there anyone who doubts their ability ever to become more self-compassionate?" At least one-third of the students will probably nod in agreement, whereupon teachers can reassure them, "This means you are making progress!"

Self-compassion training typically goes through three stages: (1) *striving,* (2) *disillusionment,* and (3) *radical acceptance.* If the group watched *The Fly* video in Session 2, teachers can refer to the video as an illustration of the three stages: Striving occurs when the martial artist is trying to kill the flies; disillusionment occurs when he breaks down in the futility of the struggle; and radical acceptance occurs when he opens his hand and a fly spreads its wings and flies away.

"Progress," for any of us, often entails dropping the goal of self-improvement. In its place is refinement of our *intention* to practice—learning to practice self-compassion for its own sake, rather than as an effort to fix ourselves or manipulate how we feel moment-to-moment. The refinement of intention that occurs as we progress toward radical acceptance is best expressed in the paradox mentioned earlier: When we struggle, we give ourselves kindness not to feel better, but *because* we feel bad.

Striving

We all start to practice self-compassion, or any self-improvement effort, with the intention to feel better. It is full of hope. Sometimes the practice bears fruit right away—for example, when we discover for the first time, "I can love myself!" This realization can be quite elevating, like the infatuation phase of a romantic relationship.

Disillusionment

Of course, as in any romantic relationship, infatuation is usually followed by disillusionment—we realize that our beloved is no longer the answer to all our problems and is, after all, a human being. In self-compassion practice, disillusionment corresponds to the discovery that "I am still the same person as before," with the same uncomfortable feelings and personal flaws. When this happens in MSC, students are likely to blame themselves or the program for failing to live up to their expectations. The problem usually lies in the intention behind the practices—the students' wish to change their personalities or how they feel, rather than accepting "what is" with an open heart. Self-compassion has been hijacked in the service of resistance. The fault is not in the *techniques,* but in the *intention* behind their use.

Consider the following example of using loving-kindness phrases to overcome insomnia. When we first learn loving-kindness and have a curious, beginner's mind, we may comfort ourselves with the phrases when we're lying sleepless in the middle of the night and easily drift off to sleep. Upon waking in the morning, we may be excited by this success and decide to use loving-kindness phrases the next night to fall asleep. Predictably, it doesn't work because the intention behind using the phrases has changed from self-comfort to a strategy for getting to sleep, and when it doesn't work, we only feel more upset. That's when we become disillusioned. Meditation teacher Bob Sharples (2003) describes these efforts to "fix" ourselves as the "subtle aggression of self-improvement"; as an antidote, he recommends that we "practice meditation as an act of love." Disillusionment is an important phase of self-compassion training because it lays bare our counterproductive striving.

Radical Acceptance

Radical acceptance is the last stage. As mentioned in Chapters 9 and 19, radical acceptance means fully embracing our *experience* and *ourselves* just as we are, from moment to moment. How do we progress toward radical acceptance? Mostly we do *less.* In radical acceptance, we are not throwing compassion at ourselves to make our pain go away; rather, we are accepting pain with a tender, soft heart. Here are some sayings that bring radical acceptance to practice:

- "The point of spiritual practice isn't to perfect yourself, but to perfect your love" (Kornfield, 2017).
- "We are not here to learn self-compassion—we are here to embrace our imperfections!"
- "I'm not okay, you're not okay . . . but that's okay!"

To repeat an earlier analogy, radical acceptance is like a parent comforting a child with the flu. The parent is not trying to drive out the flu with kindness; instead, the parent gives care and comfort as a spontaneous response to the child's suffering until the illness passes on its own. All human beings suffer in life. Can we offer *ourselves* the same kindness and affection as we might extend to a child with the flu? When we can, that's radical acceptance.

Here are some additional quotations that teachers can use to illustrate the meaning of radical acceptance:

- "We can still be crazy after all these years. We can still be angry after all these years. We can still be timid or jealous or full of feelings of unworthiness. The point is . . . not to try to throw ourselves away and become something better. It's about befriending who we are already" (Chödrön, 1991/2001, p. 4).
- "A person should not strive to eliminate his complexes but to get into accord with them" (Freud, quoted in Jones, 1955, p. 188).
- "The curious paradox of life is that when I accept myself just as I am, then I can change" (Rogers, 1961/1995, p. 17).
- "The goal of practice is to become a compassionate mess" (Nairn, 2009).

To be a compassionate mess means to be fully human—often struggling, uncertain, confused—with great compassion. This is the invitation of self-compassion.

The stages of progress do not always proceed in a linear, sequential manner. We inevitably return to striving and disillusionment when we meet formidable challenges, but the moment we *realize* we're in striving or disillusionment, with loving, spacious awareness, we return to radical acceptance. Progress is more like an upward spiral. Over years of practice, our periods of striving and disillusionment lessen, and our time in radical acceptance increases.

Teachers also go through the stages of progress on their way to becoming MSC teachers. One of the first lessons is that striving to make people more self-compassionate can be counterproductive. As teacher trainer Steve Hickman says, "People are invited in when you lean back, and people are invited out when you lean in." Teachers also go through the stages of progress *with* their students, and can be confused and uncertain about how the course is going, especially during the "muddy middle" period. At those times, it helps just to trust the curriculum and let it do the work.

How Is MSC Going for Me?
(35 minutes)

This exercise is an opportunity for participants to explore what stage of progress they may be currently in, to review how compassionately they are treating themselves in the course itself, and to see the common humanity in their struggles.

Instructions

- "Please take out a pen and paper."
- "Remembering that we cycle through the stages of progress, take a moment to reflect on when you might have experienced moments of (1) striving, (2) disillusionment, or (3) radical acceptance. Then please write them down."
- "Now please reflect on what stage you might be in *right now,* in the middle of your MSC course. If you find yourself unnecessarily *striving,* would it be possible to make a little more room for your struggle?"
- "Or if you are *disillusioned,* perhaps doubting that you could ever become more self-compassionate, can you hold your doubting heart in a tender way—perhaps offering yourself some words of comfort or encouragement?"
- "And if you are having a moment of *radical acceptance,* can you savor the experience, at least for now?"

Small-Group Discussion

Teachers now ask participants to form groups of three to discuss how the MSC course is going. The participants should take up to 5 minutes each to share whatever they feel comfortable sharing (the intervals can be signaled by a teacher ringing a bell). The task of the listeners is to pay attention without giving advice or trying to fix a problem. It helps to purposely adopt a posture that is comfortable, open, and compassionate. This discussion is an opportunity for participants to experience common humanity in the midst of struggle and human imperfection.

Inquiry

After this exercise, inquiry tends to address participants' lingering concerns about their capacity to learn self-compassion.

> BERNICE: The talk you gave on stages of progress was really helpful. I was definitely in disillusionment.
>
> TEACHER: And where are you now?
>
> BERNICE: Still disillusionment, but maybe coming out of it (*chuckling to herself*). It was helpful to know I wasn't alone when we talked together in small groups.

TEACHER: I'm glad to hear that, Bernice. Would you be willing to describe the disillusionment—perhaps what worries or frustrates you?

BERNICE: Well, I don't want to just *accept* how I am and how I feel! I was referred to this group by the therapist I'm seeing for depression because she thinks I'm too hard on myself. It depresses me to think I need to just accept how I feel.

TEACHER: So the idea of acceptance means to you that nothing will ever change?

BERNICE: Isn't that kind of what you were saying?

TEACHER: You bring up an important point, Bernice. Acceptance means opening to *this moment*—how we feel and who we are—and when we do that, we actually create new possibilities.

BERNICE: But I don't want to feel like this even for one moment! Sometimes I feel so bad inside that it's almost unbearable.

TEACHER: Do you feel like that right now?

BERNICE: No, not after speaking with the others, but it happens a lot.

TEACHER: I'm thinking, Bernice, that you are actually better at self-compassion than you think. You were relieved after hearing the talk on not trying too hard to be self-compassionate, which means something connected inside you, and then you felt the relief of common humanity with others in the small group. I also appreciate that you don't want to feel *too much* sadness. That's *wise* self-compassion.

BERNICE: You think so?

TEACHER: You're the best the judge of that, but I sense an increasing openness and tenderness toward yourself. Can we wait and see how the rest of the course unfolds for you?

BERNICE: I guess so. I'm pretty good at being a mess, maybe I can learn to be a compassionate one. (*Chuckling again*)

This inquiry could also have taken a few different directions. The teacher chose to stick with Bernice's disillusionment because that was the theme of the exercise. In the process, it quickly emerged that Bernice was cautious about opening to pain because she had a history of depression. Opening to pain is a key part of MSC, but it only becomes workable when resources are recognized and reinforced. In this case, the teacher named a few of Bernice's resources and expressed confidence in her ability to cultivate self-compassion because she was obviously engaged and learning in the group. Perhaps the only missing ingredient for Bernice was *patience,* and the teacher gently alluded to this at the end of the inquiry.

Break
(15 minutes)

Some members will continue their small-group discussions into the break. Connections between group members have been developing for 3 weeks now, so break periods tend to become increasingly relaxed and enjoyable. It is always good to have refreshments available, especially at evening programs.

Soft Landing
(2 minutes)

Teachers can guide the soft landing, or they may invite participants to practice a soft landing on their own for 2 minutes. Shifting responsibility for the soft landing to the students serves as a reminder of the practices and practice components they have learned so far:

- Inner smile
- Soothing Touch
- Kind words—"Of course you feel that way"
- Common humanity—"Just like me"
- Finding Loving-Kindness Phrases
- Rhythm of the breath
- Soles of the Feet
- Sounds in the environment
- Here-and-Now Stone (Optional)
- Compassionate Movement

When a group seems restless, a physical activity such as Soles of the Feet or Compassionate Movement might be an excellent choice for a soft landing.

Self-Criticism and Safety
(10 minutes)

This topic is designed to introduce the possibility that self-criticism serves a purpose in our lives, especially to ensure emotional safety. We have just discussed the importance of accepting all aspects of ourselves, but there is one part of ourselves that we typically don't want to accept—the inner critic. We tend to see self-criticism as a source of pain and would like to get rid of it. The following points can be used to construct a short talk on the topic of self-criticism.

Since most human endeavors are an effort to increase our sense of well-being, it makes sense to assume that self-criticism has a similar purpose. This topic can be opened with the question "What function does self-criticism serve? Is there any value in self-criticism?" Typical replies are:

- "Self-criticism motivates us to improve."
- "It helps us behave better and avoid further criticism."
- "It gives the illusion of control ('If I were better, I could avoid problems')."
- "It lowers our expectations so we don't disappoint ourselves."
- "It makes others feel better, so they like us more."

Self-criticism is usually an attempt to protect ourselves from perceived danger—to keep us safe—even if the approach appears less than productive.

In this discussion, the focus is on harsh self-criticism rather than critical discernment. It is the *tone* of the critical voice that makes all the difference. Harshness has a threatening, angry quality, whereas discernment is thoughtful and non-judgmental.

For some MSC participants, self-criticism may serve *no* useful purpose. They may have internalized self-criticism as children from abusive or neglectful caregivers ("It's all your fault," "You're a loser," or "Nobody loves you"), when it was a matter of safety and survival for them to internalize those messages. For the participants as adults, however, these messages may only cause anguish and have no safety value. It is important for students to know if their inner criticism fits into this category because if it does, intense and inexplicable fear may arise when they start being kind to themselves. Sometimes it's like breaking an invisible contract with their abusive caregivers when these students start being kind to themselves—when they begin to consider themselves *worthy* of kindness.

Conversely, some lucky students do not have a harsh inner critic. They may have occasional self-doubts, but, generally speaking, they feel internally secure. Still others cannot *recognize* a critical voice, but they feel physically or emotionally exhausted when things go wrong in their lives, reflecting discouragement or unconscious self-criticism that can be addressed with self-compassion. Teachers should remain open to all possibilities and encourage an attitude of curiosity and acceptance of whatever students uncover in the following exercise.

Motivating Ourselves with Compassion
(45 minutes)

This exercise explores the difference between motivating behavioral change with self-criticism versus self-compassion. Students will have a chance to meet the critical aspect of themselves and explore the hidden motivation behind the harsh attitude, but the main focus of the exercise is to make room for a new, compassionate voice. This is often a yang voice that motivates change from a place of encouragement and loving-kindness. Elements of this exercise were inspired by internal family systems therapy, developed by Richard Schwartz (1995). For professionals who wish to explore the clinical dimensions of working compassionately with parts, see Cornell (2013), Schwartz (1995, 2013), Sweezy and Ziskind (2013), and Chapter 20 of this book.

Motivating Ourselves with Compassion is one of the more emotionally challenging exercises in the program (i.e., it can trigger backdraft). Teachers should briefly describe the exercise and ask students to reflect whether they are emotionally open or closed, and then to choose whether they want to participate or not. Students should be advised that if self-criticism is a harsh, internalized voice of someone who traumatized them in the past, they should consider skipping this exercise. Also, anyone who starts the exercise should feel free to discontinue it if too much stress arises. The message is "Take care of yourself as we go along, giving yourself whatever you need."

The instructions for this exercise have been carefully scripted to be safe and effective for the widest range of people. The aim is also for students to have an *embodied* experience of their self-compassionate voice (Falconer et al., 2014). Teachers usually need to follow the text reasonably closely, but teachers are also encouraged to speak in an authentic voice that corresponds to the needs of the group (i.e., adjusting the tone and tempo to modulate the degree of affect experienced by the participants).

Instructions

- "Please take out a sheet of paper."
- "Think about a *behavior* that you would like to change—something you often beat yourself up about. Please choose a behavior that is actually causing problems in your life, but select a behavior that is mildly to moderately problematic, not one that is extremely harmful. And choose a behavior that is potentially changeable. (Don't choose a permanent characteristic like 'My feet are too big.') Here are some examples of behaviors that you might be criticizing yourself for and that are causing problems in your life:
  - 'I eat too much junk food.'
  - 'I don't exercise enough.'
  - 'I procrastinate.'
  - 'I'm not assertive enough.'
  - 'I become impatient too easily.' "

- "Please write down the behavior that you would like to change, but the way you usually try to change is through harsh self-criticism. Also, write down the *problems* the behavior is causing." (*Long pause*)

Finding Your Self-Critical Voice

- "Now please write down *how* you typically react to yourself when you find yourself doing this behavior. How does your inner critic express itself? Are there unkind *words* that are used? (*Pause*) Or is the *tone* of voice harsh? Sometimes it's all in the tone of voice."
- "Sometimes there are no words at all, but rather a sense of coldness or disappointment when you find yourself behaving in this way. If so, does a physical posture or image come to mind? How does a critical attitude express itself for you?" (*Pause*)

Compassion for Feeling Criticized

- "Now, switching perspectives, and taking a moment to get in touch with the part of yourself that feels criticized. Please take a moment to notice how it *feels* to receive this message. What is the impact on you?"
- "If you wish, try giving yourself compassion for how hard it is to be the recipient of such harsh treatment—taking a sympathetic moment for yourself, perhaps by validating the pain: 'This is hard,' 'This hurts.'"

Turning toward Your Inner Critic

- "Now, turning toward your inner critic with interest and curiosity. Please reflect for a moment on *why* the criticism has gone on for so long. Is the inner critic trying to protect you in some way, to keep you safe from danger, or to help you—even if the result has been unproductive? If so, please write down what motivates the inner critic." (*Long pause*)
- "If you cannot find any way that your inner critic is trying to help you—sometimes self-criticism has no redeeming value whatsoever—or if you feel your inner critic is the internalized voice of someone who abused you in some way, please just continue to give yourself compassion for how you've suffered from self-criticism in the past." (*Pause*)
- "But if you did identify some way your inner critic might be trying to keep you safe, see if you can acknowledge its efforts, perhaps even by writing down a few words of thanks. Let your inner critic know that even though it may not be serving you very well now, its intention was good, and it was doing its best." (*Long pause*)

Finding Your Compassionate Voice

- "Now that your self-critical voice has been heard, see if you can make some space for another voice: your *inner compassionate voice*. This aspect of yourself loves and accepts you unconditionally. It is also wise and clear-sighted, and recognizes how the behavior you criticize yourself for is creating problems in your life—is causing you harm. It also wants you to change, but for very different reasons."

- "Please close your eyes. Put your hands over your heart or another soothing place, feeling the warmth. Allow the compassionate side of yourself to emerge, perhaps as an image, a posture, or simply a warm feeling." (*Pause*)

- "Now reflect again on the behavior you're struggling with. Your inner compassionate self would like you to try to make a change, not because you're unacceptable as you are, but because it wants the best for you. Begin to repeat a phrase that captures the essence of your compassionate voice. Here are some examples [teachers can change the order or make up their own phrases]:

  - " 'I love you and I don't want you to suffer.'
  - 'I deeply care about you, and that's why I'd like to help you make a change.'
  - 'I don't want you to keep harming yourself. I'm here to support you.' "

  (*Pause for a full minute.*)

- "If you prefer, you can bring to mind the image of a person who cares deeply about you, or an ideal image that represents compassion to you. Imagine what this person might say to you right now."

- "Now, please open your eyes and begin to write a little letter to yourself in a compassionate voice, freely and spontaneously, addressing the behavior you would like to change. What emerges from the deep feeling and wish 'I love you and don't want you to suffer'? What words do you need to hear to make a change?" (*Pause*)

  - "If you're struggling to find words, it might be easier to write down the words that would flow from your loving heart when speaking to a dear friend who is struggling with the same issue as you." (*Give at least 5 minutes to write, if possible.*)
  - "Please wrap up your writing for now and feel free to continue writing this letter at home, or start a new letter whenever you need one."

- "If you managed to write a few compassionate words to yourself, please read them now and savor the feeling of those words flowing from your own hand. If you had difficulty finding compassionate words, that's okay too. It takes some time. The important thing is that we set our intention to try to be kinder to ourselves, and eventually new habits will form." (*Pause*)

Small-Group Discussion

Participants are now invited to form groups of three persons each to share their experience of this exercise, taking about 15 minutes total for discussion. They should be reminded that it is not necessary to share the *content* of the exercise (what they criticize themselves for), just the *process*. For example:

- "Could you connect with an inner critic or hear a self-critical voice?"
- "How did it feel to give compassion to the part of you that felt criticized?"
- "Did you discover any way your critical voice was trying to help you?"
- "Did it make sense to thank the inner critic for its efforts?"
- "What was the impact of saying the words 'I love you and don't want you to suffer'?"
- "Were you able to write from the perspective of a compassionate voice?"

During this discussion, participants should give wholehearted attention to whoever is speaking, without needing to interrupt, advise, or fix anything.

Inquiry

The focus of inquiry here is on discovering the good intentions that often drive the inner critic and making room for a compassionate voice. The following is an example of inquiry after Motivating Ourselves with Compassion.

CHANG: That was really interesting. I'm a bit blown away, to be honest. (*Pauses a moment*) I'm one of those people who constantly procrastinates, and then I beat myself up for not getting things done, which just makes me want to put things off even more. It's a vicious cycle, and my inner critic can be a bit vicious.

TEACHER: So it was pretty easy to get in touch with your inner critic? (*Said in a slightly ironic, but tender tone.*)

CHANG: Oh, yeah, that was dead easy. It's always around—calling me lazy, worthless, good-for-nothing . . . every name in the book. I've heard that voice ever since I was 14.

TEACHER: Ouch. That must be painful. Could you give yourself some compassion for the pain of that?

CHANG: Not really. I'm so used to the voice that I'm almost numb to it.

TEACHER: Right. (*Pause*) Were you able to figure out what was motivating your inner critic?

CHANG: Fear. Plain old fear. Part of me is desperately afraid of my life falling apart and keeps trying to whip me into shape.

TEACHER: So you were able to get in touch with that fear?

CHANG: Yeah. I realized *why* my inner critic is mean. It's just terrified.

TEACHER: I get it. And did you *thank* your inner critic?

CHANG: I did. I said, "Thank you for trying to protect me." And it was the weirdest thing—my inner critic felt relieved. Like it didn't have to shout so loudly because I finally listened and took in what it was saying. My inner critic actually went quiet, for the first time in a long time.

TEACHER: Wow. That must have been amazing. (*Pause*) And what happened when you tried to get in touch with your inner compassionate self? Did it have anything to say?

CHANG: Well, I couldn't get in touch with it at all at first. It felt too strange. But then, when you asked, "What would I say to a friend who had the same issue as me?", I immediately knew what to say. I'd say, "Of course you put things off; you're so busy, and you feel overwhelmed. You need some rest. But procrastinating is causing *more* stress in your life. I really care about you, and it hurts to see you struggle like this." The most amazing thing was that I realized my inner critic cared about me just as much—it just didn't know how to express it.

TEACHER: That's a pretty big realization. (*Pauses a few moments*) Is there anything you need right now?

CHANG: No, I'm good. I have hope like I haven't had for some time.

TEACHER: That's beautiful. Thanks so much for sharing your journey with us, Chang—very generous of you.

This exercise does not always unfold so smoothly, and inquiry with a single person is rarely so complete. In this case, Chang wanted to share his whole experience with the class, and the teacher was genuinely curious about what happened in the various steps of the exercise. When participants are sharing positive new insights, inquiry is mostly a matter of teachers' allowing themselves to be moved by what we hear.

This inquiry also gave the whole group a chance to review the steps of the exercise and to see the potential of a compassionate voice in their lives. The teacher could have decided to spend more time helping Chang to have compassion for the pain of his self-criticism, but the tone of Chang's voice wasn't sad, and it seemed Chang had something more important he wanted to share. A teacher might have also been tempted to explore what happened to Chang at age 14 when he started hearing the self-critical voice, but the goal of inquiry was not to delve into Chang's personal story, which could have been more like therapy. Instead, the teacher let Chang go on and validated the importance of Chang's insight that his inner critic had good intentions. The teacher didn't need to do anything else in this inquiry, other than making sure that Chang felt finished at the end.

To close the inquiry period, teachers might want to read a powerful poem by Mary Oliver (2004), "The Journey." This poem closely parallels the preceding exercise, beginning with identifying the self-critical voice and then making room for a new, more authentic, compassionate voice.

 ## Compassionate Letter to Myself
(5 minutes)

The instructions for Motivating Ourselves with Compassion include the suggestion to continue writing compassionately to oneself as a home practice whenever this kind of encouragement is needed. Teachers can offer some more specifics about compassionate letter writing, and can also cite research that supports the practice as a way to boost long-term happiness and reduce depression (Odou & Brinker, 2014; Shapira & Mongrain, 2010).

There are actually three approaches to writing a self-compassionate letter. The first, which participants have tried in Motivating Ourselves with Compassion, is writing from *the compassionate self to the struggling self* ("me to me"). The second option is writing from the perspective of a *compassionate other to oneself*—from an imaginary friend who is unconditionally wise, loving, and compassionate ("you to me"). The third option is writing from *the compassionate self to another person,* such as a dearly beloved friend who is struggling with the same concerns ("me to you"). (See Gilbert, 2012, on different ways to cultivate a compassionate self.) Some students like to write a letter to themselves and then store it away or mail it to themselves, so that they can read the letter later on and give the words a chance to soak in.

 ## Home Practice
(5 minutes)

Participants should be reminded of the two practices learned this session:

- Loving-Kindness for Ourselves
- Compassionate Letter to Myself

Students do not need to repeat the whole compassionate motivation exercise at home. Instead, when students are aware of self-criticism in daily life, they can try speaking to themselves with the attitude "I love you and I don't want you to suffer," which is supported in the Compassionate Letter to Myself practice.

In a brief discussion about home practice before ending, students can be asked, "Why do you meditate?" The usual replies are (1) "To honor my commitment," (2) "To train my brain," (3) "To have a better day," and (4) "To reduce stress." All these intentions are good, but they also bring an element of striving into the practice and reduce the inherent enjoyment of meditation. Students can be invited to consider what it would be like to meditate simply (1) to know what it is like to be alive in the moment (mindfulness) or (2) to receive love (loving-kindness and self-compassion)—perhaps even more love than they might receive from others during the entire day. The point is for students to practice in a way that is easiest and most enjoyable.

Closing
(2 minutes)

Teachers usually close the session with a short, shared group experience. If a reading seems fitting, teachers might try an excerpt from *The Velveteen Rabbit* by Margery Williams (1922/2014, pp. 5–8) that begins with "What is REAL?" and ends with "But the Skin Horse only smiled." This passage nicely captures how inner beauty emerges when we live authentically and turn toward the sharp points in our lives with kindness.

Chapter 14

Session 5

LIVING DEEPLY

Overview

Opening (Core) Meditation: Giving and Receiving Compassion

Practice Discussion

Session Theme: Living Deeply

Topic: Core Values

Exercise: Discovering Our Core Values

Informal Practice: Living with a Vow

Break

Soft Landing

Topic: Finding Hidden Value in Suffering

Exercise: Silver Linings

Topic: Listening with Compassion

Informal Practice: Compassionate Listening

Home Practice

Closing

Getting Started

- In this session, participants will:
  - ○ Learn to use breath meditation to cultivate compassion for self and others.
  - ○ Discover core values and learn to reorient to those values in daily life.
  - ○ Find hidden meaning in life's difficulties.
  - ○ Practice compassion and self-compassion while listening to others.
- These subjects are introduced now to:
  - ○ Expand self-compassion meditation to include others.
  - ○ Deepen participants' capacity for self-compassion by helping them discover what they value most.
  - ○ Enhance their ability to listen compassionately to others.
- New practices taught in this session:
  - ○ Giving and Receiving Compassion
  - ○ Living with a Vow
  - ○ Compassionate Listening

Giving and Receiving Compassion
(30 minutes)

Giving and Receiving Compassion is the third core meditation of the MSC course. It builds on the previous two core meditations, Affectionate Breathing and Loving-Kindness for Ourselves, by focusing on the breath and by layering kindness and compassion—in word, image, or felt sense—onto the breath. The new aspect of breathing in for oneself and out for others helps practitioners to stay in connection with others while practicing compassion for themselves. The in-breath may also be understood as a way of *providing* for ourselves—yang self-compassion—rather than focusing entirely on others to meet our needs.

Instructions

- "Please sit comfortably, closing your eyes—and, if you like, putting a hand over your heart or another soothing place as a reminder to bring not just awareness, but loving awareness, to your experience and to yourself."

Savoring the Breath

- "Taking a few deep, relaxing breaths, noticing how your breath nourishes your body as you inhale and soothes your body as you exhale."
- "Now, letting your breathing find its own natural rhythm. Continue feeling the sensation of breathing in and breathing out. If you like, allowing yourself to be gently rocked and caressed by the rhythm of your breathing."

Warming Up Awareness

- "Now, focusing your attention on your *in-breath* only—letting yourself savor the sensation of breathing in, one breath after another, perhaps noticing how the in-breath energizes your body."
- "If you like, as you breathe in, breathing in *kindness* and *compassion* for yourself. Just feeling the quality of kindness and compassion as you breathe in, or if you prefer, letting a word or image of kindness ride on your breathing."
- "Now, shifting your focus to your *out-breath*—feeling your body breathe out, feeling the ease of exhalation."
- "Now, calling to mind *someone whom you love* or *someone who is struggling and needs compassion*. Visualize that person clearly in your mind."
- "Begin directing your out-breath to this person, offering the ease of breathing out."
- "If you wish, sending kindness and compassion to this person with each out-breath, one breath after another."
- "If it's easier for you, you can breathe out to others in general, rather than visualizing a particular person."

"In for Me, Out for You"

- "Now, focusing again on the sensation of breathing *both* in and out, savoring the sensation of breathing in and out."
- "Beginning to breathe in for yourself and out for the other person or persons: 'In for me and out for you,' 'One for me and one for you.'"
- "And as you breathe, drawing kindness and compassion in for yourself, and sending something good out to another."
- "Feel free to adjust the balance between breathing in and out—'Two for me and one for you,' or 'One for me and three for you'—or just let it be an equal flow, whatever feels right to you at this moment."

- "Letting go of any unnecessary effort, allowing this meditation to be as easy as breathing."
- "Allowing your breath to flow in and out, like the ocean going in and out—a limitless, boundless flow. Letting yourself be a *part* of this limitless, boundless flow. An ocean of compassion."
- "Gently opening your eyes."

Settling and Reflection

We give participants some silent time for their experience to settle and be absorbed, and then we invite participants to take notice of what transpired in their inner landscapes during the meditation. Students may need to hear again that their experience of the meditation was just as it should be, no better and no worse.

Inquiry

The following inquiry unfolded with a young participant who was a new mother, Aniyah. Aniyah brought her 7-month-old daughter to the program, since the baby was nursing. It is unusual to have a baby in the classroom, but in this case the presence of the little girl was not a distraction; indeed, it seemed to warm up the atmosphere in the classroom.

> ANIYAH: This meditation was quite a surprise to me. I really let go into the rhythm of the breathing and being caressed by the breath, but when you said to focus on the in-breath, I started feeling uneasy in my stomach, almost nauseous.
>
> TEACHER: Nauseous?
>
> ANIYAH: Yeah, it was really weird. Breathing in for myself almost made me sick, like I was depriving my daughter of air. It was like I was taking all the air for myself, and there was nothing left for her to breathe. It kind of freaked me out.
>
> TEACHER: That sounds really uncomfortable. May I ask what happened next?
>
> ANIYAH: Well, the instructions were to shift the focus to another person, so I chose my daughter—breathing out for her—and I felt much better right away. I couldn't breathe in for myself, but I could breathe out for her. It was weird that it was so intense.
>
> TEACHER: I guess you were really feeling your maternal instinct! How are you feeling now?

ANIYAH: I'm okay. It does make me wonder how I will find time for myself as a new mom.

EVA: (*Raises her hand*)

TEACHER: Yes, Eva?

EVA: May I share another perspective?

TEACHER: Just a moment. (*Turning to Aniyah*) Are you good for now, Aniyah?

ANIYAH: Yes, sure.

EVA: Well, I have four children, all of whom are grown and left home, so at the end of this meditation when we could breathe in or out as much as we want for whomever we want, I just said to myself, "One for me and one for *all four of you!*"

WHOLE GROUP: (*Loud laughter*)

TEACHER: Well, that puts it in perspective, doesn't it? (*Still laughing, pausing, and then returning to Aniyah*) Aniyah, do you think this practice could help you care for yourself as a mom?

ANIYAH: I surely hope so. I think that breathing both in and out is key. Maybe just remembering to breathe in for myself sometimes?

TEACHER: I like that . . . letting your breath be your guide, so you feel connected to yourself *and* your daughter at the same time. Thanks for telling us what happened to you. That's a remarkable experience.

This inquiry with Aniyah illustrates how the direction of breathing can powerfully correlate with one's sense of self and other. In Aniyah's mind, her breathing was so blended with her infant daughter's need to breathe that she panicked when she only breathed in for herself. During inquiry, Aniyah wisely reflected on what her reaction might mean regarding her capacity to care for herself as a mother; at the end of this short inquiry, she wondered aloud whether a conscious in-breath might be a good way to begin caring for herself. The teacher also gently reoriented her to the in- and out-flow of the breath as a way to stay in connection with herself and others.

There was a short interruption in this inquiry when another participant, Eva, asked to contribute to the conversation. We usually do not encourage cross-talk during inquiry because cross-talk can slip too easily into advice giving. In this case, however, the teacher knew that Eva usually spoke from her direct experience, so she was given a chance to share her humorous observation before the inquiry returned to Aniyah and was brought to a satisfying conclusion.

Practice Discussion
(15 minutes)

The home practice discussion can begin with a one-word sharing circle before going more deeply into the details of practice. The practices from Session 4 were these:

- Loving-Kindness for Ourselves
- Compassionate Letter to Myself

Students should be quietly encouraged to share new insights as well as their challenges, to keep the practice discussion both inspiring and informative.

Some students have a tendency to offer lengthy personal stories that can take valuable time from others. At the outset of the discussion period, students can be reminded to focus their comments on their *direct experiences of the practices*—what emotions or body sensations were evoked by particular practices, and how they responded. When a teacher needs to stop a student for the sake of the group, this can be graciously accomplished by inquiring, "May I interrupt . . . ?" and then asking the student a question that shifts the conversation to a deeper level, anchors it in a practice, or elicits how the student is feeling in the present moment. Interrupting a student tends to go smoothly when the teacher has a positive, caring attitude and does not feel anxious or threatened.

Students will need support for their home practice throughout the entire course. A theme in each practice discussion is *compassionate* motivation—motivating with encouragement rather than criticism. When a student feels ashamed about not practicing during the week, the discussion can be shifted to stressful moments during the week and ways the student may have *wished* to respond to these, and then the student can be encouraged to do the same when the opportunity arises again.

Students should also be asked once again to provide weekly feedback, for their sake and for the teachers. This can be done by thanking the students as they submit written feedback, and by referencing their comments (generally and anonymously) during the practice discussion. Students are more likely to provide written feedback when they know that the information matters to the teachers.

Living Deeply
(1 minute)

This session is titled Living Deeply because participants learn to identify their core values, discover hidden meaning in their struggles, and acquire skills for listening to others in a deep, compassionate manner. In this session and the retreat that follows (see Chapter 15), teachers and participants will not explicitly connect with pain to awaken compassion. Participants get a break before they plunge into difficult emotions and challenging relationships in the last two sessions.

Core Values
(10 minutes)

The purpose of this topic is to explain core values to participants as a prelude to discovering their own core values in the next exercise. This topic and exercise are based on acceptance and commitment therapy and the work of Hayes, Strosahl, and Wilson (2012). The following points can be delivered in an interactive manner, but class discussion is usually not necessary since the subsequent exercise will answer most questions.

Why include core values in MSC? The quintessential self-compassion question is "What do I need?", and in order to answer that question, sometimes we need to know what we value most in our lives—our core values. Research has shown that affirming our core values enhances self-compassion (Lindsay & Creswell, 2014).

Human needs and *core values* are fundamental to our sense of well-being. Human needs are commonly associated with physical and emotional *survival,* such as the need for health and safety or for connection, whereas core values have more to do with *meaning,* such as the importance to us of friendship or creativity. Of course, our needs and values overlap. For example, a life without meaning is probably not worth living, so meaning is also necessary for survival. Knowing our needs and values also supports our ability to protect, provide for, and motivate ourselves to act (again, yang compassion) in important ways (McGehee, Germer, & Neff, 2017).

Furthermore, *suffering is nested in a core value,* so core values play a role in how much we suffer in life. For example, if I value outdoor recreation, then not receiving a promotion that would have demanded longer hours at the office might be a blessing, but if I need more money for my family, being passed over for the promotion could be devastating. Similarly, if I value spending time with friends, then I will be disappointed when a friend cancels a visit, but if I value time for reading and reflection, then the cancellation becomes an unexpected gift.

To clarify the meaning of core values, teachers can ask the class, "What is the difference between *goals* and *core values*?" Some points that generally come up are these:

- Goals can be achieved; core values guide us after achieving our goals.
- Goals are destinations (like Juneau, Alaska); core values are directions (like due north).

- Goals are something we do; core values are something we are.
- Goals are set by us; core values are discovered.

For example, a goal might be to finish college, with the underlying core value of "learning." Another goal might be to stay married, and the underlying core value is "loyalty." If teachers ask students to give examples of core values, they might say such things as "compassion," "generosity," "honesty," "social justice," "empowerment," "peace," "autonomy" and "connection."

There is also a difference between social norms and core values. Does a core value energize us? If it does, then it's probably an authentic core value and not simply a social norm. Research has shown that self-compassion fosters authenticity, embracing who we are rather than who we are supposed to be (Zhang et al., 2019). Teachers can also offer students a list of core values to help them uncover their own, such as the Personal Values Card Sort by Miller, Matthews, C'de Baca, and Wilbourne (2011).

Discovering Our Core Values
(25 minutes)

This exercise helps students uncover their own core values, so that they can wisely and compassionately care for themselves. The exercise also explores internal and external *obstacles* that might interfere with participants' living in accord with their core values. Finally, participants will have a chance to consider whether self-compassion could help them to live in accord with their core values (or help them deal with the reality that sometimes they can't).

The following quote from Thomas Merton (1975) helps set the stage for this exercise: "If you want to identify me, ask me not where I live, or what I like to eat, or how I comb my hair, but ask me what I am living for, in detail, and ask me what I think is keeping me from living fully for the things I want to live for" (pp. 160–161).

Instructions

- "This is a written reflection exercise, so kindly take out a pen and paper."
- "Now, please close your eyes, and in your mind's eye, find yourself in the room. If you can, smiling at yourself in welcome."
- "Placing your hand over your heart or elsewhere and feeling your body. This body has been with you for many years, working hard to live a happy life."

Looking Back

- "Imagine that you are in your elderly years. You're sitting in a lovely garden as you contemplate your life. Looking back to the time between now and then, you feel a deep sense of satisfaction, joy, and contentment. Even though life hasn't always been easy, you have managed to stay true to yourself to the best of your ability."

- "Which core values are represented in that life? For example, happiness, peace, compassion, equity, inclusivity, loyalty, adventure, hard work? Please write down your core values."

Not Living in Accord with Values?

- "Now drop back inside and ask yourself if there are any ways that you are currently *not living in accord with your core values,* or ways in which your life seems to be out of balance with your values—especially personal ones. For example, perhaps you are too busy to spend much quiet time in nature, even though nature is your great love in life." (*Pause*)

- "If you have several values that feel out of balance, please choose one that is especially important for you to work with for the remainder of this exercise, and write it down."

Obstacles

- *External.* "We all have obstacles that prevent us from living in accord with our core values. Some of these may be *external* obstacles, like not having enough money or time, power or privilege, or having too many conflicting obligations. Please reflect on this for a moment, and then write down any external obstacles." (*Pause*)

- *Internal.* "There may also be some *internal* obstacles getting in the way of your living in accord with your core values. For instance, are you afraid of failure, do you doubt your abilities, or is your inner critic getting in the way? Please drop inside and reflect, and then write down any internal obstacles." (*Pause*)

Could Self-Compassion Help?

- "Now consider if *self-compassion* could help you live in accord with your true values—for example, by helping you deal with internal obstacles like your inner critic. Or is there a way self-compassion could help you feel safe and confident enough to take new actions, or risk failure, or let go of things that aren't serving you? Again, taking time to reflect, and then writing down what you discover." (*Pause*)

Compassion for Insurmountable Obstacles

- "Finally, if there are *insurmountable* obstacles to living in accord with your values, can you give yourself compassion for that hardship? Let's take a moment and try this out—perhaps offering yourself some words of appreciation and respect for your core values." (*Longer pause*)
- "Is there some way you can express this core value in your life that you haven't considered before, even if this expression is incomplete?" (*Pause*)
- "And if the insurmountable problem is that you are imperfect, as all human beings are, can you forgive yourself for that, too?" (*Pause*)

Settling and Reflection

Students usually need a little time to settle and reflect on this exercise before speaking about it. Teachers can remind participants of what they just experienced:

- "Did you discover any core values? Did one in particular rise to the top?"
- "How did it feel to name internal and external obstacles to living your life in accord with your core values?"
- "What happened when you brought compassion to yourself in light of those obstacles?"
- "Could you forgive yourself for being imperfect?"

Discussion in Pairs (Optional)

If there is time, ask participants to discuss in pairs, for 5 minutes per person, what they learned. This is usually a robust conversation, and talking about core values helps participants strengthen their commitment to them.

Inquiry

Discussing participants' core values tends to empower them rather than making them feel vulnerable. Many participants—notably men, this time—are willing to share their experience of this exercise. The following inquiry also illustrates the close relationship between core values and human needs.

JAMAL: I came up with a few core values that were important to me, but they seemed to be in conflict with each other. For example, I really want to be a good father, and I also want to be a good lawyer. Those were the life goals that pointed me to the core values of being a good man and also being successful. I notice that these values often come into conflict, such as when I need to stay late at the office to work on a case, when I really want to be home and put my kids to bed.

TEACHER: Thanks for analyzing the situation so thoughtfully, Jamal. The example you gave makes the situation quite clear, and you're probably not alone with that dilemma.

JAMAL: I know (*smiling*). It came up in the discussion, too.

TEACHER: Sometimes it's hard to prioritize our values since there are many different parts to our lives—home life, work life, and so on.

JAMAL: So how do we deal with that? I'm always feeling deficient in one area or the other.

TEACHER: Can we take a closer look at the obstacles, Jamal?

JAMAL: Sure.

TEACHER: For example, are there any *external* obstacles?

JAMAL: Yes, *time*. There's not enough time in the day to do everything I want to do.

TEACHER: That's a good one. And *internal* obstacles?

JAMAL: Yeah. I guess I want to be perfect—an amazing lawyer and an awesome father.

TEACHER: I'm wondering if you have a core value that is underlying your desire to be perfect?

JAMAL: It sounds pathetic, but perhaps I just want everyone to like me. No, to be honest, I'd like everyone to *love* me. That's not really a core value, is it? (*Smiling sheepishly*)

TEACHER: Well, it's a pretty basic human need, Jamal. How do you think you would feel if everyone loved you?

JAMAL: I'd feel safe, relaxed. I wouldn't be running around trying to prove myself all the time.

TEACHER: That seems like an important insight, Jamal. I just heard you say that being loved by everyone would make you feel safe. Would it be possible, Jamal, to feel safe and loved even now, even if you aren't perfect?

JAMAL: Oh, geez! Okay, I get it . . . *self-compaaasssssion* (*stretching out the word in a mischievous manner*).

TEACHER: There's a *proooogram* for that (*also smiling puckishly*). Seriously, Jamal, what might you say to a friend, heart to heart, who confided in you that he was running himself ragged trying to be perfect?

JAMAL: Men don't usually talk like that, especially not in my world, but I'd say to him, "Bro, you aren't perfect, but you are a good person."

TEACHER: And what do you think would happen if you occasionally said that to *yourself*?

JAMAL: It just might help me. I know it's true—I just need to be reminded.

TEACHER: Thanks for being so candid in front of everyone. That takes a lot of courage.

JAMAL: Sure. I'll keep you posted about how it goes.

It's a fairly common theme that we experience conflict between our core values. It's also a common theme that being imperfect gets in the way of our being able to live in accord with all our core values. To help resolve the conflict for Jamal, the teacher brought the conversation into his emotional needs that were lying beneath his core values. Then the teacher used the device of "What would you say to a friend?" to help Jamal activate compassion for himself, especially for his human imperfection.

In Jamal's case, his core values depended on his needs. Sometimes it's the opposite: For example, a person's *need* to spend time in nature may be related to a *core value* of protecting the earth. Values tend to have a more conceptual flavor, whereas needs tend to be more emotional. Needs (especially universal human needs) and values can also be identical, such as needing and valuing connection, autonomy, authenticity, or safety. In MSC, the meanings of needs and values are less important than facilitating deeper insight into what matters for each individual and meeting conflict with compassion.

Living with a Vow
(5 minutes)

This informal practice augments the Discovering Our Core Values exercise by inviting participants to remember to apply their core values in daily life. Often our feelings of dissatisfaction, frustration, and anxiety arise out of an awareness that we are not living in accord with our core values. When we discover that we're in the wrong place, at the wrong time, doing the wrong thing, with the wrong people, it's time to remember our core values. We need to draw on the action side of self-compassion to make a change in our lives. A vow can help us do that.

What's a *vow*? A vow is an *aspiration* to which we continually reorient ourselves when we notice that our behavior is not in accord with our core values. A vow functions like the breath in meditation; it's a refuge to which we can return in the chaos of daily life. We need to be compassionate with ourselves when we notice we've strayed (no shame or recrimination), just as in meditation. Loving-kindness phrases themselves can be vows if the phrases reflect core values, such as "May all beings be happy and free from suffering," or "May I learn to love all beings."

Instructions

- "Please select a core value that you may like to manifest for the rest of your life."
- "Write it in the form of a vow: 'May I . . . ' or 'I vow to . . . as best I can.' "
- "Close your eyes and repeat your vow silently. How does it feel when you set your intention in this direction? Does it feel right?"

Teachers can suggest to participants that they can begin repeating their vows first thing in the morning, before they get up, or create a little ritual such as lighting a candle when they say their vows. Starting the day with a vow can keep a student headed in the right direction throughout the day. Or students can remind themselves of their vows before they go to sleep, especially remembering small ways that they behaved consistently with their core values (Jinpa, 2016).

Before closing this topic, teachers may want to read a poem about core values, "The Way It Is," by William Stafford (2013).

Break
(15 minutes)

As usual, students need a chance to stretch and refresh themselves before becoming reimmersed in additional experiential exercises. The break in Session 5 separates two different topics—core values and compassionate listening.

Soft Landing
(2 minutes)

After students are seated, teachers can lead a soft landing themselves, or invite group members to practice on their own for 2 minutes; the latter encourages participants to apply short practices in their daily lives.

Finding Hidden Value in Suffering
(5 minutes)

Compassion is a resource when we struggle because it allows us to turn toward suffering with kindness and understanding. This topic helps us turn toward suffering by bringing *curiosity* to it. Although most of us are afraid of failures and hardships, they often teach us lessons we would not have learned otherwise. As the meditation teacher Thich Nhat Hanh (2014) has said, "No mud, no lotus." The beautiful lotus flower draws its nutrients from the muddy bottom of a lake.

Challenges also force us to go deep inside and discover resources or insights that we may not have known. Teachers can give personal examples to their students or can share this one: MSC is unlikely to have been created, at least in its present form, if one of us co-developers (Chris) had not suffered for decades from public speaking anxiety. Self-compassion allowed him to accept himself as a flawed human being, which in turn made it possible to see and accept the shame that lay beneath his public speaking anxiety (see the Preface). Self-compassion helps us all to feel safer, and it gives us the courage to turn toward suffering, linger with it, and learn from it.

Silver Linings
(10 minutes)

Students now have a chance to identify one past event in each of their lives that was very difficult to bear yet offered invaluable life lessons. In MSC, we refer to these events as "silver lining stories." The term *silver lining* comes from the English proverb "Every dark cloud has a silver lining." A second purpose of the Silver Linings exercise is to provide content for participants to share in the next informal practice, Compassionate Listening. Silver lining stories contain both pathos and epiphanies that make for a compelling listening experience.

Instructions

- "This is a pen-and-paper reflection exercise."
- "Please close your eyes and think of a struggle in your own life that seemed very difficult or even impossible to bear at the time, but that, as you look back, taught you an important lesson. Please choose an event that is far enough in the past that it is clearly resolved and you learned what you needed to learn." (*Pause*)
- "Not every dark cloud has a silver lining. Sometimes we learn nothing from suffering, and our triumph is simply to return to ordinary life. That's okay, too. However, for the sake of this exercise, please choose a challenging event that had a silver lining."
- "What was the situation? What was the challenge? Please write it down. We will be sharing these experiences in small groups later on, so please think of an incident that you might feel comfortable sharing with others." (*Long pause*)
- "If you wish, please write down some kind words that validate what you endured, such as 'That was hard!' or 'This was not your fault . . . you just

didn't know enough to avoid the situation,' or 'I'm so proud of you for having the strength to get through it.' "

- "Now, what deeper lesson did the challenge or crisis teach you that you probably would never have learned otherwise? Please write that down, too." (*Long pause*)

- "Soon we will have a chance to use our silver lining stories as opportunities to practice compassionate listening with one another."

It is usually not necessary to conduct inquiry after this exercise. Teachers can go straight to the next topic, Listening with Compassion, and the next informal practice, Compassionate Listening. The Compassionate Listening practice usually provides sufficient opportunity for participants to share and digest their Silver Linings stories.

Listening with Compassion
(3 minutes)

This topic introduces another aspect of living deeply—the ability to sustain connection with others in their experience of suffering. Teachers can ask their students, "Have you ever tried to tell someone about a struggle you were having, and the listener jumped in too soon with advice on how to fix it? How does it feel when this happens?" Participants usually respond that it feels frustrating and that they don't feel heard or validated. Then teachers can humorously add, "I wonder if any of *us* have ever done that?"

Why do we interrupt someone who wants to share a difficult experience? One reason is that it is difficult to listen to the suffering of others because we empathically share their suffering; it feels like our own, and it is real suffering. By speaking, we reduce the intensity of what we're hearing. Sometimes we go into our heads and try to find a solution to the speaker's problem, which may be more about how we regulate our own emotions than what the speaker needs. Unfortunately, jumping in with advice on how to fix a problem often breaks the emotional connection with the speaker. The speaker is hoping, consciously or unconsciously, to receive compassion, and compassion alone is a powerful vehicle for transforming suffering.

How do we stay in connection with another person whose pain is almost too much for us to bear? First, we need to stay in connection with *ourselves*. That is, we need to be aware of our own empathic pain and be compassionate with ourselves. When we are open and accepting of our ongoing reactions to the speaker, including feeling overwhelmed or triggered, then we can allow the other person to speak without trying to stop or shape what is being said.

Compassionate Listening
(40 minutes)

This practice provides skills for listening compassionately during difficult conversations. Participants will discover how to listen *from the neck down*—what we call "embodied listening" in MSC—and how to apply the Giving and Receiving Compassion meditation as a way to return to connection when the mind wanders.

Participants form groups of three persons each, and every member of the group gets a chance to share their silver lining story. Since there are many elements to this exercise, teachers should thoroughly familiarize themselves with the instructions before proceeding. This practice can be quite poignant, so tissues should be available for tearful participants. Even though participants are asked to choose silver lining stories that are clearly in the past, these stories often carry emotional residue that emerges during the telling of them.

Instructions

- "We're going to use our silver lining stories to practice compassionate listening. This means we are going to listen with our hearts, offering each other our supportive presence, rather than giving advice as we often do."

- "In a moment, we will get into groups of three people. Each person will take about 5 minutes to share their silver lining story, as well as the lesson learned. Feel free to take a pass—to not share your story, or to sit out the practice altogether—if you need to close at the moment. Now please form groups of three persons and wait for further instructions."

Teachers wait for participants to get into their groups of three before continuing with the instructions. If a group has four persons, one person in the group can be asked to volunteer to be a listener only.

Embodied Listening

- "This is a social experiment of sorts: listening without speaking. While one person is telling a story—what happened and what was learned from it—the others are invited to listen carefully to what is being said. The listeners are not allowed to speak, however, and are not allowed to touch, but should otherwise look and behave normally and compassionately."

- "As a listener, instead of formulating what you are going to say, you have the opportunity to listen from the neck down—feeling in your body what the speaker is saying, as well as listening with your ears and with your eyes. [Teachers can also offer a relevant quote: "Most people do not listen with the intent to understand; they listen with the intent to reply" (Covey, 2013, p. 251).]

- "Let yourself be touched or moved by what you hear. This practice is a chance to physically experience common humanity in our shared stories of suffering and redemption."

- "Not only are we practicing embodied listening, but also loving, connected presence—that is, compassion. Therefore, please allow warm feelings for the speaker to arise within you, and feel free to express compassion with your face and eyes."

- "Please note your posture or body language and purposely adopt a comfortable, open, and compassionate posture."

Giving and Receiving Compassion

- "In a moment, we will start to share our stories. As you listen, let your breathing occur quietly in the background of your awareness. Of course, your mind will naturally wander from time to time. For example, if you find yourself emotionally hooked or overwhelmed by what you hear, you may become distracted by your own story as it relates to what you are hearing, or you may feel an urgent need to speak. That's when we can begin practicing Giving and Receiving Compassion."

- "Focus on your breath for a while, breathing compassion in for yourself and out for the speaker. Breathing in for yourself will reconnect you with your body, and breathing out will connect you with the speaker. Continue breathing compassion in and out until you feel reconnected and can listen again in an embodied way."

- "The physical activity of breathing in and out helps us maintain loving, connected presence. It also satisfies the urge to speak because it gives us something to do rather than thinking about what we need to say."

- "Please let this practice be easy, just listening and breathing, and see what happens. There is no need to do this perfectly. Just embodied listening and breathing."

- "Each person will have 5 minutes to speak, and I will ring the bell at 5-minute intervals. If the speaker has finished early, please sit silently together, with closed eyes, until the bell rings. The speaker should feel free to add anything that comes to mind during the silence. If the speaker still has more to say when the 5-minute bell rings, please take a moment to conclude your story, especially by sharing the silver lining."

- "There will be a 1-minute period of silence between 5-minute sharings. During this time, everyone please close your eyes and let what you said or heard settle inside you." Teachers can remind participants of the instructions during the silent period, such as connecting with the in- and out-breath when distracted. "After 1 minute, you will hear another bell, and the next speaker can begin to share a silver lining story."

- "Each small group will have an additional 5–10 minutes at the end of the sharing period to honor each person's story, and to reflect together on the experience of listening and speaking under these conditions."

- "Does anyone have questions about how to do this? I know the instructions are somewhat complicated, so I will remind you of them as we go along."

- "Now, please decide who will be the first speaker, the second speaker, and the third speaker. For instance, this time the first speaker can be the one with the *shortest* first name."

A teacher now rings a bell to start the exercise. (It helps to use a stopwatch to keep track of time.)

Small-Group Discussion

After each person has spoken, a teacher rings the final bell and gives another minute for all participants to reflect with closed eyes on what they have just experienced. The teacher then invites the small-group members to discuss this experience among themselves—honoring what each person has shared, avoiding the tendency to advise or fix, and reflecting on these two questions:

- "What was it like to listen in this way?"
- "What was it like to be listened to in this way?"

Inquiry

There is usually no shortage of volunteers willing to discuss their experience of Compassionate Listening. One participant shared the following experience of being both a listener and a speaker.

RUTH: This totally worked for me. I really liked the experience of just listening and not feeling compelled to say anything. That way I wasn't planning what I would say next, and I just kept listening to what the speaker was trying to say.

TEACHER: So you were off the hook to give a reply?

RUTH: Yes, and the breathing part helped with that. I'm not sure I did it right because I was feeling my breath the whole time. Sometimes I felt the urge to speak, especially when someone teared up—but then focusing on the breath gave me something else to do, and I discovered I didn't need to speak after all.

TEACHER: It seems the breath was always in the background, but you focused on it when you needed to.

RUTH: Yes, that's how it happened. I have one question, though: Should we be listening like this *all* the time?

TEACHER: What do *you* think would be best?

RUTH: Well, I'm a therapist, and I think it would be good, at least a little more. When others were listening to *me* in this practice, I didn't feel like they should be talking more. I rather liked that I didn't have to entertain them and I could really get into my own experience. It was a case of "less is more." I felt the generosity and love of people listening to me in rapt attention (*giggling self-consciously*). I guess it felt like this practice reboots the system—gets us listening in a way that we were taught to listen in graduate school, but may have forgotten. It's so hard *not* to speak when a person is struggling.

TEACHER: That's for sure!

RUTH: Anyhow, thanks. Lots of food for thought here.

Ruth touched upon key points that participants tend to share after this practice—namely, that it was a relief just to listen without an obligation to speak, that the breath helped her *not* to speak, that speaking without interruption helped her find her own answers, and that she didn't need others to speak more. Most participants feel touched and grateful when they are heard in this way, but not all do. For example, one participant said that she felt ashamed and isolated when she told an embarrassing story and no one in her group spoke up to support her. Therefore, teachers should be open and welcoming toward all reactions to this "social experiment."

Compassionate Listening presupposes that, as listeners, we focus as much on the *speaker* as on what is being *spoken*. We can only do this when we abandon the urge to fix the person or the problem, restrain our own minds from wandering and our tongues from speaking, and sense deeply what is happening for the person. The ability to listen compassionately is also what makes the inquiry process work. We implicitly teach others how to be *self*-compassionate by listening compassionately to them.

Home Practice
(5 minutes)

The new practices in this session were:

- Giving and Receiving Compassion
- Living with a Vow
- Compassionate Listening

As an additional homework assignment during the coming week, students can extend the Silver Linings practice by considering whether there is a *current* difficulty in their lives that might also have a silver lining. If so, they can reflect on what hidden lesson could be contained in the current dilemma and how might self-compassion help them learn this lesson.

Students should be reminded to take notice when an MSC practice is easy, pleasant, or especially meaningful to them. Those are the practices that participants are most likely to stick with over time. Students should also be encouraged, yet again, to provide weekly feedback. Finally, they should be told about the upcoming retreat.

Retreat

A 4-hour silent retreat typically occurs on a weekend day after Session 5, usually from 1:00 to 5:00 P.M., after lunch. Teachers often like to schedule the retreat for a separate week and hold off on Session 6 until the following week. To prepare students for the retreat, teachers can share the following information:

> "The retreat is a special opportunity to deepen mindfulness and self-compassion—to practice what we have already learned, to learn a few new practices, and especially to have 4 hours of uninterrupted immersion in the practices. The retreat is held in silence (except for guidance by the teachers), and most participants find that the time passes quickly and easily. The teachers are available to talk if anyone feels the need. You are encouraged to wear casual clothing and to bring a cushion or yoga mat, if you like. Finally, you should arrange for a quiet evening *after* the retreat, in order to digest and savor the retreat experience."

Closing
(2 minutes)

Teachers can close Session 5 any way they like. A poem by Rosemerry Wahtola Trommer (2013), "One Morning," illustrates what it means to be present with another person without an agenda or need to fix anything.

Chapter 15

Session R

RETREAT

Overview

Getting Started

- In the retreat, participants will:
  - Experience mindfulness and self-compassion practices as an integrated whole.
  - Savor the experience of mindfulness and self-compassion.
  - Discover the power of a silent meditation retreat.
- The retreat happens now to:
  - Give participants a deeper understanding of the practices they already know.
  - Provide an opportunity for practicing in a more spacious, relaxed atmosphere—less new learning and fewer group exercises.
- Core meditations:
  - Affectionate Breathing
  - Loving-Kindness for Ourselves
  - Giving and Receiving Compassion
- New practices taught:
  - Compassionate Body Scan
  - Sense and Savor Walk
  - Savoring Food
  - Compassionate Walking (Optional)

Introduction to the Retreat
(15 minutes)

The purpose of the 4-hour retreat is to give participants an opportunity to immerse themselves in the experience of mindfulness and self-compassion. The retreat should take place in a setting where participants feel safe and have privacy. The specific practices taught in the retreat, and the sequence of the practices, can be determined by the needs of the group. Typically, the three core MSC meditations (Affectionate Breathing, Loving-Kindness for Ourselves, and Giving and Receiving Compassion) are included in the retreat, and some new practices are introduced. Sitting meditation generally alternates with movement practices to keep participants comfortable and alert. Teachers should be warm and allow themselves to be playful, so that participants have a positive experience. As always, it is more important to create a relaxed atmosphere than to squeeze a lot of practices into the available time.

Instructions

Teachers can begin by asking these questions:

- "For whom is this your first meditation retreat?"
- "Has anyone been on one or more weeklong retreats?"

They can then make the following points as they introduce participants to the retreat:

- "Don't worry if this is your first retreat. Our intention is to make it a rewarding experience for everyone. We'll be practicing mindfulness and self-compassion together, mostly in silence, for the next 4 hours. The time generally passes quickly, and the teachers are available if anyone feels the need to talk."
- "This retreat is an opportunity to bathe in mindfulness and compassion. It helps to let go of expectations about how the retreat should go for you or how you should feel. All we'll be doing is opening to our moment-to-moment experience and giving ourselves kindness and compassion . . . and seeing what happens."
- "We will maintain *companionable silence* throughout the retreat, without the discussion periods that usually following each practice. Some of you may have been on retreats where *noble silence* is practiced, meaning that people keep their gaze down and don't make eye contact, in addition to being silent. In companionable silence, we can make eye contact, smile, and connect with others, but all without speaking."
- "Silence draws our attention inward—some people say that it's the main vehicle by which retreats work. Therefore, while you can be friendly toward others, please do not try to engage them with your words. Let others have their own experience. Also, let yourself be free from the obligation to pay attention to others." [To illustrate the uniqueness of silence, teachers can read the poem "The Silence," by Wendell Berry (2012), or read part of an essay by Barbara Hurd (2008) that begins with "To Aquinas's wisdom I'd add that silence arrests flight . . ." (p. 47).]
- "We will have at least two walking periods during the retreat. When you need to use the bathroom, please try to do so during a walking period. Of course, you can also use the bathroom any time you wish."
- "Most meditations will be 20–30 minutes in length. We'll practice the three core meditations of the MSC program—Affectionate Breathing, Loving-Kindness for Ourselves, and Giving and Receiving

Compassion—as well as some new practices. There will be fewer instructions than usual during meditation, to give more space for your own experience. Also, feel free to disregard the meditation instructions and practice along the lines already familiar to you."

Compassionate Body Scan
(40 minutes)

The Compassionate Body Scan is an opportunity to enhance mindfulness of the body, and also to nurture a more warm, compassionate attitude toward the body, especially when there is physical or emotional discomfort. The body scan was popularized by Jon Kabat-Zinn (1990) in the MBSR program. The following version of the body scan is explicitly designed to cultivate an attitude of warmth and goodwill toward the body in a variety of ways:

- Inner smile (friendly inclination)
- Soothing touch (comforting the body)
- Safe place (returning to an emotionally neutral body part)
- Loving-kindness (kind words and attitude)
- Compassion (when there is discomfort in the body)
- Appreciation (for the gifts of each body part)

This Compassionate Body Scan is an exercise in loving, spacious *awareness* of the body, along with *appreciation* when there is ease and *compassion* when there is discomfort. It is a way of making friends with the body, embodying the yin qualities of comforting, soothing, and validating our experience.

Instructions

Introduction

- "Please find a comfortable position, resting on your back with your hands about 6 inches from your sides and your feet shoulder-width apart. Then place one or two hands over your heart (or another soothing place), doing this as a reminder to bring loving, connected presence to your body throughout this exercise. Feel the warmth and gentle touch of your hands. Take three slow, relaxing breaths, and then return your arms to your sides, if you like."
- "In this meditation, we will be bringing warmhearted attention to each part of the body in a variety of ways—moving from one part to another,

practicing how to be with each part of the body in a kind and compassionate way. We will be inclining our awareness toward the body with curiosity and tenderness, perhaps as you might incline toward a young child."

- "If you feel ease and well-being in a particular body part, you can invite some appreciation or gratitude to arise within you toward that part of your body. If you have judgments or unpleasant sensations regarding a body part, perhaps you can let your heart soften in sympathy for the struggle—you can also place a hand on that part of your body as a gesture of compassion and support, imagining warmth and kindness flowing through your hand and fingers into your body."

- "And if any area of your body is too difficult to stay with, feel free to move your attention to another body part for a while, especially a body part that is emotionally or physically neutral, allowing this exercise to be as comfortable as possible."

Body Scan

- "Starting with the *toes on your left foot,* and beginning to notice if there are any sensations in your toes. Are your toes warm or cool, dry or moist? Just feeling the sensations in your toes—ease, discomfort, or perhaps nothing at all—and letting each sensation be just as it is. If your toes feel good, perhaps giving your toes a wiggle and a smile of appreciation."

- "Then moving to the *sole* of your left foot. Can you detect any sensations there? Your feet have such a small surface area, yet they hold up your entire body all day long. They work so hard. Feel free to send your left sole some gratitude if that feels right. If there is any discomfort, opening to it in a tender way."

- "Now sensing your *whole foot.* If your foot feels comfortable, you can also extend gratitude for the discomfort that you *don't* have. If there *is* any discomfort, allowing that area to soften as if it were wrapped in a warm towel. If you like, validating your discomfort with kind words, such as 'There's a little discomfort there; it's okay for now.' "

- "Gradually moving your attention up your leg, one part at a time, noticing whatever body sensations are present, sending some appreciation if the part feels fine, and sending compassion if there is any discomfort. Moving slowly though the body, still focusing on your left side, to your . . .
  - "ankle."
  - "shin and calf."
  - "knee."

- "When you notice your mind has wandered, as it always will, just returning to the sensations in the part of your body you were attending to."

- "You might also wish to add some words of kindness or compassion, such as 'May my [knees] be at ease. May they be well.' Then returning your attention to the simple sensations in each body part."

- "Allowing this entire process to be exploratory, even playful, gently working your way through your body. Moving on to your . . .
  - "thigh."
  - "hip."

- "If you feel uneasy or judgmental about a particular body part, try putting a hand over your heart and gently breathing, imagining that kindness and compassion are flowing through your fingers into your body."

- "Or if you feel ease, offering an inner smile of appreciation, if that feels right to you."

- "Now bringing loving awareness to your entire *left leg*, making room for whatever you may be sensing or feeling."

- "And moving on to the *right leg*, to your . . .
  - "right toes."
  - "right sole."
  - "right foot."
  - "ankle."
  - "shin and calf."
  - "knee."

- "Feel free to skip any part of the body if too much physical or emotional discomfort arises. Now on to your . . .
  - "thigh."
  - "hip."
  - "entire right leg."

- "Now bringing your awareness to your *pelvic area*—the strong bones that support your legs, and also the soft tissue in your pelvic area. Perhaps feeling your buttocks on the floor or on the chair—large muscles that help you climb stairs and also allow you to sit softly and comfortably."

- "And now your *lower back*. A lot of stress is stored in the lower back. If you notice any discomfort or tension, you might imagine your muscles relaxing, melting with tenderness."

- "Feel free to shift your posture a little if an adjustment will make you more comfortable."

- "And then your *upper back*."

- "And now moving your attention to the front of your body, to your *abdomen*. Your abdomen is a very complicated part of the body, with many organs and body functions. Perhaps sending some gratitude and appreciation to this part of the body. If you have judgments about your belly, seeing if you can say some words of kindness and acceptance."

- "Then moving up to your chest. The center of your breathing, also your heart center. Infusing your chest with awareness, appreciation, and acceptance. Perhaps putting a gentle hand on the center of your chest, allowing yourself to feel whatever it is you're feeling right now."

- "You should feel free to touch any part of the body as we go along, even gently stroking that part, whatever feels right to you."

- "Continuing to incline your awareness toward your body with the same quality of warmth you might have toward a young child, feeling the sensations in your . . .
  - "left shoulder."
  - "left upper arm."
  - "elbow."

- "Bringing tender awareness to each part of your body. Your . . .
  - "left lower arm."
  - "wrist."
  - "hand."
  - "fingers."

- "Feeling free to wiggle your fingers, if you like, savoring the sensations that arise when you move your fingers. Your hands are uniquely designed to hold and move fine objects, and are very sensitive to touch."

- "And now scanning your whole left arm and hand with loving and compassionate awareness."

- "And moving to your right side, to your . . .
  - "right shoulder."
  - "right upper arm."
  - "elbow."
  - "lower arm."
  - "wrist."
  - "hand."
  - "fingers."
  - "whole right arm and hand."

- "And now proceeding with awareness toward the head, beginning with the *neck*. If you like, touching your neck with your hand, remembering how the neck supports your head throughout the day, how it is a conduit for blood to the brain and air to the body. Offering appreciation and kindness to your neck if it feels good—either mentally or with physical touch—or sending compassion if there is any tension or discomfort there."

- "Finally, moving on to your *head*, beginning with the back of the head, the hard surface that protects your brain. If you like, gently touching the back of your head with your hand, or simply touching it with your awareness."

- "And then your *ears*—those sensitive organs of perception that tell you so much about your world. If you are glad for the capacity to hear, allowing appreciation to arise in your heart. If you are worried about your hearing, perhaps putting a hand over your heart and giving yourself some compassion."

- "And then offering the same loving or compassionate awareness to your other organs of perception, such as your . . .
  - "eyes."
  - "nose."
  - "lips."

- "Don't forget to recognize your *cheeks, jaw,* and *chin* for how they help you eat and speak and smile."

- "And finally, your *forehead* and the *crown of your head,* and underneath . . . your *brain.* Your tender brain is composed of billions of nerve cells that are communicating with each other all the time to help you make sense of your world. If you like, saying 'thank you' to your brain for constantly working on your behalf."

- "When you have finished giving kind and compassionate attention to your whole body, try offering your body a final shower—from head to toe—of appreciation, compassion, gratitude, and respect."

- "And then gently open your eyes."

After finishing these instructions, teachers give students some time to stretch, and perhaps to roll onto one side and gradually bring themselves into a sitting position. Then we move directly to the next exercise without discussion or inquiry.

Sense and Savor Walk
(30 minutes)

The Sense and Savor Walk is a mindfulness practice—*mindfulness of positive experience.* This practice is particularly uplifting when it takes place in a beautiful, natural setting. However, it can also take place indoors if there is sufficient room for everyone to walk around. (A public space is not ideal for the Sense and Savor Walk because participants are likely to feel self-conscious.) The Sense and Savor Walk was adapted from a field experiment designed to study savoring by psychologists Bryant and Veroff (2007).

To complete this practice within 30 minutes, teachers need to allow participants at least 5 minutes to get outside and 10 minutes to return. Therefore, students are allotted 15 minutes to do the practice itself. The following instructions can be delivered when everyone has gathered at the practice location.

Instructions

- "*Savoring* is mindfulness of pleasant experience. Savoring refers to *recognizing* pleasant experience, *allowing* ourselves to be drawn into it, *lingering* with it, and *letting it go* when the time is right."
- "We will not be *trying* to enjoy ourselves—just *allowing* ourselves to notice, linger with, and enjoy whatever calls to us."
- "We will be *silently* walking around for about 15 minutes. The goal of the walk is to notice any pleasurable objects, slowly, one after another, using all your senses—sight, smell, hearing, touch, and maybe even taste. (But please avoid taking photos with your smartphone!)"
- "What do you find beautiful, attractive, enjoyable, or inspiring while you are walking? Do you enjoy the scent of fresh air, the warm sun, a beautiful leaf, the shape of a stone, a smiling face, the song of a bird, the feeling of the earth under your feet?"
- "When you find something delightful or pleasant, let yourself go into it. Really savor it. Feel a tender leaf or the texture of a stick, if you like. Feel free to *give yourself over* to the experience, as if it is the only thing that exists in the world."
- "When you are ready to discover something new, let go and wait until something else appears that is pleasurable and delightful to you. Be like a honeybee going from one flower full of nectar to another. When you are full with one, go on to another."
- "Take your time and see what happens."

After 15 minutes, teachers can ring a bell to let students know that it is time to return to the retreat space. When everyone has gathered and settled down, teachers may read the poem "Aimless Love" by Billy Collins (2014). This poem describes the free-floating, tenderhearted awareness that the Sense and Savor Walk often evokes.

Posture Instruction
(10 minutes)

Most students will be sitting in a chair or on the floor for the remainder of the retreat, except during movement practices. Participants should feel free to sit any way they like, or to stand up or lie down when they need to. Lying down is likely to make the mind wander or put a student to sleep, which is also okay if the student needs to rest the body or even take a nap. However, if a student wishes to be alert during meditation, the best posture is upright yet relaxed.

For those sitting either on the floor or in a chair, the following suggestions may help students find a comfortable position:

- "Flatten and drop your shoulder blades."
- "Tip your pelvis forward."
- "Lift the crown of your head."
- "Tuck your chin slightly."
- "Find a balancing point."

Participants sitting on the floor can experiment with raising their buttocks on a cushion or placing pillows under their knees. If their hips are tight, participants can place a cushion between their legs and bend their legs backward at the knees. Teachers can go from one student to the next and adjust their posture if they feel competent to do so.

Affectionate Breathing
(20 minutes)

Please refer to Session 2 (Chapter 11) for the instructions on how to lead Affectionate Breathing, the first core meditation in MSC.

Savoring Food
(15 minutes)

Students are encouraged to practice continuous mindfulness during the retreat, moving seamlessly from one activity to the next. One such activity is eating. Many participants are familiar with mindful eating—being aware, moment by moment, of the myriad sensations associated with the act of eating. The Savoring Food practice is mindful eating with the added invitation to *enjoy* the sensations of eating. Teachers should bring snacks for students for this practice. They can ask students to choose their snacks and return to their seats for the following instructions.

Instructions

- "Please take a moment and enjoy how the food *looks* to you. (*Pause*) Then enjoying the *smell* and perhaps how it *feels* to the touch."
- "Giving yourself a chance to reflect on the many hands that were involved in bringing this food to your mouth—the farmer, the trucker, the grocer . . ."
- "Now, getting ready to eat your snack *very slowly*—noticing first how you may be salivating before reaching for the food, bringing it to your mouth, noticing when it crosses your lips and when you bite down, appreciating the first splash of flavor, swallowing with awareness of the sensation of swallowing . . ." (*Pause*)
- "Continue eating in this way, giving yourself permission to notice, and particularly to enjoy, the act of eating, one sensation after another." (*Long pause*)
- "When you have finished eating, are there any lingering sensations to remind you that you have just eaten?"
- "Now opening your awareness to your entire body. How do you feel in your body right now?"

Soles of the Feet
(15 minutes)

Please refer to Session 2 (Chapter 11) for instructions for Soles of the Feet. This practice is a form of mindful walking, specifically focusing on the soles of the feet while walking. The retreat provides an opportunity to walk for a longer period of time. Students can practice with a minimum of guidance, perhaps with only a few words from teachers every now and then.

Loving-Kindness for Ourselves
(20 minutes)

Please refer to Session 4 (Chapter 13) for instructions for Loving-Kindness for Ourselves, the second core meditation of MSC. Remind participants to decide in advance which phrases they would like to use in this meditation, so they do not use the time to search for new phrases.

Compassionate Movement
(5 minutes)

Please refer to Session 3 (Chapter 12) for instruction on how to lead Compassionate Movement. It is an optional practice; teachers can lead the practice whenever it appears that students need to move their bodies. Compassionate Movement is a *physical* expression of self-compassion.

Giving and Receiving Compassion
(15 minutes)

Please refer to Session 5 (Chapter 14) for instructions for Giving and Receiving Compassion, the third core meditation in MSC. Again, teachers are encouraged to give students more silence than usual during this meditation, depending on the needs of the group.

Compassionate Walking (Optional)
(20 minutes)

This informal practice builds on the earlier practices of Soles of the Feet (mindful walking), Loving-Kindness for Ourselves (using loving-kindness phrases), and Giving and Receiving Compassion (breathing compassion in and out).

Compassionate Walking is an *optional* practice because it can be stressful for some participants to look into the eyes of other group members. There are also cultures where gazing into the eyes of another person is inappropriate. To ensure everyone's comfort, teachers can describe the practice beforehand and let group members decide if they want to participate. Teachers can also mention different reactions that people may have, such as nervousness about making eye contact or disappointment if there is too little eye contact. Participants should be encouraged to engage in this practice to whatever extent they feel comfortable, noting that after some initial nervousness, most participants find the practice quite valuable. Compassionate Walking can also be taught without the instruction to make eye contact.

Instructions

- "Let's start by standing up and clearing the space of chairs and cushions, so we can walk around freely for the next 15 minutes."
- "When you're ready, please find a spot and stand still, feeling the soles of your feet on the floor. Slowly rocking forward and backward, making little circles with your knees, feeling the soles of your feet."

- "Now returning to stillness, and with a modest gaze directed toward the floor, noticing your breathing in your body, feeling your body breathing in and breathing out."

- "When you are ready, beginning to silently offer yourself kindness and compassion, perhaps as a phrase (such as 'May I be happy and free from suffering'), a breath, or an inner smile."

- "Then slowly begin milling around the room in a random way, still gazing toward the floor, offering yourself kindness and compassion, over and over."

- "You will notice that there are many others moving with you. If it feels right, focusing your attention on another person as you walk by, still with a modest gaze, silently offering kindness and compassion to the other person just as you offered it to yourself. For example, 'May *you* be happy and free from suffering,' or sending a breath or an inner smile in the direction of the other person." (*Pause*)

- "Knowing you can return your attention to yourself whenever you like." (*Pause*)

- "Finally, raising your gaze and making eye contact—taking a moment together—silently offering kindness and compassion in the manner most comfortable for you." (*Pause*)

- "Letting your eyes do the work rather than talking, touching, or hugging, even if you have the impulse to do so."

- "If it makes sense to you, allowing yourself to see *beyond* the physical eyes in front of you, perhaps even sensing something in common—our common humanity."

- "Making space for whatever arises for you, letting yourself *feel* and *be* just as you are, right here and right now. Knowing you can return to kindness and compassion to yourself whenever you need to—'May *I* be happy and free from suffering.'"

Teachers should give students 4–5 more minutes to practice, occasionally offering guidance and encouragement. A teacher then gently rings a bell to end the practice and invites participants to take their seats.

Coming Out of Silence
(15 minutes)

This exercise gently eases participants out of silence and into conversation. Teachers should ask participants to pair up and sit side by side, ear to ear, facing in opposite directions. Each person is given 5 minutes to whisper to the partner something about the personal experience of the retreat, and then they exchange roles. Teachers can keep time with a bell. When both partners have finished speaking, they can take a moment to thank one another and rejoin the whole group.

Group Discussion
(15 minutes)

Teachers can facilitate a general discussion (using the inquiry method) about what participants experienced during the retreat:

- "What did you notice?"
- "What challenged you?"
- "How did you respond?"
- "What did you learn?"

Below are two examples of inquiries that could occur at the end of the retreat.

PAWEL: To be honest, I was a bit worried about this retreat. The thought of sitting for 4 hours and not speaking sounded like torture to me. That's not my thing. I'm always on the move . . . I think that's why I'm a good salesman.

TEACHER: So what *was* it like, sitting for so long?

PAWEL: It was really pretty easy. The practice I liked most was the Sense and Savor Walk. It was almost trippy. Like how I imagine it would be taking psychedelics. I kept saying, "Oh, wow! Oh, wow!" The bark of a tree looked amazing. The ants were like little moving miracles. The bird songs were happening inside me almost as much as they were outside. (*Tearing up a little*) It was so beautiful.

TEACHER: (*Smiling and feeling Pawel's joy*)

PAWEL: I think I will never forget that. What I also realized was that we can be mindful and compassionate any time, not just in meditation. This may make others in the room say, "Duh!," but I really understand now that mindful self-compassion isn't about meditation or any *practices,* for that matter—it's about what your mind is doing—and we can meditate any time and anywhere. We can become free any moment of the day by a simple inner shift.

TEACHER: I think this is very important, Pawel. I wonder if you could say a little more about that inner shift. I'm really curious, if you don't mind saying a little more.

PAWEL: It's hard to say. (*Pause*) It feels more like a gift, like grace. I'm not sure I can do it on purpose. Maybe on purpose, but not with too much effort. I think I just need to give it some time, and also let go and open up. Yes, that's it. The thing about the Sense and Savor Walk was that I didn't try to do anything except be very receptive. I think that's the shift. I'm really grateful for this. Thanks so much.

TEACHER: Thank *you*, Pawel!

And the inquiry that followed Pawel's:

DANIELLE: I appreciate a lot what Pawel was saying. My experience was similar. For me, perhaps the main take-home message of the retreat is *patience*. We did a lot of practices, but they all seemed to flow into each other, like it was one single practice. I got to feel what it was like to just open up, and to be super-kind to myself when I got stressed out. Like Pawel was saying, it's not the technique—it's a state of mind.

TEACHER: And you said you learned about patience?

DANIELLE: I think what helped is that we didn't have anywhere to go and nothing to do. And our phones were turned off! That's pretty rare. I think that rushing around, always planning and strategizing, really blocks mindfulness and self-compassion. Before this retreat, I have been squeezing meditation practice into my day but not really being self-compassionate, I'm sorry to say. This was different. It's like what Pawel was saying. We have to stop rushing around and open up, and then the magic happens.

TEACHER: So slowing down helped you to drop into the actual experience of mindfulness and self-compassion, rather than *working* at self-compassion?

DANIELLE: Yes, that's it. Practices are one thing and the experience is another. (*Short pause*) I guess we really need both. I think, for me, I need to remember to be patient when I practice.

TEACHER: I think I understand, Danielle. This is an important take-home message indeed—actually, for all of us.

DANIELLE: I'll try to remember patience.

TEACHER: Not so easy in our busy world, but worth remembering. Thanks, Danielle.

Pawel and Danielle discovered key insights that are likely to arise during the retreat—namely, that striving and haste are impediments to mindfulness and self-compassion. These insights can be communicated in words (see also the "Insights from Practice" section of Chapter 7), but they do not transform lives until they are directly experienced. The retreat provides an excellent opportunity to have this kind of deeper engagement with the practices and reach new understanding.

Closing
(5 minutes)

Teachers can end the retreat with a poem or a moment of silence, or perhaps by playing the song "Japanese Bowl" by Peter Mayer (see Mayer, 2010, for the song on CD, or find the YouTube video online with the search words "Mayer" and "Japanese Bowl"). Using the metaphor of repairing ceramic bowls with gold resin (*kintsugi*), Mayer's song expresses how inner beauty arises when we honor the cracks and bruises sustained in the course of a lifetime.

Before leaving the retreat, participants should be reminded that they will probably be more emotionally open than usual, and that they should take good care of themselves, allowing themselves to relax and savor the retreat experience, for the remainder of the day.

Chapter 16

Session 6

MEETING DIFFICULT EMOTIONS

Overview

Opening (Core) Meditation: Loving-Kindness for Ourselves

Practice Discussion

Session Theme: Meeting Difficult Emotions

Topic: Stages of Acceptance

Topic: Strategies for Meeting Difficult Emotions

Informal Practice: Working with Difficult Emotions

Break

Soft Landing

Topic: Shame

Informal Practice (Optional): Working with Shame

Home Practice

Closing

Getting Started

- In this session, participants will:
  - Learn to meet difficult emotions by using mindfulness and self-compassion.
  - Understand the meaning of shame, and learn how self-compassion is an antidote to shame.
- These subjects are introduced now to:
  - Strengthen previously learned skills in more challenging situations.
  - Help participants apply mindfulness and self-compassion in a targeted manner to a common source of suffering—difficult emotions.
- New practices taught this session:
  - Working with Difficult Emotions, which includes three components: (1) labeling emotions, (2) mindfulness of emotion in the body, and (3) soften–soothe–allow (SSA)
  - Working with Shame (Optional)

Loving-Kindness for Ourselves
(20 minutes)

Instructions for Loving-Kindness for Ourselves can be found in Session 4 (Chapter 13). If teachers plan to teach the optional practice in this session, Working with Shame, they will need to limit this meditation to 15 minutes, including inquiry.

Practice Discussion
(15 minutes)

Participants may want to reflect on their retreat experience, or on how their home practice was influenced by the retreat. New practices learned at the retreat were these:

- Compassionate Body Scan
- Sense and Savor Walk
- Savoring Food
- Compassionate Walking (Optional)

And new practices taught in the previous regular session (Session 5) were as follows:

- Giving and Receiving Compassion
- Living with a Vow
- Compassionate Listening

Below is an inquiry with a participant who was still having difficulty finding time to meditate.

MARTINA: I'm still having a lot of trouble meditating. I like it when I actually meditate—I like it a *lot*—but I just don't seem to get to it. I'd really like some help with that. The program is almost over, and I'm still not meditating regularly!

TEACHER: How long do you *want* to meditate, Martina?

MARTINA: Oh, maybe 30 minutes each morning. Now it's only 15 minutes every couple of days. That's ridiculous.

TEACHER: So you're saying that you like it when you meditate, but getting *started* is the problem?

MARTINA: Yes.

TEACHER: And what do you think is the main obstacle to getting started?

MARTINA: Emails! It's a nasty habit. As soon as I turn on my computer, the morning is gone. (*Pause*) Thinking about it, I guess I like doing emails because it makes me feel productive, to be perfectly honest with you.

TEACHER: I get that. I'm wondering, though: What goes through your mind when you think about meditating?

MARTINA: Oh, I think I *should* meditate, or else I will never make any progress.

TEACHER: Sounds like one more "should" in the morning. Who needs that?

MARTINA: Yeah, I guess.

TEACHER: But when you say you *like* to meditate, what do you like about it?

MARTINA: I really like the sense of being in touch with myself and also giving myself love, or *opening* to love, whenever I want. It's a luxury. After that, the day is all work.

TEACHER: It sounds to me, Martina, like you really *get* meditation. That's great to hear. I especially appreciate the aspect of "being" with yourself, rather than "doing" meditation, which is work all over again.

MARTINA: I only wish I could remember that—being with myself! When I *think* about meditating, it's yet another task to accomplish in the morning.

TEACHER: What do you think would help you remember, Martina?

MARTINA: (*Long, thoughtful pause*) Maybe if I started my phrase, "I love you and don't want you to suffer," *before* I turn on my computer. I'd rather hear that phrase than anything I'm likely to read in my emails, that's for sure! And then I could just close my eyes, right there on the spot, and let the words really wash over me.

TEACHER: And then you're already meditating!

MARTINA: Right! Maybe this will help. I'll try and let you know.

TEACHER: Please do, Martina. I think we'd *all* like to know how it goes for you. I'm going to try what you said myself—saying the phrases just before I switch on my computer. What a great idea!

Teachers will need to support their students' meditation practice throughout the entire program. New habits develop slowly, and 8 weeks is a relatively short period of time to develop a meditation habit. The inquiry with Martina shows how a teacher can focus on a student's moment-to-moment experience, to help the student realize that mindfulness and self-compassion actually bring *relief* from daily stress rather than creating an additional burden. When students discover the pleasures of practice, and savor those moments afterward, they encourage themselves to practice in creative ways. Remember: If it's a struggle, it's not self-compassion.

Meeting Difficult Emotions
(1 minute)

To begin this session, Meeting Difficult Emotions, teachers can explain to participants that they have now learned a wide variety of mindfulness and self-compassion skills and will begin applying them to more challenging situations. This session shows how to bring mindfulness and self-compassion to *difficult emotions,* and the next session will address *challenging relationships.* This session also takes a closer look at *shame,* the most difficult emotion of all.

Stages of Acceptance
(5 minutes)

The Stages of Acceptance topic is designed to encourage participants to be more self-compassionate in their approach to difficult emotions—to approach them with caution and respect. It is not self-compassionate for any of us to overwhelm ourselves with difficult emotions, with a distant vision of making them go away. As the saying goes, "Walk slowly, go further." The following talking points can be summarized in the teacher's own words and embellished with examples from the teacher's own experience.

What *are* difficult emotions? Difficult emotions are emotions that cause us pain, such as anger, fear, and grief. Sometimes when we turn toward difficult emotions, even with mindfulness and compassion, our pain temporarily increases. Meditation practitioners often wonder how much emotional distress they should allow into their practice. The meditation teacher Thich Nhat Hanh once answered that question succinctly: "Not much!" When we want to build the resource of self-compassion, we only need to *touch* emotional pain as a catalyst for compassion to arise.

To illustrate a more radical approach to confronting emotional pain, teachers can read "The Guest House" by 13th-century Persian poet Rumi (1999) to their students. This beautiful poem describes how when a difficult emotion comes knocking at our door and we let it in—even when it's so strong that it clears our house of its furniture—the emotion may be making room for some new understanding. The poem offers reassurance that our capacity to endure and transform emotional turmoil may be greater than we currently know. Given the choice, however, we should probably titrate the amount of suffering we allow into our lives, to keep from becoming overwhelmed. Sometimes we aren't ready to have our homes violently swept of their furniture by surprise visitors. The art of self-compassion involves inclining *gradually* toward emotional discomfort.

We can learn to accept difficult emotions in stages. Five stages of acceptance (Germer, 2009) are described below and can be illustrated by extending Rumi's guest house metaphor, as described by MSC teacher Christine Brähler (2015):

- *Resisting*—struggling against what comes; hiding in the house, blocking the door, or telling the visitor to go away.
- *Exploring*—turning toward discomfort with curiosity; peeking through the peephole in the door to see who has arrived.
- *Tolerating*—safely enduring, holding steady; inviting the guest in but asking him to remain in the entry hall of the house.
- *Allowing*—letting feelings come and go; allowing the guest to go wherever she wants to in the house.
- *Befriending*—seeing the value in all experience; sitting down with the guest and listening to what the guest has to say.

Each successive stage corresponds to a gradual release of emotional resistance to difficult emotions.

Strategies for Meeting Difficult Emotions
(10 minutes)

Three strategies for working with difficult emotions are offered in Session 6:

- *Labeling emotions*—identifying and validating the emotions.
- *Mindfulness of emotion in the body*—feeling emotions as body sensations, versus thinking about them.
- *Soften–soothe–allow (SSA)*—caring for and comforting ourselves because we have difficult emotions.

These practices are not strategies to *alleviate* difficult emotions, but just to meet them and be with them—yin self-compassion. We are establishing a new *relationship* to emotional suffering that keeps us from feeling overwhelmed and, over time, leads us to feel better.

Labeling Emotions

Naming or labeling difficult emotions helps us to disentangle, or "unstick," ourselves from them. If we can say, "This is anger," or "Fear is arising," we get perspective on the emotion rather than being engulfed by it. This gives us some emotional freedom. Creswell, Way, Eisenberger, and Lieberman (2007) discovered that when we label difficult emotions, activity in the amygdala—a brain structure that registers danger—becomes less active and less likely to trigger a stress reaction in the body. "Name it and you tame it."

How we label emotions is important. There is a difference between *validating* how we feel, as we would for a loved one, and labeling an emotion in a monotone, robotic manner. We should try labeling our emotions in a warm, compassionate tone. For example, we might say, "Oh, dear, you are feeling so *sad* right now," or "I see how *hurt* you are."

Mindfulness of Emotion in the Body

Emotions have mental and physical components—thoughts and body sensations. Research suggests that emotions are associated with distinct, yet culturally universal, parts of the body (Nummenmaa, Glerean, Hari, & Hietanen, 2014). For example, the emotion of disgust is usually associated with sensations in the gut and throat, and sadness is felt in the center of the chest. When we feel an emotion like sadness or disgust, we also have thoughts and images related to those emotions. Emotions actually constitute a *network* of neurological, physiological, muscular, and hormonal components (Damasio, 2004; Scherer, 2005). When one component changes, the whole network is affected.

Body awareness is an important factor in emotion regulation (Füstös, Gramann, Herbert, & Pollatos, 2013). Thoughts arise and disappear so quickly that it is difficult to work with them. The body, in contrast, is relatively slow-moving. When we find the physical component of an emotion and hold it in mindful awareness, we are in a better position to change our relationship to the entire emotion. "Feel it and you can heal it."

Soften–Soothe–Allow

SSA constitutes a kind and compassionate relationship to difficult emotions, and to ourselves:

- *Softening*—physical self-compassion
- *Soothing*—emotional self-compassion
- *Allowing*—mental self-compassion

SSA allows us to stop resisting difficult emotions, and giving up resistance means that we suffer less from difficult emotions. (The sequence of softening, soothing, and allowing can be changed according to the personal preference of students or teachers.) The first two strategies—labeling emotions and becoming mindful of emotions in the body—help us to *disentangle* from difficult emotions, and SSA helps us *warm up* our experience.

 ## Working with Difficult Emotions
(30 minutes)

Working with Difficult Emotions is a multicomponent informal practice. It is introduced here in a meditative way in order to help teachers and students explore the nuances of each component, but once the practice becomes familiar, it can be applied quickly and easily. In everyday life, the different components of Working with Difficult Emotions can be practiced singly or in combination, and in any sequence that feels right at the time. Working with Difficult Emotions is one of the most popular informal practices in MSC, especially the SSA component.

Participants should be advised that this practice involves bringing a current life dilemma to mind, and that they should engage in the practice as much or as little as they like, depending on how emotionally open or closed they may feel at the moment. Teachers can remind students, "If you are closing, please let yourself close." Teachers should also provide sufficient pauses between instructions for students to mindfully feel their way into their bodies and their emotions.

Instructions

- "Please find a comfortable position, sitting or lying down. Then close your eyes and take three relaxing breaths. You should be very comfortable when you are practicing with difficult emotions."

- "Place your hand over your heart, or another soothing and supportive place, for a few moments to remind yourself that you are in the room, and that you, too, are worthy of kindness."

- "Let yourself recall a *mildly to moderately difficult situation* that you are in right now—perhaps a health problem, stress in a relationship, a microaggression, or a work issue. Do not choose a very difficult problem, or a trivial problem. Please choose a situation that generates some stress in your body when you think of it, but doesn't overwhelm you. Also, because this practice emphasizes the yin qualities of softening and soothing, it is better not to choose a situation that makes you feel angry or feel that you need to protect yourself."

- "Clearly visualize the problem. Who was there? What was said? What happened? Or what *might* happen?"

Labeling Emotions

- "As you relive this situation, notice if any emotions arise within you. (*Pause*) And if so, seeing if a *label* for an emotion comes up—a *name*. Here are some examples:
  - "Worry?"
  - "Sadness?"
  - "Grief?"
  - "Confusion?"
  - "Fear?"
  - "Longing?"
  - "Despair?"

- "If you are having many emotions, seeing if you can name the *strongest* emotion associated with the situation."

- "Now, repeating the name of the emotion to yourself in a tender, understanding voice, as if you were validating for a friend what the friend was feeling: 'That's longing,' 'That's grief.' "

Mindfulness of Emotion in the Body

- "Now expanding your awareness to your body as a whole." (*Pause*)

- "Recalling the difficult situation again (if it has begun to slip out of your mind), naming the strongest emotion you feel, and scanning your body for where you feel it most easily. In your mind's eye, sweeping your body from head to toe, stopping where you can sense a little tension or discomfort. Just feel what is 'feel-able' in your body right now. Nothing more." (*Longer pause*)

- "Now, if you can, please *choose a single location in your body* where the feeling expresses itself most strongly—perhaps as a point of muscle tension in your neck, a painful feeling in your stomach, or an ache in your heart."

- "In your mind, inclining gently toward that spot."

- "See if you can experience the sensation directly, as if from the inside. If that's too specific or feels too strong, see if you can just feel the general sense of discomfort."

Soften–Soothe–Allow

- "Now begin *softening* into that location in your body. Letting the muscles soften and relax, as if in warm water. Softening . . . softening . . . softening . . . Remember that you're not trying to *change* the feeling— you're just *holding* it in a tender way. If you wish, just softening a little around the edges."

- "Now, *soothing* yourself because of this difficult situation. If you wish, placing a hand over the part of your body that feels uncomfortable, and just feeling the warmth and gentle touch of your hand. Perhaps imagining warmth and kindness flowing through your hand into your body. Maybe even thinking of your body as if it were the body of a beloved child. Soothing . . . soothing . . . soothing."

  - "And are there some comforting words that you might need to hear? For instance, you might imagine if you had a friend who was struggling in the same way. What would you say to your friend? Maybe 'I'm so sorry you feel this way,' or 'I care deeply about you.'"

  - "Can you offer *yourself* a similar message? Maybe 'Oh, it's so hard to feel this,' or 'May I be kind to myself.'"

- "If you need, feel free to open your eyes whenever you wish, or let go of the exercise and just feel your breath."

- "Finally, *allowing* the discomfort to be there. Making room for it, releasing the need to make it go away."

- "And allowing *yourself* to be just as you are, just like this, if only for this moment."

- "Softening . . . soothing . . . allowing. Softening . . . soothing . . . allowing. Taking some time and going through the three steps on your own." (*Pause*)

- "You may notice that the feeling starts to shift or even change location. If so, that's okay. Just stay with it. Softening . . . soothing . . . allowing."
- "Now letting go of the practice and focusing on your body as a whole. Allowing yourself to feel whatever you feel, to be exactly as you are in this moment."
- (*Gently ring the bell.*)

Settling and Reflection

Some participants who chose a very tough situation in their lives may still be experiencing difficult emotions after this practice. Therefore, teachers should give participants a minute to settle, and then prime the inquiry period with the following questions:

- "Were you able to find a *label* for the most difficult emotion?"
- "What was it like to *explore your body* for a physical sensation associated with the emotion? Were you able to locate where you *felt* the emotion, at least in a general way?"
- "Did the emotion change when you *softened* that part of the body, *soothed* yourself, and *allowed* it to be there?"
- "Did you encounter any difficulties with this practice?"

Teachers can also invite students into discussions in pairs (10 minutes total), if it seems that students would benefit from discussing their experience together.

Inquiry

Working with Difficult Emotions tends to be very moving for participants, and a typical inquiry might go like this.

AISHA: That was something I didn't expect. I started out with what I thought was a straightforward, minor misunderstanding with my boss for something that happened at work. I could name it and felt it as a pulsing in my gut. It was hard to soften around it at first, I must admit—but when I just went to the edges, I could do it. I put a hand there and soothed myself and allowed the sensation to be there.

TEACHER: Right, so it sounds like you were able to follow along with the practice. You said something unexpected happened?

AISHA: Well, the pulsing in my stomach began to move. It went straight to my throat. Then I felt a strong constriction there, almost like I was choking. I had to open my eyes for a moment.

TEACHER: Thanks for doing that—opening your eyes.

AISHA: Yeah, well, I realized what was underneath the misunderstanding. I was actually feeling humiliated, disrespected. *That* was hard to feel. But it's not a new feeling for me. I suffered a lot in public school because I was one of only a handful of black kids. Mostly microaggressions—subtle and indirect comments, you know.

TEACHER: Oh, I'm so sorry about that, Aisha. That hurts. (*Pause, as everyone feels Aisha's pain*) Did you continue with the practice?

AISHA: Yeah, kind of, but it was pretty intense.

TEACHER: Do you mind if I ask a question? Are you still feeling those emotions in your body?

AISHA: (*Tearing up*) Yeah, I am.

TEACHER: Would anything be a comfort to you right now? Any words of kindness, or some physical gesture?

AISHA: My soothing touch is to cradle my face, like my mom used to do when I was little. (*Cradling her face*) That feels better. (*Nodding*) I'm okay. I'll be okay.

TEACHER: Okay, but please let me know if you want to talk more about this. We all have deep wounds, and this practice can tap into them. Thanks for having the courage to share your experience.

During this practice, it is common for emotions to shift and for deeper, more difficult emotions to be discovered. In Aisha's case, she had already felt the more difficult emotion in her body, so the focus of inquiry was then to *name* the emotion—"humiliation"—and to evoke the resource of self-compassion to *hold* it. In other words, the teacher repeated some steps of the exercise to address the new emotion during the inquiry. The teacher resonated with Aisha's painful history of discrimination and chose to refocus on the practice itself and Aisha's present-moment experience. It may have been more helpful to stay longer with the content of Aisha's pain and validate it more fully, but the teacher was also cautious about overexposing Aisha in the group. In the end, the inquiry allowed everyone to stay connected with Aisha's experience, and her resource of soothing touch (cradling her face) was reinforced in the inquiry.

Although most MSC practices require some degree of body awareness, Working with Difficult Emotions focuses more than usual on *sensory* experience. Therefore, an inquiry like the following is also likely to occur.

JOY: Is it possible to practice SSA even if a person is unable to feel emotions in the body?

TEACHER: May I ask, Joy, if you are asking for someone else or for yourself?

JOY: For me, I guess. When you said to scan your body for where you felt the emotion the most, I started spacing out and really couldn't do it.

TEACHER: If you don't mind, could we back up a bit?

JOY: Sure.

TEACHER: Were you able to *name* the strongest emotion in the situation?

JOY: Yes, I could. It was "grief." My difficult situation was that I had to put my cat to sleep last week, and I'm still upset about it.

TEACHER: Oh, I'm really sorry to hear that, Joy. Those feelings must still be pretty raw. But nonetheless you wanted to work with that situation?

JOY: Yes, perhaps I shouldn't have, but I did.

TEACHER: Okay, but then you found yourself spacing out when you tried to find the emotion of grief in your body? Can you say more about that?

JOY: Yeah, I guess I just kinda checked out.

TEACHER: Do you think you checked out for a reason? For example, maybe your body was protecting you from the full impact of your grief?

JOY: Could be.

TEACHER: Could we try a little experiment together?

JOY: Yes.

TEACHER: Could you tell me right now if your body is relaxed, or if there is some stress in your body?

JOY: There's some stress, partly from speaking and partly from the practice.

TEACHER: That's good, thanks. And how do you *know* that you feel stress?

JOY: Well, there's some uneasiness in my chest and stomach—some tension.

TEACHER: What would you say . . . more in the chest or more in the stomach?

JOY: That's hard to say . . . perhaps more in the chest.

TEACHER: (*Puts hand on his own chest, with a long exhalation.*) It seems you actually have all it takes to do this practice. For self-compassion training, we only need to touch pain . . . and then we can give ourselves compassion.

JOY: Thank God!

TEACHER: Yes, indeed. (*Smiling*) I'm also curious, Joy: Were you feeling tired before we started this practice?

JOY: I was exhausted, really, but I didn't want to miss the practice.

TEACHER: We're more likely to space out when we feel tired, and also when we choose a tough situation to work with. Seems you had both. But you were able to identify generally where you felt the tension, which is all you need.

JOY: Yeah, I guess so.

TEACHER: And remember, you don't need to do *every* practice that we try in class, just do what feels right to you, okay? (*Pause*) Thanks for raising this important subject, Joy.

There are many reasons why participants may not have much body awareness. Some people are "heady" types and don't live in their bodies; some have trauma histories (physical or emotional) and have learned to stay out of their bodies; some have strong emotions like shame that drive their awareness out of their bodies; and some people just don't like their bodies and don't want to inhabit them. In Joy's case, she may have had a trauma history that the teacher didn't want to explore in public (she said she "checked out" of her body, suggesting dissociation). However, she also tried to complete this practice when she was emotionally closed (she was exhausted), and she chose a very tough situation to explore, so her ability to focus on her body was compromised. Nonetheless, most MSC participants have sufficient body awareness to do all the practices because all they need is a *general* sense of physical or emotional uneasiness to activate self-compassion.

Inquiry tends to be most interesting for the whole group when a participant is willing to discuss an obstacle or struggle, so teachers should occasionally ask if anyone experienced difficulty during a practice. At the end of this particular inquiry, Joy felt comforted by knowing that she could indeed practice Working with Difficult Emotions, and that she was not to blame for her struggle during the practice (fatigue and intense emotions affected her focus). Most importantly, she learned that she didn't need to push herself so hard to learn self-compassion, and that she could let the practices do the work for her. This last theme cannot be stated often enough in an MSC class.

At the end of inquiry, teachers can read the poem "Allow," by Danna Faulds (2002), which eloquently describes the process of opening to difficult emotions.

Break
(15 minutes)

Students will need a good break before shifting their attention to the second half of the session—the topic of shame. As participants become more familiar with one another and with their teachers, they are more likely to seek out their teachers during the break. Teachers may need to take special care that they themselves also get a break.

Soft Landing
(2 minutes)

Teachers can lead the soft landing themselves, ask a student to lead it, or invite participants to practice on their own. Teachers can remind students of what they have learned so far that can be adapted into a 2-minute soft landing:

- Soothing Touch
- Gentle vocalizations
- Self-Compassion Break
- Loving-kindness phrases
- Affectionate Breathing
- Soles of the Feet
- Labeling emotions
- Soften-Soothe-Allow
- Asking, "What do I need?"
- Living with a Vow
- Compassionate Body Scan
- Compassionate Movement
- Giving and Receiving Compassion

Below is an example of a teacher-led soft landing, this time with more than one element, since students have become more proficient with different practices during the course.

- "Let's take a couple of minutes together to land softly in the present moment, perhaps by simply closing our eyes and noticing how our bodies feel at this moment. (*Pause*) Do you feel fatigued or energetic? Are there any points of tension in your body? And what emotions might be present in your body?"
  - "Now connecting with the natural rhythm of your breathing, how your body rhythmically breathes in and out." (*Pause*)

- "And asking yourself, perhaps in the same tone as you might speak to a dear friend, 'What do I *need* right now?'" (*Pause*)
- "And when something comes to mind, beginning to inhale that quality for yourself, naturally and easily with each in-breath, and then gently exhale, one breath after another." (*Longer pause*)
- "And finally, when it feels right, slowly opening your eyes."

Shame
(15 minutes)

Self-compassion is uniquely helpful for dealing with shame (Gilbert & Procter, 2006; Johnson & O'Brien, 2013), which is perhaps the most difficult human emotion. This topic takes a look at shame through the eyes of compassion—the meaning of shame, its component parts, the ways it is created and sustained—and underscores why self-compassion is an antidote to shame. The purpose is to "de-shame" shame.

The topic of shame naturally follows Working with Difficult Emotions because students are likely to encounter shame in that practice and to have questions about it. A discussion of shame also serves as an introduction to the next practice, Working with Shame. Working with Shame is a variation on Working with Difficult Emotions and is an *optional* practice. It should only be taught if there is sufficient time left in the session, as well as enough energy in the group to do so. If not, students can still work with the emotion of shame in the practice they have already learned, Working with Difficult Emotions.

Shame is a taboo word; the mere mention of it scares some people (Scheff & Mateo, 2016). Therefore, the topic should be presented in a reassuring, matter-of-fact manner. The tone of a teacher's delivery helps to regulate how deeply participants connect with and engage their own shame experiences.

The Meaning of Shame

A formal definition of *shame* is "a complex combination of emotions, physiological responses and imagery associated with the real or imagined rupture of relational ties" (Hahn, 2000, p. 10). For more on shame, please see Chapter 20, as well as Dearing and Tangney (2011); DeYoung (2011); Gilbert and Andrews (1998); Nathanson (1987); and Slepian, Kirby, and Kalokerinos (2019).

Seen through the eyes of compassion, there are three paradoxes that can take the sting out of shame:

- Shame feels *blameworthy,* but it is an *innocent* emotion.
- Shame feels *isolating,* but it is a *universal* emotion.
- Shame feels *permanent,* but it is *transitory,* like all emotions.

These paradoxes are also insights that correspond to the three components of self-compassion—self-kindness, common humanity, and mindfulness—respectively. When we are in the grip of shame, it becomes workable when we remember these insights.

First, shame is an *innocent* emotion. In using the word *innocent,* we are not denying that shame may have tragic consequences, such as violence to self and others. We are merely suggesting that shame arises from the universal wish to be loved. Shame and the wish to be loved are two sides of the same coin. Reminding ourselves that shame arises from the wish to be loved opens the door to exploring and managing shame.

To illustrate our need for love, teachers can read a poem by Hafiz, a 14th-century Persian mystic, "With That Moon Language," loosely translated by Daniel Ladinsky (Hafiz, 1999). This poem describes the universal pull in us to connect. Teachers can also ask their groups, "How many of you wish you were a little less approval-seeking?" The majority of participants in an MSC group usually raise their hands, further suggesting that we all wish to be loved.

The wish to be loved starts at birth. A child has many needs and is completely helpless to meet those needs. However, when newborn children manage to get someone to love them, the basic necessities of life are usually provided (Lieberman, 2013). And we never grow out of the wish to be loved. As adults, we still need others to protect us from danger, to help provide for our physical needs, and to support our efforts to raise our own children. Shame is the emotion that arises when we believe we are too flawed to be loved and accepted by others. Shame can make us feel truly desperate, as if we are fighting for our lives, because being loved by others is essential for human survival.

In addition to remembering that shame is an innocent emotion, shame becomes workable when we realize we are not alone when we feel shame; it is a *universal* emotion. It also helps us to realize that shame is a burden carried by only *part* of ourselves for a *limited* period of time, not a permanent characteristic of who we are. MSC participants can directly experience the three insights in the practice that follows this topic.

Sources of Shame

Shame is a more difficult emotion for some people than others. For example, people are more likely to struggle with shame when they suffered from *childhood neglect* (Bennett, Sullivan, & Lewis, 2010; Claesson & Sohlberg, 2002) or *abuse* (Kim, Talbot, & Cicchetti, 2009); grew up in a *critical household* (Gilbert & Irons, 2009); or suffered from *social oppression* and a narrative of inferiority by the dominant culture (e.g., due to race, ethnicity, gender, religion, sexual orientation) (Bessenoff & Snow, 2006). Some shame is *intergenerational,* based on suffering that was experienced in previous generations (Rothe, 2012; Weingarten, 2004). Shame probably also has *genetic* and *neurological* aspects, as evidenced by the psychopathic personality, which lacks empathy and normal shame (Larsson, Andershed, & Lichtenstein, 2006; Seara-Cardoso & Viding, 2015). Since the experience of shame is so multidetermined, it is usually "not our fault, but it is our responsibility" (Gilbert & Choden, 2014, p. xv).

Shame and Other Emotions

There is a difference between *guilt* and *shame* (Tangney & Dearing, 2002; Whittle, Liu, Bastin, Harrison, & Davey, 2016). Guilt refers to feeling bad about something we *did*; shame is feeling bad about something we *are*. To illustrate this point, teachers can give a personal example. One of us (Kristin) likes to tell the story of when she was singing along with the radio in the car while her autistic son, Rowan, then 10 years old, sat in the passenger seat. During one song, Kristin abruptly stopped and exclaimed, "I'm such a terrible singer!" and without missing a beat her son replied, "You're not a terrible singer, Mommy, you just *sing terribly*." Ever so sweetly, Rowan shifted the burden of criticism from herself to the action—from *being* bad to *doing* something badly.

Shame may underlie many difficult emotions, such as anger, grief, and fear. When difficult emotions become "sticky" and we can't let them go, there is often a vein of shame running through them. For example, persistent anger may arise from feeling disrespected and ashamed; in other words, the sense of "self" is under attack. Persistent grief may arise after the death of a loved one if we feel we were not "good enough" while the person was alive. The reason that public speaking anxiety persisted so long for one of us (Chris) was that he first needed to address shame before he could accept the anxiety that arose out of shame. Emotions and behaviors associated with shame are difficult to manage unless we directly address their root cause.

There is also a difference between *adaptive* and *maladaptive* shame (Greenberg & Iwakabe, 2011). Adaptive shame enhances functioning, whereas maladaptive shame reduces functioning. Adaptive shame says, "I feel bad about myself and I will take steps to correct the situation," whereas maladaptive shame just says, "I'm bad." Self-compassion helps us move from maladaptive shame to adaptive shame.

Shame is likely to emerge in any one of us when things go very wrong in our lives. For example, when we lose our health, wealth, love, or work, we ask, "Why me?!" Intense and disturbing emotions are likely to trigger the following chain reaction:

- "I *feel* bad."
- "I don't *like* this feeling."

- "I don't *want* this feeling."
- "I *shouldn't* have this feeling."
- "Something's *wrong with me* to have this feeling."
- "I'm *bad!*"

We move quickly from "I *feel* bad" to "I'm *bad!*" Therefore, the seeds of shame can sprout in us even when the conditions of our lives are otherwise optimal.

Negative Core Beliefs

Specific, repetitive thoughts go through our minds when life becomes very difficult—lingering self-doubts, sometimes originating in childhood, that seem patently obvious and true. These are our *negative core beliefs* (Dozois & Beck, 2008; Young, Klosko, & Weishaar, 2003). Teachers can provide the following examples of negative core beliefs and solicit additional ones from the class:

- "I'm defective."
- "I'm unlovable."
- "I'm helpless."
- "I'm inadequate."
- "I'm a failure."

Just as every emotion has a mental and a physical component, one or more negative core beliefs are the mental component(s) of the emotion of shame. They arise from the wish to be loved.

The negative core beliefs that human beings have about themselves are not unlimited in number, perhaps one or two dozen. Since there are over 7 billion people on the planet, we can conclude that whatever imperfection we think separates us from the rest of the humanity is probably shared by half a billion people! Therefore, although the experience of shame may make us feel desperately alone, it is actually a sign of our common humanity.

Self-Compassion as an Antidote to Shame

Self-compassion is a healthy response to shame. The alternative is to resist and avoid shame, which inevitably makes it worse. When the sense of "self" is under attack, we need self-compassion—we need to hold ourselves in a loving embrace. Self-compassion is a way of finding self-worth without depending on external approval. Self-kindness counters the self-judgment of shame; common humanity counters the feeling of isolation in shame;

and mindfulness counters the tendency to over-identify with our behavior ("I'm bad").

Shame and Silence

What sustains shame? Trying to hide our shame behind a veil of silence can make the shame persist for a very long time. "We are only as unlovable as our secrets." Mostly we fear that our unlovable qualities (i.e., negative core beliefs) will be exposed, and we will be rejected when they become known. Ironically, shame points to our common humanity—our shared negative beliefs about ourselves and the universal human wish to be loved. To loosen the grip of shame, first we have to *admit* to ourselves that we have these beliefs; then we need to *bring compassion* to ourselves for suffering in this way; and, finally, we need to *share* our self-doubts with others when we feel safe enough to do so.

Compassion for the Whole Self

As human beings, we have many aspects, or parts (Cornell, 2013; Schwartz, 2013). We have wounded parts and compassionate parts, lovable parts and unlovable parts, strong parts and weak parts—the list is endless. When we are engulfed in shame and believe that we are fundamentally unlovable, our awareness is inevitably absorbed in only one small part of who we are. Self-compassion embraces *all* aspects of ourselves.

Working with Shame (optional)
(45 minutes)

Working with Shame is an adaptation of Working with Difficult Emotions. It contains the same steps of labeling (i.e., identifying negative core beliefs), mindfulness of emotion (i.e., shame) in the body, and SSA (responding with compassion). Labeling negative core beliefs and finding shame in the body provide "handles" that make shame more tangible and workable.

Additionally, our experience of shame can be transformed by remembering the three insights: that shame is innocent (self-kindness), universal (common humanity), and transitory (mindfulness). Teachers should keep these elements in mind and gracefully reiterate them while leading the following practice.

Working with Shame is likely to activate some backdraft in participants. Teachers should carefully consider the members of their group before leading this practice, especially if shame is a key issue for some of them. Teachers should also be very familiar with this practice before proceeding, and have at least 45 minutes remaining in the session. Before starting, teachers can briefly describe Working with Shame to their students and offer the usual safety caveats, including that participants should feel free to skip the practice or disengage from it whenever they wish. Again, if the safety caveats are delivered in a relaxed, matter-of-fact manner, students are more likely to participate and discover the richness of the practice. Tissues should be made available for tearful participants.

Instructions

- "In this practice, we will be thinking of a situation in which you felt somewhat ashamed or embarrassed. You will be encouraged to focus more on embarrassment than on shame. However, if you go from 0 to 10 on the intensity scale when you start to feel embarrassed, please give yourself the freedom to disengage from the practice, open your eyes, focus on your breath, take a bathroom break, or attend to yourself in some other way."
- "Please find a comfortable position, sitting or lying down. Close your eyes, partially or fully, and take a few deep, relaxing breaths."
- "Then, placing your hand over your heart or another soothing place, reminding yourself that you are in the room, perhaps allowing kindness to flow through your hand into your body."
- "Now, please bring an event to mind that made you feel *embarrassed* or *somewhat ashamed*. Let it be a past event that is over and done. For example: You may have overreacted to something; maybe you said something dumb at a work meeting; perhaps you made a culturally clueless remark and you still feel a bit ashamed about it; or maybe you flubbed a shot and lost an important game for your sports team." [If it suits a particular group, a teacher can add something humorous, such as "You may have passed gas in church or on a silent meditation retreat."]
  - "Please choose an event that is upsetting enough that you can feel it in your body. If it doesn't make you feel uneasy, please choose another, but no more than a 3 or 4 on an intensity scale from 1 to 10."
  - "Let it be an event that *you would not like anyone to hear about or remember* because if they did, they would probably think less of you."
  - "Please choose a situation that makes you feel bad about yourself, but not one in which you hurt someone and feel the need to make amends."
  - "Also, please do *not* choose a situation that involves someone from whom you still need to protect yourself." (*Long pause*)
- "No one will know what you are thinking about during this practice. After the practice is completed, we will have small discussion groups, but you will *not* be asked to share the *content* of your reflection—only the *process,* such as what you noticed or felt. Therefore, this practice is a private exploration in the safe container of your own mind."
- "Please feel your way into the embarrassing situation, remembering the

event in some detail. This takes some courage. Use all your senses, especially noting how shame or embarrassment feels in your body."

Labeling Core Beliefs

- "Now, please reflect for a moment and see if you can determine precisely *what you are afraid others might discover about you* if they knew about the event. Can you give it a name? Perhaps 'I'm defective,' 'I'm unkind,' or 'I'm a fraud.' These are examples of negative core beliefs."

- "If you found more than one negative core belief, please choose the one that seems to carry the most weight."

- "As you go into this, you may already be feeling alone. If you are feeling this way, recognize that we are 'alone together': Everyone in this room has feelings very similar to yours right now. Shame is a universal emotion."

- "Now name the core belief for yourself in a compassionate voice, perhaps as you might name it for a friend. For example, 'Oh, you've been thinking that you are *unlovable*. That must be so painful!' Or just say to yourself in a warm, compassionate voice: 'Unlovable. I think I'm unlovable.'"

- "Remembering that when we feel embarrassed or ashamed, it is only *part* of us that feels this way. We don't *always* feel like this, although the feeling may seem very old and familiar."

- "And our negative core beliefs arise out of the wish to be loved. We are all innocent beings, wishing to be loved."

- "As a reminder, please know that you can open your eyes at any time during this practice if it becomes uncomfortable, or otherwise disengage any way you like."

Mindfulness of Shame in the Body

- "Now, expanding your awareness to your body as a whole."

- "Recall the difficult situation again (*pause*), and scan your body for where you feel embarrassment or shame most readily. In your mind's eye, sweeping your body from head to toe, stopping where you can sense a little tension or discomfort."

- "Now, please *choose a single location in your body* where shame or embarrassment expresses itself most strongly—perhaps as a point of muscle tension, hollowness, or heartache. You don't need to be too specific."

- "Please raise your hand if you need more time to find a place in your body where shame or embarrassment resides."

- "Again, please take good care of yourself as we do this practice."

Soften–Soothe–Allow

- "Now, in your mind, gently inclining toward that location in your body."
- "*Softening* into that area. Letting the muscles soften, letting them relax, as if in warm water. Softening . . . softening . . . softening . . . Remember that we're not trying to change the feeling; we're just holding it in a gentle way. If you wish, just softening a little around the edges.'"
- "Now, *soothing* yourself because of this difficult experience. If you wish, placing your hand over the part of your body that holds embarrassment or shame, and just feeling the warmth and gentle touch of your hand—acknowledging how hard that part of our body has been working to hold this emotion. Perhaps imagining warmth and kindness flowing through your hand into your body. Maybe even thinking of your body as if it were the body of a beloved child. Soothing . . . soothing . . . soothing.'"
- "And are there some comforting words that you might need to hear? If so, imagine you had a friend who was struggling in the same way. What would you say to your friend, heart to heart? Perhaps 'I'm so sorry you feel this way,' or 'I care deeply about you.' What would you want your friend to know, to remember?
- "Now, try offering yourself, or the suffering *part* of yourself, the same message: 'Oh, it's so hard to feel this,' or 'May I be kind to myself.' Letting the words in, to whatever extent possible."
- "Again, remembering that when we feel embarrassed or ashamed, it is only *part* of us that feels this way. We don't *always* feel like this."
- "Finally, *allowing* the discomfort to be there, letting your body have whatever sensations it is having and your heart to feel as it does. Making room for everything, and releasing the need to make anything go away."
- "And allowing *yourself* to be just as you are, just like this, if only for this moment."
- "Softening . . . soothing . . . allowing. Softening . . . soothing . . . allowing."

Common Humanity

- "Every person in this room has been feeling some sort of embarrassment or shame. We're all human, with strengths and weaknesses. Right now, we're connected in the universal emotions of embarrassment or shame . . . *and the wish to be loved*."
- "Now, letting go of the practice and focusing on your body as a whole. Allowing yourself to feel whatever you feel in this moment."
- (*Gently ring the bell.*)

Settling and Reflection

After giving participants a chance to settle, teachers can ask the following questions:

- "Were you able to identify a *negative core belief* in the experience of embarrassment or shame?"
- "Could you find embarrassment or shame in your body? If so, where?"
- "What was your experience of softening? Soothing? Allowing?"

Small-Group Discussion

Group members now form small groups of three persons each and take 15 minutes total for informal discussion of this practice. Teachers should remind participants that they do not need to share the details of their embarrassing or shameful situation, and to try not to offer any advice—just to listen. Also, students who do not want to share their experiences right now are welcome to sit out the discussion, but these groups are usually quite lively and engaging for those who participate.

Inquiry

Most participants will have a positive experience of Working with Shame if it is guided in a warm, encouraging tone, and if there is enough time to discuss the practice in small groups. Here is a typical inquiry following the practice and small-group discussion.

NATHAN: This was an important practice for me. It was uncanny how the experience of embarrassment took me to a core belief I have struggled with my whole life. The embarrassing situation for me is not remembering names. (*Older group members chuckle sympathetically.*) I know I'm not alone, especially in my generation, but I think I worry about this more than others.

TEACHER: Would you be willing to name the core belief behind it? And please don't feel any obligation to do so!

NATHAN: No problem at all. My core belief is that I'm *stupid*! That's an old one for me. I *know* I'm not stupid, but I had a younger brother who was very smart, and I always felt dumb in comparison. It's no surprise that I freeze up when I can't remember names . . . I'm stupid all over again!

TEACHER: Thanks for being so candid, Nathan. I wonder what happened next in the practice, after you discovered the negative core belief? Were you able to feel the shame in your body?

NATHAN: I noticed that the shame of being stupid takes my breath away. It felt in my body like breathlessness. I think I hold my breath when I feel shame.

TEACHER: (*Puts a hand on his own chest, pauses. and takes a deep breath.*) And then? What happened next?

NATHAN: Then I sent some love through my fingers into my chest, and that felt good. I started breathing again. (*Pause*) What was really interesting was the next part of the exercise, when we talk to ourselves. I said to myself, "You just want to be loved. You think that forgetting names will make you unlovable. It's awkward, I know. But even when you can't remember a name, you're still the same person, you're just as lovable . . . in an awkward kind of way!" (*Chuckling now*)

TEACHER: I love your cheeky compassionate voice, Nathan! So I wonder, what is your take-home message from this practice?

NATHAN: I guess it's giving myself love when I feel stupid and ashamed. That never occurred to me before. Probably *necessary*, too . . . because at my age it's all downhill from here! (*Smiling*)

TEACHER: Thanks, Nathan. I think we're all on the same train!

This inquiry had a lot of humor in it, as well as a sense of common humanity about aging and the universal wish to be loved. The inquiry unpacked key aspects of the practice itself without much assistance from the teacher. Nathan readily shared his core belief of being "stupid," even though he was told he didn't need to. The teacher didn't dwell on the content, however. Instead, he pointed Nathan to the process of the practice—finding feelings of shame in the body, giving himself compassion—and then helped him crystallize what he had learned so that he could use it as a resource in the future.

Home Practice
(5 minutes)

Teachers should remind students that if they found something difficult during the session that is lingering with them, they should not forget to use the skills they have learned so far in the course—or, more specifically, the skills that have been taught in the session itself.

The new practices learned in this session were as follows:

- Working with Difficult Emotions, including (1) labeling emotions, (2) mindfulness of emotion in the body, and (3) SSA
- Working with Shame (Optional)

Participants are encouraged to apply the three elements of Working with Difficult Emotions in their daily lives, but not necessarily as formal home practice. This is because teachers do not want students unnecessarily reminding themselves of difficulties in their lives. Participants are also encouraged to apply the insights they have learned about shame—it arises from the *wish to be loved*, it's a *universal* emotion, and it is *temporary*—if shame arises during the week.

Teachers can give students the following additional reminders:

- "Please keep practicing those skills that you find most enjoyable and beneficial."
- "Cultivate the *intention* to be compassionate, but *drop the effort.* Practice in a way that is a pleasure and not a chore—not like work."
- "Connect via email with others in the group—sharing insights, challenges, inspirations, or questions."
- "Reflect upon your weekly practice and provide written feedback."
- "We only have 2 more weeks left to practice together. MSC is almost over."

Teachers can also ask if there is sufficient interest among some group members to extend the next session by 30 minutes to address unanswered Parking Lot questions (see Chapter 10), or if the group would like their questions to be addressed via email. Alternatively, participants who would like personal responses to their questions can stay after class for a conversation with a teacher.

Closing
(2 min)

The session may be closed by simply ringing a bell or perhaps by reading the poem "Wild Geese" by Mary Oliver (2004), which eloquently describes a compassionate response to shame and illustrates the three components of self-compassion. Another option is to play the Peter Mayer (2010) song "Japanese Bowl" or show the music video featuring the song, if neither was done during the retreat (see Chapter 15). This song is particularly poignant after the topic of shame.

Chapter 17

Session 7

EXPLORING CHALLENGING RELATIONSHIPS

Overview

Opening Meditation: Compassionate Friend

Practice Discussion

Session Theme: Exploring Challenging Relationships

Topic: Pain of Disconnection

Exercise: Meeting Unmet Needs

Exercise (Optional): Silly Movement

Topic (Optional): Forgiveness

Break

Soft Landing

Topic: Pain of Connection

Informal Practice: Self-Compassion Break in Relationships

Topic: Caregiving Fatigue

Informal Practice: Compassion with Equanimity

Home Practice

Closing

Getting Started

- In this session, participants will:
  - Meet unmet needs in relationships with self-compassion.
  - Combine self-compassion and equanimity to manage caregiving fatigue.
- These subjects are introduced now to:
  - Help participants apply the resources of mindfulness and self-compassion in a highly challenging context—personal relationships. Relationships tend to lie at the heart of everyone's emotional life.
- New practices taught this session:
  - Compassionate Friend
  - Self-Compassion Break in Relationships
  - Compassion with Equanimity

Compassionate Friend
(30 minutes)

The purpose of the Compassionate Friend meditation is to help participants discover a wise and compassionate presence, or part, within themselves. The compassionate friend can be a source of comfort (yin) or encourage us when we need to take action (yang). This meditation is taught at the start of Session 7, so that participants feel emotionally supported before addressing challenging relationships.

Compassionate Friend is derived from the Compassionate Image meditation of Paul Gilbert (2009). It is a secular adaptation of Tibetan visualization meditation that helps a practitioner to connect with the true Self—the person's innately wise and compassionate nature. However, in this meditation, it isn't necessary to believe in a compassionate Self to discover hidden resources of wisdom and compassion within oneself.

Some participants have rich imaginations and enjoy visualization practices, and some do not. Previous meditations have included some visualization, but have been based mostly on sensory experience (Affectionate Breathing) or language (Loving-Kindness for Ourselves). Teachers should advise their group members to practice in a relaxed manner with a minimum of expectations, allowing the meditation to unfold by itself and letting images come and go. If no images arise, that is also fine, and the participants can simply linger with any supportive feelings that might be present. If an image arises that causes distress, participants can choose to change the image or disengage from the meditation and nourish themselves in some other way.

Instructions

- "Please find a comfortable position, either sitting or lying down. Gently close your eyes. If you like, taking a few deep breaths to settle into your body. Perhaps putting one or two hands over your heart or another soothing place, to remind yourself to give yourself *loving* attention."

Safe Place

- "Now imagining yourself in a place that is safe and comfortable—as comfortable as possible. It might be a cozy room with a fireplace, or a peaceful beach with a warm sun and a cool breeze, or a forest glade. It could also be an imaginary place, like floating on clouds . . . anywhere you feel reasonably peaceful and safe. Letting yourself enjoy being in this place." (*Pause*)

Compassionate Friend

- "Soon you'll receive a visitor, a warm and compassionate presence—a compassionate friend—who embodies the qualities of wisdom, strength, and unconditional love."
- "This being may be a spiritual figure; a wise, compassionate teacher; or a person from your past, like a grandparent. Or the being may have no particular form—perhaps it is more like light, or a warm presence."
- "Your compassionate friend cares deeply about you and would like you to be happy and free from unnecessary struggle."
- "Please allow an image or being to come to mind." (*Pause*)

Arrival

- "You have a choice to go out from your safe place and meet your compassionate friend, or to invite the friend in. (*Pause*) Please take that opportunity now, if you like."
- "Placing yourself in just the right position in relation to your compassionate friend. You may have some respectful distance, or you may be very close—whatever feels right. Imagining your compassionate friend in as much detail as possible, especially allowing yourself to *feel* what it's like to be in the friend's presence. There is nothing you need to do except experience the moment." (*Pause*)

Meeting

- "Your compassionate friend is wise and all-knowing, and understands exactly where you are in your life journey. Your friend might want to tell you something—something that is *just what you need to hear right now*. Please take a moment and listen carefully to what your compassionate friend might have to say. (*Pause*) If no words come, that's okay, too—just continue to experience the good company. That's a blessing in itself." (*Pause*)

- "And perhaps *you* would like to say something to your compassionate friend. Your friend listens deeply, and completely understands you. Is there anything *you'd* like to share?" (*Pause*)

- "Your friend may also like to leave you with a gift—a material object. The object might simply appear in your hands, or you can put out your hands and receive one—something that has special meaning to you. (*Pause*) If something appears, what is it?" (*Pause*)

- "Now taking a few more moments to enjoy your friend's presence. (*Pause*) And as you continue to enjoy the good company, allowing yourself to realize that your friend is actually a *part of yourself*. (*Pause*) All the compassionate feelings, images, and words that you are experiencing flow from your own inner wisdom and compassion."

Return

- "Finally, when you're ready, allowing the images to dissolve gradually in your mind's eye, remembering that compassion and wisdom are always within you, especially when you need them the most. You can call on your compassionate friend any time you wish."

- "Settling back into your body and letting yourself savor what just happened, perhaps reflecting on the words you may have heard or the object that may have been given to you." (*Pause*)

- "And finally letting go of the meditation and allowing yourself to feel whatever you feel and to be exactly as you are."

- "Gently opening your eyes."

Settling and Reflection

This meditation can be deeply moving for participants, so teachers should allow a minute of silence to allow the meditation to settle and be absorbed, and for participants to reflect on what they have just experienced.

Inquiry

During inquiry, some participants may feel inclined to share their entire meditation experience, and others may not know where to begin. Here are some examples of questions to facilitate inquiry:

- "Would anyone be willing to share what you experienced—perhaps a *touching moment* or a particular *challenge?*"
- "Could you visualize a reasonably *safe* and *peaceful* place?"
- "Did a *compassionate friend* come to mind?"
- "Did you *hear* something that was meaningful for this time in your life?"
- "What was the quality of the message? Soothing? Encouraging?"
- "Did you have anything you wanted to *say* to this being?"
- "Did you *receive* anything with special meaning?"
- "How was it to discover that this warm, compassionate friend is actually a *part of you*, accessible whenever you need it?"

Sometimes participants are surprised by the message given by the compassionate friend. Consider this inquiry:

TISHA: Wow. I wasn't expecting that. My compassionate friend was a talk show host I particularly admire. Silly, I know, but it's who showed up.

TEACHER: Interesting.

TISHA: I got the strong message that I need to change my job. It's a toxic work environment, and even though the pay is good I'm not happy there. Because I'm a single mother I haven't seriously considered leaving, but she helped me realize that my happiness matters. It really matters. My friend told me that I can find another good-paying job that is a better fit, but that I have to start actively looking. It makes me scared to think about it, though. I'm not sure I'm ready to make that leap.

TEACHER: Are you feeling scared now?

TISHA: Yeah.

TEACHER: Is there anything you can do to support yourself as you think about the message you received? Maybe drawing on some yang self-compassion to give you strength and courage?

TISHA: I think so. I hope so. I don't know.

TEACHER: Well, just take it slowly. Remember you can call on your compassion friend whenever you need her, even if she is busy hosting a talk show (*smiles*).

This inquiry shows how participants can be guided to ask themselves what they need, with perhaps a little encouragement in the direction of yin or yang. Framing the question in this way often provides a context that is helpful for participants to make sense of their experience.

The following inquiry illustrates an experience that is likely to occur for at least one person in the group during the Compassionate Friend meditation—reconnecting with someone who has passed away.

JESS: (*Wiping away tears*) This was a big one for me. My mother died when I was 14 years old, around a time when we were fighting a lot. I really didn't expect her to show up, but there she was.

TEACHER: Oh, my.

JESS: I felt robbed when my mother died, but I also felt bad about how I behaved during the last year of her life. I have always wanted to make it right, almost like she would be alive again if I could make it right. I know it sounds crazy.

TEACHER: Not crazy, Jess.

JESS: Well, there she was, just standing in my room at the foot of my bed radiating love to me. She didn't say anything, but I had the sense that she had been loving me all these years, and I didn't know it. (*Wiping tears again; pause*) That was it, really.

TEACHER: (*Pause*) Sounds like she didn't *need* to say anything.

JESS: No, wait . . . she *did* say something.

TEACHER: Is it something you could share, or would you rather keep it to yourself?

JESS: It was kind of like she was speaking inside me, and she said, "I'm soooo proud of you. Just keep doing what you're doing. I'm so proud of you."

TEACHER: How beautiful. (*Smiles and pauses*) How does it feel inside when you remember what you heard?

JESS: Really good . . . strong. I'm feeling loved.

TEACHER: That's lovely. I'm wondering if I could ask you one more question?

JESS: Sure.

TEACHER: At the end of the meditation, we say something like this: "Allow the image to gradually dissolve in your mind, and remember that the love and wisdom have always been inside you, and you can call on them whenever you wish." How was that part for you?

JESS: I knew it was true. Whenever I thought of my mother, I only felt regret about my behavior toward her. But now it's like I found my mother again! (*Many tears are flowing, also among the group members.*)

TEACHER: (*Holding her hand over her heart*) You and your mother have given a gift to all of us, Jess. (*Pause, with a silent nod of appreciation*)

When a participant reconnects with someone who is deceased in the Compassionate Friend meditation, the teacher's purpose is mainly to bear witness to the experience. In this inquiry, the teacher asked Jess to share the words she heard and how she felt in her body, to help her more fully absorb what happened. The key insight of the Compassionate Friend meditation comes at the end, when participants realize that the image, the wisdom, and the compassion all come from within. Therefore, it is instructive for the entire group when that component of the meditation is highlighted during inquiry.

Participants can have a wide range of experiences with Compassionate Friend. When teachers are working with emotionally fragile or traumatized populations, they may change the instructions to evoke an *ideal* compassionate image, such as a spiritual figure or an imaginary figure, rather than a real person with whom the participant may have unresolved emotional conflict. Commonly, however, when participants connect with the compassionate side of a real person, they may also begin to reconcile themselves with that person.

Participants who have a powerful experience with this meditation wonder why it is not a core meditation and comes so late in the program. The reason is that visualizations are difficult for many people (Duarte, McEwan, Barnes, Gilbert, & Maratos, 2015). However, participants who resonate with the Compassionate Friend meditation can be invited to make it a core practice of their own.

Practice Discussion
(15 minutes)

This is the last time during the course that participants will be able to discuss their home practice. For this reason, participants should be encouraged to share any experiences or lingering questions that have been on their minds, as well as discussing the new home practices from last session:

- Working with Difficult Emotions, including these three components: (1) labeling emotions, (2) mindfulness of emotion in the body, and (3) soften–soothe–allow (SSA)
- Working with Shame (Optional)

Even if the Working with Shame practice was not included in Session 6, teachers can ask students whether they were aware of any point when shame arose in their lives during the week, and, if so, how they responded to it.

Now is also a good time to ask participants how mindfulness and self-compassion practice may have affected their lives over the past 6 weeks: "Have you noticed any changes in your life since the course began?" For example, one participant who had diabetes told the group that she measured her blood glucose every day, and that she needed less insulin during each successive week of the program. Most participants who are still in the program will have success stories to share with others.

Participants should be invited to share their difficulties as well. Here is an example.

> ANDRE: I think that many people know by now that I joined this MSC class because my wife asked me to. I don't want to get into the details of why, but I just don't trust her; she hurt me deeply. She's a psychologist and thinks I need more self-compassion to get over my suspiciousness. I think she's right, but I have not learned to trust her any more since the MSC program started.
>
> TEACHER: So you were hoping to trust your wife more. How does it feel to still not trust her?
>
> ANDRE: Really bad. I don't like being suspicious, and I know that she resents how I feel because there's nothing she can do.
>
> TEACHER: So are you trying to be less suspicious, or would you like to be kind to yourself *because* you are suffering from suspiciousness?
>
> ANDRE: Probably both, but I'm afraid to let down my guard.
>
> TEACHER: That's a very important point, Andre, and I'm glad you mentioned that. Maybe you need to stay vigilant so that you're not hurt again. Maybe you need to stay alert rather than comforting and soothing yourself for the pain you felt, or the anguish you feel about your wife. Self-compassion is also a force for protection.
>
> ANDRE: Hmmm. Now that you mention it, maybe so.
>
> TEACHER: I also appreciate that you bring up this topic, Andre, because today we will explore challenging relationships. The key message of this session is that all relationships have pain in them, and we will begin to experiment with what happens when we meet the pain with mindfulness and compassion. You can try this approach during today's session without having to change how you do things at home.
>
> ANDRE: Thanks.
>
> TEACHER: Thank *you*, Andre.

In this short inquiry, Andre and the class were reminded that self-compassion isn't a clever new strategy to feel better; rather, it is a healthy alternative to berating ourselves or trying in vain to manipulate our emotions. This is a core message of MSC and cannot be restated frequently enough.

Finally, there may be questions in the Parking Lot (see Chapters 10 and 16) that need attention before the program ends. Most questions answer themselves as participants gain experience with mindfulness and self-compassion, but if some class members expressed interest last week in extending this session by 30 minutes to address questions, they can be told now if that option is available.

 ## Exploring Challenging Relationships
(1 minute)

Since Session 7 is an emotionally demanding session, with a new opening meditation as well (Compassionate Friend), teachers may wish to give the class a short stretch break before introducing the topic of the day.

After sharing the title of this session, Exploring Challenging Relationships, teachers can point out that most emotional pain is created in the context of relationships and can also be alleviated in relationships, including the relationships we all have *with ourselves*. This session shows how to apply skills participants have already learned to explore relational pain, and also teaches new skills.

 ## Challenging Relationships
(5 minutes)

All human relationships include pain from time to time. As adults, we can learn to respond to relational pain in a new way. Since we know better than anyone else *what* we need and *when* we need it, we can and should try to meet our own needs directly.

When relational pain is difficult to bear, we instinctively try to block it out, work hard to lessen it (unfortunately, even with mindfulness and self-compassion practices!), or try to change the relationship or the person who causes us pain. Teachers need to establish themselves firmly in the understanding that in Session 7, participants are only learning to *meet* relational pain with mindfulness and self-compassion, rather than using these tools to *fix* relationships. The aim of this session is to help participants plant seeds of kindness and understanding, especially toward themselves, and then for everyone to be patient and see what happens. If teachers imply to their students that the practices in this session will improve their relationships, everyone will feel frustrated. Relational improvement is a likely consequence of self-compassion, but it occurs as a side effect of practice rather than by pursuing it directly.

We are all more likely to open to relational pain when we realize its universality. Here are two relevant (comic, ironic) quotes:

- "Hell is—other people!" (Sartre, 1989).
- "Every marriage is a mistake. Some people just cope with their mistakes better than others" (Minuchin, quoted in Pittman & Wagers, 2005, p. 140).

Teachers can also read a description of Schopenhauer's "porcupine dilemma," various versions of which are easily found online. This dilemma refers to a situation in which porcupines want to huddle together in the cold, but they hurt each other with their sharp quills or spines. The point is that conflict and pain are inevitable in relationships.

This session focuses on two broad categories of relational pain: (1) the pain of *disconnection* (when we are rejected by others, experience loss, or have a sense of distance or separation) and (2) the pain of *connection* (empathic distress, when we experience the difficulties of others as our own).

Pain of Disconnection
(10 minutes)

This session first examines the pain of *dis*connection because disconnection tends to be more emotionally activating than the pain of connection, and teachers don't want students to leave the session right after being stirred up.

Feeling disconnected—rejected, betrayed, lost, or alone—can cause a host of difficult emotions to arise. *Anger* is a common reaction because disconnection hurts and makes us feel unsafe. Anger is a natural form of self-protection (yang), but it can also persist for years after it no longer serves a helpful function. In Session 7, the focus is on anger that arises from disconnection, as an example of how to respond to disconnection with mindfulness and self-compassion.

Anger isn't necessarily "bad." Like all emotions, anger has positive functions. Teachers can solicit suggestions from the group about how anger might be *useful* in relationships. Here are some possible responses:

- "Anger gives us information that someone has overstepped our boundaries and hurt us in some way."
- "Anger can provide us with the energy needed to protect ourselves or take action to make a change." Teachers can ask the class for examples, such as how anger may motivate someone to escape domestic abuse or fight for social justice.
- "Anger can be wise if it reduces harm to others." Teachers can ask for examples, such as speaking sharply to a child who is

endangering herself. This is known as *fierce compassion,* or yang compassion.

- "Anger can support our general well-being if we don't turn it against ourselves in harsh self-criticism."

As with all emotions, our *relationship* to anger is what determines whether it is helpful or harmful.

Next, teachers can ask the group how anger can be *harmful.* Here are some examples:

- "Anger can be bad for our physical health [by raising blood pressure, etc.]."
- "Anger can destroy relationships."
- "Anger can take us out of the present moment."

If we continually harden our emotions in an attempt to protect ourselves against attack, over time we may develop bitterness and resentment. Anger, bitterness, and resentment are "hard feelings" (Christensen, Doss, & Jacobson, 2014). Hard feelings are resistant to change, and we can carry hard feelings around for a long time, even when we don't need them anymore. Some relevant sayings are these:

- "Anger corrodes the vessel that contains it."
- "Anger is the hot coal we pick up to throw at another person."
- "Anger is the poison we drink to kill someone else."

Meeting Anger with Mindfulness and Self-Compassion

If we decide that anger is *not* helpful to us any longer, that it isn't protecting us but has hardened into bitterness, we can explore it and learn to respond in new ways. The following sequence can open the door to self-compassion when we experience unhelpful anger or bitterness in relationships.

- *Validating anger.* First, we need to fully validate our anger before we can do anything about it. Many people know that they are angry, but they still subtly criticize themselves for being angry. This is especially true for women, and other groups that experience discrimination, for whom anger can come at a high price. *Validating* anger has a yang-like quality—supporting the truth of our anger and the worth of ourselves when we are angry.

- *Soft feelings.* The next step is to identify *soft feelings* behind the hard feeling of anger. Often anger is protecting more tender, sensitive emotions. Teachers can ask students for examples of soft feelings against which anger might serve as protection, such as feeling scared, lonely, or lost. Leaning into soft feelings has a yin-like quality.

- *Unmet needs.* Behind soft feelings are usually *unmet needs* (Rosenberg, 2015). Examples of unmet needs are the needs to be seen, heard, validated, connected, respected, or known. The most universal need is the need to be loved. A teacher can read a nuanced re-visioning of anger in David Whyte's (2015) essay on anger from his book *Consolations*, beginning with these words: "Anger is the deepest form of compassion." Students should be invited to reflect on their own need to be loved, and to consider how their lives might be different if they saw that need in themselves and others. Students typically note that they might feel less afraid of others and feel less alone if they were continuously aware of the need in all of us to be loved.

- *Self-compassion.* Validating anger, finding soft feelings, and discovering unmet needs are all mindfulness skills that enable the last step—a *compassionate response*. It is easier to evoke compassion for ourselves when we are no longer frozen in anger and we understand that our unmet needs are universal, legitimate, and worthy. Self-compassion is finally giving ourselves the love and compassion we may have been yearning to receive from others for many years.

Meeting Unmet Needs
(30 minutes)

The purpose of this exercise is to validate the experience of anger and to meet underlying needs with self-compassion, carefully blending the qualities of yin and yang. It is taught as an exercise during class because it has many stages that may make it difficult even for reasonably alert participants to work their way through. Teachers should be aware that a key aspect of the exercise comes at the end—meeting unmet needs with compassion. At that stage, participants can still meet their pain with compassion, even if they are not entirely clear about the unmet needs or soft feelings that lie beneath their anger.

To make this exercise easier and safer, we ask participants to focus on a *past* relationship in which their anger no longer serves a protective function. Nonetheless, the exercise is designed so that participants can still connect with the protective side of self-compassion if they need to. It is also essential that participants choose a mildly to moderately difficult relationship for this exercise, not a traumatic relationship, or they will be unable to complete the exercise. Even when a student selects a reasonably benign relationship for this exercise, it may still trigger old wounds or needs. Therefore, as with all challenging exercises and other practices, participants should feel free to skip this exercise or disengage from it if they become emotionally overwhelmed during the exercise. There are points throughout the exercise where teachers can help participants decide whether or not to proceed to the next stage.

Instructions

- "Please close your eyes and think of a *past relationship* that you still feel angry or bitter about—a relationship that was mildly to moderately disturbing, but not traumatizing. Try to choose a relationship in which your anger *no longer serves a* purpose—is not protecting you—and you're ready to let it go." (*Pause for reflection*)
- "Now choose a *specific event* in that relationship that troubles you. You are more likely to stay alert and follow this exercise if you pick an event and a relationship that were not too easy, but also not too tough." (*Longer pause for reflection*)
- "Remember the details as vividly as possible, getting in touch with your anger and feeling it in your body."

Validating Anger

- "Know that it's completely natural for you to feel as you do. Let the anger flow freely as an energy in your body, without trying to control or suppress it, perhaps saying to yourself, 'It's completely okay to feel angry,' or 'My anger is trying to protect me,' or 'I am not alone. Lots of people would feel this way in this situation.' "
- "*Fully validate* the experience of being angry, while trying not to get too caught up in who said or did what to whom."
- "There is no need to move on from here, if validating your anger is what you need the most right now. Maybe you have suppressed your anger in the past and need to fully feel it right now. If that is the case, just let the remaining instructions slip into the background and allow the anger to flow through your body, without judgment. If you like, you can offer yourself a supportive gesture, such as placing a fist over your heart (a sign of strength) and covering it with the other hand (a sign of warmth)."

Finding Soft Feelings

- "If you are sure that your anger is no longer protecting you, and you want to release it, let's begin to see what's underneath. Are there any soft feelings behind the hard feeling of anger?
  - "Hurt?"
  - "Frightened?"

- ○ "Lonely?"
- ○ "Sad?"
- ○ "Ashamed?"

- "If you can identify a soft feeling, try naming it for yourself in a gentle, understanding voice, as if you were supporting a dear friend: 'Oh, that's sadness,' or 'That's fear.' " (*Pause*)
- "Again, if you need to, you can stay right here. What feels right to you?"

Discovering Unmet Needs

- "If you feel ready to move on, see if you can release the storyline of this hurt, if only for a while. You may have thoughts about right and wrong. See if you can set those thoughts aside for a moment, asking yourself, 'What *basic human need* do I have, or did I have at the time, that was not met?' The need to be . . .
  - ○ "seen?"
  - ○ "heard?"
  - ○ "safe?"
  - ○ "connected?"
  - ○ "valued?"
  - ○ "special?"
  - ○ "respected?"
  - ○ "loved?"
- "Again, try naming the need in a gentle, understanding voice." (*Pause*)

Responding with Compassion

- "If you wish to move on, try putting one or two hands on your body in a supportive way if you are not doing that already. The hands that have been reaching outward—longing to receive compassion from others— can become the hands that give you what that you need. Even though you wished to receive kindness or understanding from another person, that person was unable to do so for a variety of reasons."
- "But you have another resource—your own compassion—and you can start to meet your needs more directly. What did you want to *hear*? Can you begin to say that to yourself? For example:
  - ○ "If you needed to be seen, the compassionate part of you can say to the hurt part, 'I see you!' "
  - ○ "If you needed to feel connected, your compassionate part can say, 'I'm here for you,' or 'You belong.' "

    ○ If you needed to be respected, you can say, 'May I know my own value.' "

    ○ If you needed to feel loved, perhaps you can say, 'I love you,' 'You matter to me,' or 'I see you.' "

"In other words, you can say to yourself, or a part of yourself, right now what you may have been longing to hear from someone else—perhaps for a long, long time." (*Pause*)

- "And how did you want to be *treated* by this other person? Would it make sense to commit to taking action, however small, to care for yourself as you always wanted to be treated by others?" (*Pause*)

- "If you're having trouble giving yourself compassion for your unmet needs, or if you feel confused and can't identify an unmet need, can you give yourself compassion for *that* difficulty?"

- "Now letting go of the exercise, and simply resting in your experience, letting this moment be exactly as it is, and yourself exactly as you are."

- "And gently opening your eyes."

Settling and Reflection

Students may feel tired by the end of this challenging exercise. Teachers should validate their students' efforts, and also invite them to let the experience settle and to reflect on what they have just experienced. In preparation for inquiry, teachers may ask the following questions:

- "How did it feel to *validate* your anger?"
- "Could you find *soft feelings* behind the anger? If so, which ones?"
- "Did you discover an *unmet* need?"
- "How did it feel to try to *meet* the unmet need with self-compassion?"
- "How do you feel now?"

Inquiry

Meeting Unmet Needs is likely to elicit more diverse responses during inquiry than any other MSC exercise. Some participants feel like it is the first time in their life they have received permission to be angry and are transformed just by letting their anger flow without judgment. Others who want to let go of their anger move smoothly to the end of the exercise and experience the emotional release that each stage has to offer. Some participants get to the end of the exercise, but can't let go of the old wish for the other person to meet their needs. Still others get distracted or fall asleep.

It's very important that MSC teachers don't subtly give the message that anger is bad, especially to female participants and members of other groups who are disempowered or discriminated against. Validation from the teacher is essential. Consider this example:

ALICIA: I'm shaking.

TEACHER: Are you okay?

ALICIA: Yeah. Actually, I'm great. And I'm pissed off!

TEACHER: Can you explain?

ALICIA: My whole life I've been told that women shouldn't be angry. It makes them ugly. I got that message from my mother very strongly. My boyfriend did something recently that made me angry, and I've been trying to forgive him and understand him and have compassion for him, but you know what? I'm angry!

TEACHER: So did you stay with the first part of the exercise and just validate and feel your anger?

ALICIA: I did. For the first time in my life I just allowed my anger to flow, without judging it or suppressing it. I realized I needed this anger! He shouldn't have done what he did, and I need to draw a boundary and say no.

TEACHER: Wow, that's beautiful.

ALICIA: It is isn't it? I'm not sure what I'm going to do, but I feel like my anger is a life force flowing through me, that I need it. That it's a good thing.

TEACHER: When yang self-compassion arises to protect us, it is a good thing, an essential aspect of caring for ourselves.

ALICIA: I'm going to need to sit with this for a while. And probably better to think carefully about how to talk with my boyfriend about it.

TEACHER: Yes, just sit with it. No need to change anything. And when it comes time to talk with your boyfriend, I'm sure you can use your inner wisdom to decide the best way to express your feelings.

ALICIA: Thank you. What a gift.

For many participants, the main point of this exercise is to help them feel and embrace their anger, especially if it's serving a protective function. It's difficult to apply tender yin compassion to a feeling like anger, so if strong anger is arising it's better for participants to stay in the validating stage, letting their anger move freely through the body. This exercise can help participants tap directly into the protective and empowering aspects of self-compassion, and with the help of a teacher who validates their anger, it can be transformative.

Other participants may get a bit lost in this exercise, and find it easier to navigate through Meeting Unmet Needs when engaged in inquiry with a teacher who keeps them focused and provides support and encouragement. If a student loses the thread of the exercise, the teacher can take the student back to the point where the student became distracted and then accompany the student to the next stage (or stages) of the exercise, as in this example.

JIM: This exercise didn't work so well for me. When we got to the part where we were supposed to meet our unmet need with self-compassion, I just got upset because I really don't want to give myself compassion for what my ex-wife did to me. I need an apology.

TEACHER: I can see that you were hurt. I'm sorry to ask this, but do you think you will ever get an apology?

JIM: No, not really. She's too messed up to apologize . . . okay, I *am* angry!

TEACHER: *Of course* you are. It also looks like you chose a rather tough relationship for this exercise, but now that we're into it, may I ask you a question?

JIM: Sure.

TEACHER: Were you able to find a soft feeling behind your anger?

JIM: No, not really.

TEACHER: Do you think that it's important to stay angry at your ex right now—is it protecting you in some way? Or would you like to let go of some anger?

JIM: I'd like to let it go because I spend too much time thinking about it. Like they say in AA, "She's taking space in my head without paying rent!" It also gives me bad dreams. It just hurts, and we broke up ten years ago!

TEACHER: Okay, then the first step might just be to find where it hurts . . . can you feel that in your body, even right now?

JIM: Yes, my stomach is all cramped up. I feel like I was kicked in the stomach.

TEACHER: Would you be willing to put your hand on your stomach and just be with your feelings in a tender way for a moment? (*Jim and the teacher do the gesture together.*) Relationships can hurt like this.

JIM: (*Keeps his hand on his stomach.*)

TEACHER: Now, if it feels okay, I wonder if you would be willing to try putting your other hand over your heart or some other soothing place . . . because not only is your stomach suffering, *you* are suffering.

JIM: (*Puts one hand over his heart and leaves the other on his stomach.*)

TEACHER: As you do this, can you connect with some other emotional pain behind your anger—a *soft* feeling?

JIM: Yes, all alone. I'm feeling lonely, I guess.

TEACHER: (*Pausing to give time to Jim to feel his loneliness*) And is there a particular place in your body where you feel the loneliness?

JIM: Yes, it's hollowness in my chest. I know that feeling very well.

TEACHER: And what do you need when you feel lonely like that . . . even now . . . what do you need in a moment like this?

JIM: (*Pause*) I just need to know that I'm loved. (*Starting to tear up*)

TEACHER: You are brave to say that out loud, Jim. If you look around, I think you will notice that you touched a nerve in many of us.

JIM: (*Looks around and sees many moist eyes.*) Thank you . . . everyone.

TEACHER: I wonder what you could say to yourself the next time you feel like this—something kind and understanding?

JIM: Maybe just "It's not a crime to want to be loved."

TEACHER: Thank you, Jim. And how do you feel right now?

JIM: A bit better. Thanks.

Jim was one of those students who went along with the whole exercise, but didn't feel it very deeply the first time. This is likely to happen when a student chooses a very challenging relationship and also wants to fix it in the exercise. Jim and the teacher repeated most of the exercise during inquiry, but this time, with the support of the teacher and the group, Jim connected more intimately with his experience. His emotional honesty resonated with other group members, and he received, in real time, the acceptance he longed to receive from his ex-wife. By unpacking the whole Meeting Unmet Needs exercise, the teacher was also able to remind everyone in the group of the different elements of the exercise, each of which can be applied in daily life.

One way of bringing this emotionally charged exercise to a close is by reading a passage in "Being Direct" by Mark Nepo (2000) that begins with these words: "We waste so much time trying to cover up who we are"

(p. 158). This passage points to wounds behind our anger, as well as our universal wish to be loved.

Silly Movement (Optional)
(5 minutes)

At this point in the session, teachers can come up with a Silly Movement routine to introduce a playful attitude into the room. Some examples are starting a simple dance step and gradually making it faster and faster, or inviting participants to make up their own Monty Python "silly walk" routine (to find videos of this, use the search terms *silly walk* and *Monty Python*).

The following are instructions for an example of Silly Movement, suggested by MSC participant Larry Butler. This exercise can be presented in a humorous manner, perhaps introduced as an "esoteric practice" transmitted to a very few special individuals. Such an introduction builds interest before the exercise descends into hilarity. Teachers should demonstrate this exercise while they deliver the instructions.

Instructions

- "Everyone, please stand up. If you can't stand, please join in from a sitting position. Let's begin by *shaking our hands* toward the floor, as if shaking water off our hands." (*One or both teachers begin.*)
- "Now notice how the *whole body* moves with your hands, bouncing up and down, rhythmically, each time you shake your hands." (*Teachers start bouncing.*)
- "Perhaps noticing odd and unusual *sounds* coming out of your mouth with every shake." (*Teachers grunt and whoop.*)
- "And now noticing that your feet might even *lift off the floor*—levitate!—all by themselves. That's the esoteric part." (*Teachers begin to jump up and down.*)
- "And now your *arms*—it's like they have a life of their own." (*Teachers throw their arms in the air.*)
- "And your *legs*, watch them go!" (*Teachers begin kicking up their legs, continuing to make noises.*)
- "And maybe your body even starts to *spin around*." (*Teachers spin around with flailing arms while making funny sounds.*)

Soon everyone is laughing. When the teachers notice that the group is slowing down, they can initiate a round of applause and say to the group, "And that, ladies and gentlemen, is 'Shameless Qigong'!" (Teachers can come up with other names, such as "Silly Yoga," "Shake and Bake," etc.)

Forgiveness (Optional)
(10 minutes)

The topic of Forgiveness naturally follows the Meeting Unmet Needs exercise when students find it difficult to forgive someone who has caused them pain. It outlines a five-step process for forgiving *others* for the pain they have caused us, as well as forgiving *ourselves* for pain we may have caused others. Forgiveness is not an entirely new topic in the MSC course because it has been introduced in Session 1 when teachers noted how we all unwittingly hurt one another because of our differences (especially unseen differences), and offered forgiveness phrases in behalf of themselves and the group.

The Forgiveness topic is optional because there is usually not enough time before the break to complete it. However, when students raise the issue, teachers can offer the following points in a concise manner, or they can share the following information with students after the session via email. (For more on forgiveness, see Aktar & Barlow, 2018; Enright & Fitzgibbons, 2000; McCullough, Pargament, & Thoresen, 2001.)

The central point of forgiveness practice is that we cannot forgive others or ourselves without first opening to the hurt that we have experienced or caused to others. To forgive *others,* we must first face the simple fact that we were hurt. To forgive *ourselves,* we must first open to guilt or shame for hurting others. As the saying goes, "Forgiveness is giving up all hope for a better past."

Forgiveness doesn't mean accepting bad behavior or resuming a relationship that caused us harm. We cannot forgive anyone if we remain in a state of anxiety or fear. In other words, if we are being harmed in a relationship, we need to protect ourselves before we can forgive. This is especially true for cultural harm; we need to feel safe before we can see the humanity in our oppressors and begin to forgive.

Even when the harm we experience from others feels personal and intentional, it is usually the product of a universe of interacting causes and conditions stretching back through time. For example, the offending persons may have partly inherited their temperament from their parents and grandparents, and their actions may have been shaped by their personal history, cultural identity, health status, current events, and so forth. Therefore, they have limited knowledge and control over precisely what they say and do from one moment to the next. This is the same for everyone, including ourselves.

Sometimes we hurt others without intending to do so, and we still feel regret for causing such pain. An example is when a lover chooses to be with a person more suitable for her, or when a young adult leaves home and his parents feel bereft and alone. This kind of pain is not the fault of anyone, but it can still be acknowledged and healed with self-compassion.

As noted above, there are five steps to forgiveness. Teachers can summarize these steps for students, perhaps illustrating each step with a personal example:

1. *Opening to pain*—reliving the pain of what happened.
2. *Self-compassion*—allowing our hearts to melt with sympathy for the pain, no matter what the causes and conditions might have been.
3. *Wisdom*—beginning to recognize that the situation wasn't entirely personal, but was the consequence of many interdependent causes and conditions.
4. *Intention to forgive*—"May I begin to forgive myself (or others) for what I (they) did, wittingly or unwittingly, to have caused this person (me) pain."
5. *Responsibility to protect*—committing ourselves to not repeating the same mistake, or to staying out of harm's way, to the best of our ability.

If there is time in the session, teachers may guide students through an exercise in which these five steps are practiced. Teachers can invite students to think of a person they would like to forgive—someone who has caused them mild to moderate pain, and from whom they no longer need to protect themselves—and then go through the stages together.

Timing is everything. Instead of guiding a forgiveness exercise, teachers may prefer to read a prayer by Bishop Desmond Tutu and his daughter Mpho (Tutu & Tutu, 2015), titled "Prayer before the Prayer." This prayer helps the reader understand the natural ambivalence about reliving old pain—ambivalence that is a precursor to genuine forgiveness.

Break
(15 minutes)

As usual, teachers should give participants a chance to refresh themselves and to connect informally with one another. The break is especially important in Session 7 because it is a challenging session.

Soft Landing
(2 minutes)

Teachers can customize a brief soft landing from anything learned so far, or read the following list of practices and invite participants to give themselves their own soft landing:

- Soothing Touch
- Gentle vocalizations
- Self-Compassion Break
- Loving-kindness phrases
- Affectionate Breathing
- Soles of the Feet
- Labeling emotions
- SSA
- Asking, "What do I need?"
- Living with a Vow
- Compassionate Body Scan
- Compassionate Friend
- Compassionate Movement
- Giving and Receiving Compassion

Pain of Connection
(10 minutes)

The second half of Session 7 focuses on the other type of pain experienced in relationships—the pain of *connection*. This is the pain we all feel when someone close to us is suffering. The pain of connection is based on our human capacity to resonate empathically with others.

Teachers should make this topic interesting by using personal anecdotes, by citing research literature, or by using other teaching modalities such as videos or poetry. The following points provide a conceptual framework for exploring the pain of connection.

The human brain is highly social (Adolphs, 2009; Lieberman, 2013). We appear to have neurons dedicated to feeling in our own bodies what others are feeling—*mirror neurons* (Gallese, Eagle, & Migone, 2007; Rizzolatti, Fadiga, Gallese, & Fogassi, 1996). Furthermore, similar neural circuits are stimulated when people watch others express emotion as when they experience their own emotions (Decety & Lamm, 2006; Keysers, Kaas, & Gazzola, 2010; Lieberman, 2007). For example, witnessing another person in pain activates similar brain structures in the observer as in the person in pain (Bernhardt & Singer, 2012; Decety & Cacioppo, 2011; Saarela et al., 2007).

Our capacity to resonate empathically with others is evolutionarily adaptive. Not only do we require this capacity to raise our young, but we also need to understand and cooperate with one another to survive. Although the expression "the survival of the fittest" is generally attributed to Charles Darwin, he actually considered *cooperation* to be the key factor that helped a species to survive—"survival of the kindest" (Keltner, 2009, p. 52).

Emotions are contagious (Hatfield, Cacioppo, & Rapson, 1993; Nummenmaa, Hirvonen, Parkkola, & Hietanen, 2008; Wild, Erb, & Bartels, 2001). (Teachers can show their students a humorous video of empathic resonance, which can be found on the Web with the search term *talking twin babies*.) Most parents have seen how their children mirror their moods, and they can also regulate their children's emotions by changing their own emotions (Calkins, 1994; Morris, Silk, Steinberg, Myers, & Robinson, 2007). Note that empathy occurs on a preverbal level, which is how parents and infants emotionally communicate before children have language.

Emotional resonance also occurs in intimate partner relationships. For example, imagine that your partner has returned home in a good mood, but you are in a bad mood. You try to hide your mood and don't say anything about it. "What's the matter?" your partner asks, now grumpy. And you say, "*Me?* What's the matter with *you?*" Despite our best efforts, it is difficult to hide how we really feel, or to inhibit emotional contagion. We are influenced by a wide variety of subtle communications, such as a twinkling eye, a long sigh, or a slight shift in the tenor of a person's voice. Therefore, we are inevitably responsible for the moods of others (at least partly), but they are also responsible for how *we* feel.

Our contagious emotions can send us into a *downward spiral,* in which negative emotions trigger negative thoughts and appraisals in one person that can lead to similar or worse thoughts and feelings in another person (Fredrickson, Cohn, Coffey, Pek, & Finkel, 2008). The good news is that self-compassion can interrupt a negative cycle and start an *upward spiral* instead. When we cultivate compassion—engendering feelings of kindness and concern for ourselves or others—our improved attitude can lead to positive thoughts and interactions with others.

Self-Compassion Break in Relationships
(1 minute)

Rather than getting caught in a downward spiral, applying the Self-Compassion Break (taught in Session 1; see Chapter 10) within a relationship is a way to change the tone and direction of a conversation. Teachers can remind participants to take a Self-Compassion Break the next time they are in a heated argument. For example, participants can excuse themselves from the interaction, put a hand over the heart or elsewhere as an expression of self-kindness or self-protection—reminding themselves that their needs count too—and then silently repeat, "This is a moment of suffering. . . .

Suffering is part of any relationship. . . . May I be strong. . . . May I give myself the compassion that I need." The conversation can be continued when one or both persons feel they have shifted from feeling threatened to feeling some degree of care and concern. If it appears that the compassionate frame of mind will be lost immediately upon seeing the other person, it can help to practice Giving and Receiving Compassion (taught in Session 5; see Chapter 14) for a while after returning to the conversation.

Caregiving Fatigue
(15 minutes)

Caregiving fatigue is another example of how human connection can become painful. Most participants in MSC courses are personal caregivers in some capacity, such as caring for children, elderly parents, or spouses; many are also professional caregivers in a field such as medicine, mental health, or education. To keep this topic interesting and interactive, teachers may introduce each point with a question, beginning with these two:

- "How many people here are caregivers in their professional lives—doctors, nurses, therapists, or the like?"
- "And how many people are caregivers in their personal lives—taking care of children, elderly parents, friends, spouses, or others?"

Teachers can then discuss how empathic resonance is a key feature of *all* caregiving relationships, and how caregiving can become overwhelming, leading to exhaustion, when we feel the pain of others for an extended period of time.

Teachers can next ask, "What are some signs of caregiving fatigue?" Students usually identify signs and symptoms such as frustration, irritability, absent-mindedness, lack of interest, avoidance, loneliness, worry, and poor sleep. Teachers can then make the point that caregiving fatigue is not a weakness; it is a sign of being human. We all have our limits as to how much empathic distress we can bear. When it's too much, and we resist the experience, we become fatigued and shut down. The result is that we may begin to resent the very people we are supposed to care for. This shift in attitude can be doubly disconcerting for people who consider themselves to be naturally compassionate.

Teachers can continue by asking, "What are we encouraged to do when we suffer from caregiving fatigue?" The usual advice is self-care—exercising, spending time with friends, or going on a vacation.

"What is the main limitation of these self-care strategies?" The primary limitation is that self-care tends to happen off the job. We need something that can help us *on* the job. The challenge is to find a way to be in the caregiver role itself that is less depleting.

"Does anyone feel that the problem is having *too much* compassion, which means we should learn to toughen up?" This is a common misconception based on confusion between the terms *empathy* and *compassion*. What is the difference? Carl Rogers (1961/1995) defined *empathy* as "an accurate understanding of [another's] world as seen from the inside. To sense [another person's] world as if it were your own" (p. 248). *Compassion* is the capacity to empathize, with the addition of warmth and kindness. If we just feel the suffering of others without having the emotional resources to hold it, we will eventually burn out. Compassion is a sense of care that *embraces* suffering rather than fighting it (Bloom, 2017). Empathy says, "I *feel* you." Compassion says, "I *hold* you."

Compassion is a positive emotion and is inherently energizing. Neuroscientists Tania Singer and Olga Klimecki (2014) trained two groups of people for several days to experience either empathy or compassion, and then showed them a short film depicting others' suffering. The film activated distinctly different brain networks in the two groups of trainees. Empathy training also led to self-reported negative affect, whereas compassion training generated positive affect. Therefore, what is commonly called "compassion fatigue" might be more accurately described as "empathy fatigue" (Klimecki & Singer, 2012; Stebnicki, 2007). A compelling video about this research can be found online by using the search terms *Matthieu Ricard* and *empathy fatigue*. Paradoxically, we need *more* compassion, not less, to alleviate caregiving fatigue.

Next, teachers can ask, "How can we grow in compassion for others who are already exhausting us?" The answer is "self-compassion!" Empathic distress is just another source of emotional pain for which a healthy response may be self-compassion. This can be done in the caregiving situation itself. We can say to ourselves, "This is so stressful; I'm feeling overwhelmed," and give ourselves kindness right then and there. In our roles as caregivers, we often believe that we should only be concerned with the needs of others and are self-critical when we think we aren't giving enough. However, when we don't attend to our own emotional needs as well, we will become depleted and unable to give to others (Egan, Mantzios, & Jackson, 2017; Mills & Chapman, 2016).

Importantly, we need to remember that the individuals we care for are empathetically resonating with our own mind-states. Empathy goes both ways. If we are frustrated and exhausted, others resonate with these negative feelings, but if our mind-states are ones of kindness and compassion, others resonate with these positive feelings. In this way, having self-compassion in caregiving situations is actually a *gift* we give to others. It is not selfish. Teachers can give personal examples to illustrate this point, perhaps from their own experiences of raising children or caring for a sick spouse.

The following quote from a teaching by the Dalai Lama (2012b) illustrates the importance of self-compassion as a foundation for sustaining and expanding our compassion for others: "For someone to develop genuine compassion towards others, first he or she must have a basis upon which to cultivate compassion, and that basis is the ability to connect to one's own feelings and to care for one's own welfare. . . . Caring for others requires caring for oneself."

Equanimity

Another important skill for dealing with caregiver fatigue is *equanimity*. This term refers to maintaining mental balance in the midst of opposites, such as pleasure and pain, success and failure, or joy and sorrow. It is a spacious attitude that naturally develops with sustained mindfulness practice. Equanimity is not cold detachment, but arises from deep understanding of the transient, interdependent nature of reality. It is a different kind of caring, based on both emotional intimacy and wise discernment.

Equanimity can be cultivated by using language that helps us to emotionally disentangle from a challenging situation long enough to see ourselves and others with more perspective. An example is the "Serenity Prayer" penned by Reinhold Niebuhr (1943, p. xxiv): "God, give us grace to accept with serenity the things that cannot be changed, courage to change the things that should be changed, and the wisdom to distinguish the one from the other."

Equanimity gives us the emotional space to *choose* to be compassionate and remain in connection with others. For example, participants in MSC who are also psychotherapists can probably relate to how quickly they become emotionally entangled when clients mention suicide, even if they have just met them. From that moment onward, the therapists' attention is wrapped up in preventing suicide or extracting a promise from such clients that they will not commit suicide before the next session. Equanimity practice can help clinicians to step back from their natural fear reaction in such situations, stay in empathic connection with the clients, and work together toward meaningful safety planning.

Compassion with Equanimity
(25 minutes)

Compassion with Equanimity is an informal practice that can be applied in the midst of caregiving situations as a self-compassionate response to empathetic distress and fatigue. It is introduced now as a guided practice that combines equanimity phrases with the Giving and Receiving Compassion (Session 5) meditation.

Instructions

- "Please find a comfortable position, and take a few deep breaths to settle into your body and into the present moment. You might like to put your hand over your heart, or wherever it feels comforting and supportive, as a reminder to bring affectionate awareness to your experience and to yourself."

- "Bring to mind someone you are caring for who is exhausting you or frustrating you—someone you care about who is suffering. For this introductory practice, please choose someone who is *not* your child, as this can be a more complicated dynamic. Visualize the person and the caregiving situation clearly in your mind, and feel the struggle in your own body."

- "Now please listen carefully to these words, letting them gently roll through your mind:
  - 'Everyone is on their own life journey.' (*Pause*) 'I am not the cause of this person's suffering, nor is it entirely within my power to make it go away, even though I wish I could.' (*Pause*) 'Moments like these can be difficult to bear, yet I may still try to help if I can.' "

- "Aware of the stress you are carrying in your body, inhale fully and deeply, drawing compassion inside your body, filling every cell of your body with compassion. Letting yourself be soothed by inhaling deeply, and by giving yourself the compassion you need." (*Pause*)

- "And as you exhale, sending out compassion to the person who is associated with your discomfort." (*Pause*)

- "Continue breathing compassion in and out, allowing your body to gradually find a natural breathing rhythm—letting your body breathe itself."

- " 'One for me, one for you.' 'In for me, out for you.' "

- "Occasionally scanning your inner landscape for any distress and responding by inhaling compassion for yourself and exhaling compassion for others."

- "If you find that anyone needs *extra* compassion, directing your breath in that direction."

- "Noticing how your body is being caressed from the inside as you breathe."

- "Letting yourself float on an ocean of compassion—a limitless ocean that embraces all suffering." (*Pause*)

- "And listening to these words once again:
  - 'Everyone is on their own life journey.' (*Pause*) 'I am not the cause of this person's suffering, nor is it entirely within my power to make it go away, even though I wish I could.' (*Pause*) 'Moments like these can be difficult to bear, yet I may still try to help if I can.' "
- "Now letting go of the practice and allowing yourself to be exactly as you are in this moment."
- "Gently open your eyes."

Settling and Reflection

Teachers give participants a minute or two to let the practice settle, especially allowing them to linger with any words, sensations, or feelings that have provided a sense of relief or freedom.

Inquiry

Caregivers generally appreciate the permission that Compassion with Equanimity gives them to see their limits and attend to their own needs (yang self-compassion) during caregiving. This may be especially challenging for women, who are socialized to subordinate their needs to those of others. Some participants bring their children to mind when they do this practice, even though they have been advised against it. We discourage working with one's children the first time around because parents of young children tend to believe they are indeed the *sole* causes of their children's suffering. However, even parents of young children can derive great benefit from the practice after they understand the wisdom of equanimity—namely, that how we think and feel is the result of an infinite array of interdependent factors, most of which are beyond our understanding or control. This insight releases the heart and mind to be compassionate in a realistic, sustainable manner. Consider the following inquiry.

> BARBARA: I am taking care of both of my elderly parents at the moment. They are still living in their home, but my father is often incontinent, and my mother is refusing to put him in assisted living or to go into assisted living with him. I can see that it's taking a toll on her. We never had a great relationship, but now she's angrier than ever.
>
> TEACHER: It sounds like you are in a very tough position, Barbara. May I ask what it was like when you heard the equanimity phrases during the practice?
>
> BARBARA: What a relief! I think I let out a loud sigh. I hope I didn't disturb anyone!

TEACHER: Was there some part of the phrases that spoke to you the most?

BARBARA: Yes, just reminding myself about our different life journeys. I could see the whole trajectory of my mother's life, and how she survived by being tough, principled, and often angry. I realized that's just the way she is, and I'm not to blame when she's angry at me.

TEACHER: That sounds important to know, Barbara. And what was it like to breathe in for yourself and out for your mom?

BARBARA: I guess the breathing came pretty easy. I really wanted to breathe in for myself because I felt sorry about my pain—sorry for how I have been treated by my mother. And then I started feeling sorry about her pain. It was kind of like feeling compassion for myself opened my heart more to her. I was really breathing out for her, for her sad situation. It really isn't fair that people have to suffer so much in old age.

TEACHER: Yes, it's not fair. And I'm appreciating how opening to your own sadness allowed you to see what may be behind your mother's anger. That's compassion. You seem to have experienced the essence of this practice the first time around. Do you think you can bring what you learned here to your visits with your parents?

BARBARA: Yes, I believe so. I want to write the equanimity phrases on a card and keep them in my car, and I also want to breathe in and out when I'm there. I'll see how it goes.

TEACHER: Yes, let's see. Thank you, Barbara.

This inquiry flowed smoothly because Barbara simply wanted to share her process and the relief it brought. Barbara might have been tempted to share more of her story, but the teacher elegantly redirected her to the practice itself, and Barbara unpacked for the whole group how the equanimity phrases created space for her to understand her mother better, as well as to be kinder to herself. This was the intention of the practice, which Barbara illustrated by sharing her experience. Finally, the teacher validated Barbara's capacity for compassion and helped Barbara create a bridge between her classroom experience and her daily life.

Some caregivers do not feel entitled to breathe in for themselves. They can be reminded of the oxygen mask metaphor in an airplane: "When the air pressure in the cabin drops, put on your own oxygen mask first before assisting others." Teachers can also point out that a newborn baby has to breathe in before it can breathe out, and that everyone in the delivery room is waiting anxiously to see the child breathe in. Not only is inhalation necessary for survival, but others *want* us to breathe in for ourselves, even as adults!

Home Practice
(5 minutes)

The new practices learned in this session were:

- Compassionate Friend
- Self-Compassion Break in Relationships
- Compassion with Equanimity

In addition, some participants may want the instructions for the Meeting Unmet Needs exercise. This exercise can be found in *The Mindful Self-Compassion Workbook*.

Students who have emotional residue from this exercise are advised to apply the skills they have learned so far—not to make the difficulty go away, but simply because compassion is a healthy way to respond.

The next session is the last meeting in the MSC course. The coming week is a good time for participants to review all the practices they have learned during the course, and to note down what practices they might like to continue after the course ends. Participants are also invited to bring anything they might like to share at the last class, such as a poem, a short story, or a personal reflection. Students should not feel obligated to bring anything to the last class because the closing ceremony provides an opportunity for each person to contribute.

Closing
(2 minutes)

Teachers can close Session 7 with one-word shares, with a moment of silence, or with the poem "Compassion" by Miller Williams (1997). This poem has also been set to music and recorded by his daughter, Lucinda Williams (2014). Some teachers like to adapt Miller Williams's poem for *self*-compassion by changing a few key pronouns to refer to oneself.

Chapter 18

Session 8

EMBRACING YOUR LIFE

Overview

Opening Meditation: Compassion for Self and Others

Session Theme: Embracing Your Life

Topic: Cultivating Happiness

Topic: Savoring and Gratitude

Informal Practice: Gratitude for Small Things

Topic: Self-Appreciation

Informal Practice: Appreciating Our Good Qualities

Break

Soft Landing

Exercise: What Would I Like to Remember?

Topic: Tips for Maintaining a Practice

Closing

Getting Started

- In this session, participants will:
  - Learn to practice savoring, gratitude, and self-appreciation, to correct the human negativity bias.
  - Reflect on key insights and practices that each participant might like to remember after the course ends.
- These subjects are introduced now to:
  - Help participants cultivate happiness as a support for compassion training.
  - Encourage ongoing practice *after* the MSC program.
  - Close the program in a positive, uplifting manner.
- New practices taught this session:
  - Compassion for Self and Others
  - Gratitude for Small Things
  - Appreciating Our Good Qualities

 ## Compassion for Self and Others
(25 minutes)

This new meditation expands the use of loving-kindness and compassion phrases to include any sentient beings that may arise in a participant's mind, one after another, thereby making the mind a friendly, compassionate place to inhabit. Participants are invited to extend their compassion practice to others after their own need for compassion is met.

Teachers can make the point that even if the world does not change, we can still live happy lives by cultivating a kind and compassionate attitude toward every living being who appears in our minds.

Instructions

- "Please sit in a comfortable position, close your eyes, and take three, deep, relaxing breaths."
- "Placing a hand over your heart or another soothing place, and letting yourself feel the gentle touch or the warmth of your hand."
- "Then opening to the world of sensation in your body—the pulsations and vibrations—noticing how it feels to have a human body right now." (*Pause*)
- "Beginning to connect with your breathing, feeling the sensation of breathing in and breathing out." (*Pause*)

- "Now beginning to offer yourself some kindness—perhaps just breathing in for yourself again and again, or offering yourself an inner smile with each breath, or letting some words ride on your breathing, such as 'May I be happy and free from suffering.'" (*Long pause*)

- "When you are ready, allowing yourself to be aware of any persons or other living beings that may enter your mind. When someone appears, sending something good to that person—perhaps a relaxing out-breath, an inner smile, or words such as 'May *you* be happy and free from suffering.'" (*Long pause*)

- "Lingering with this being for a while and offering good wishes for as long as you like, any way you like, and then waiting for the next being to appear in your mind."

- "Letting the process be slow and easy, lingering for at least a few breaths with each being."

- "Returning at any time to *yourself*—returning to home base—whenever you need to, for as long as you like." (*Long pause*)

- "And then opening again to whoever appears in your mind."

- "Finally, letting go of the meditation and allowing yourself to feel exactly what you are feeling and to be just as you are, if only for this one moment."

Settling and Reflection

As usual, teachers should give their participants a chance to absorb their experience of this meditation, and then to reflect on what they just experienced.

Inquiry

Depending on how much time is available, teachers should feel free to skip inquiry on this meditation and go straight to the topic of the day. If inquiry is conducted, however, it might go something like this:

> ZOE: Well, that was pretty intense.
>
> TEACHER: Would you like to share?
>
> ZOE: The meditation started out pretty easy. My kids popped up, and I sent them loving-kindness. My friends came to mind, and I sent them loving-kindness. I was having a lovely time. But then all these people started showing up that I didn't like very much. My ex-boss. A political figure who shall remain unnamed. I tried to send them loving-kindness, but I couldn't. I just felt numb. So then I did what you said and returned to myself, for feeling numb.

That's when things started to shift, and believe it or not, I actually started to feel some goodwill even toward the politician. I said, "May you grow in wisdom and compassion." But it wasn't snarky; I actually *felt* it. I wasn't expecting that. Then my heart just expanded—like it had no boundaries. It was amazing.

TEACHER: Right now your face is so radiant. It's beautiful to see. Thank you for sharing, Zoe.

In this inquiry, the teacher's only task was to be present for Zoe's experience and to share her joy.

In addition to being a loving-kindness and compassion meditation, in some ways Compassion for Self and Others is also a mindfulness meditation—*mindfulness of living beings*—because we bring loving awareness to any sentient beings that arise in our minds, one after another. Inevitably, challenging persons will show up in our minds, providing an opportunity to practice switching between compassion for others and compassion for ourselves (recharging our batteries), depending on what is needed to maintain a kind and compassionate state of mind.

Embracing Your Life
(1 minute)

Session 8, Embracing Your Life, contains practices that help participants to recognize and enjoy the *positive* aspects of their lives, including themselves. It also prepares students to embrace their lives *after* the course has ended by encouraging ongoing mindfulness and self-compassion practice.

Cultivating Happiness
(5 minutes)

Over the past seven sessions, the MSC curriculum has focused primarily on *negative* experiences and on the potential of mindfulness and self-compassion to transform these into something positive. After all, compassion is a positive emotion. However, life is a mixture of good and bad, bitter and sweet. This session focuses on how to get the most out of the *positive* experiences in our lives, and our positive qualities, so that we can enjoy *all* the moments of our lives more fully. It is also necessary to savor the good in our lives in order to sustain the energy and optimism required for compassion training.

As discussed in Session 2 (Chapter 11), the mind is evolutionarily predisposed to focus on problems. The psychological term for this tendency is the *negativity bias* (Rozin & Royzman, 2001). As Rick Hanson (2013, p. xxvi) has quipped, we are "Velcro for bad experiences and Teflon for good ones." Negative emotions (e.g., fear, anger, shame) also narrow our perceptual field, whereas positive emotions (e.g., joy, peace, love) broaden our awareness (Fredrickson, 2004a). Helen Keller (2000, p. 25) wrote, "When one door of happiness closes, another opens, but often we look so long at the closed door that we do not see the one that has been opened for us."

In this session, we teach three ways to cultivate happiness by correcting for the negativity bias:

- Savoring
- Gratitude
- Self-appreciation

Teachers may wish to read the poem "The Word," by Tony Hoagland (2011). This poem illustrates the importance of including pleasure in our lives, among the many other items on our to-do lists.

Savoring and Gratitude
(10 minutes)

Savoring

Savoring is mindfulness of positive experience. It refers to *recognizing* pleasant experience, *allowing* oneself to be drawn into it, *lingering* with it, and *letting it go*. Research indicates that this simple practice can greatly increase happiness and life satisfaction (see Bryant & Veroff, 2007; Quoidbach, Berry, Hansenne, & Mikolajczak, 2010). Savoring (of positive memories) has also been shown to increase activity in brain areas (striatum and medial prefrontal cortex) associated with positive emotions and resiliency (Speer, Bhanji, & Delgado, 2014).

Two examples of savoring have already been introduced during the MSC retreat: the Sense and Savor Walk, and Savoring Food. In both of these practices, the instruction is to "give yourself permission" or "allow yourself" to enjoy the experience, rather than to "try to enjoy yourself." The simple pleasure of lingering with positive sensations and emotions can be a radical discovery for striving mindfulness and compassion practitioners. The following instructions can be given as an example of savoring:

- "Any pleasant experience can become a savoring exercise. For example, we can rub our hands together and simply notice the sensations in the hands as we do this." (*Demonstrate the motions.*)
- "Or we can slowly and gently rub our hands together, allowing ourselves to *enjoy* the sensations of rubbing our hands together." (*Continue to demonstrate.*)
- "Does this little shift in intention—the intention to savor—alter your experience in any way?"

Teachers can then solicit comments from the class. In this session, the teachers only need to point out that most mindfulness exercises can be practiced as savoring exercises, rather than introducing new savoring practices.

Gratitude

Gratitude means appreciating the good things that life has given us. If we just focus on what we want but *don't* have, we'll remain in a negative state of mind. Abundant research shows that gratitude practice enhances physical and emotional well-being (Dickens, 2017; Emmons & McCullough, 2004; Jackowska, Brown, Ronaldson, & Steptoe, 2016; Wood, Froh, & Geraghty, 2010).

Gratitude is also a *wisdom* practice. One component of wisdom is understanding the complexity of a situation, or recognizing how every event is interdependent with other events (Olendzki, 2012). When we practice gratitude, we are acknowledging the many factors, large and small, that contribute to our lives. We can say that gratitude is the *texture* of wisdom; it is how wisdom feels. Moreover, gratitude is a *relational* practice and a *connection* practice. The joy that arises from gratitude may be attributed, in part, to freedom from the illusion of separateness and insight into interdependence.

Teachers can show a video to their students to illustrate the power of gratitude. Here are two options:

* David Steindl-Rast, a Benedictine monk, speaking about "gratefulness." To access this video, go to *https://gratefulness.org* and click first on "Practice" and then on "A Good Day" for the 5-minute video.
* Selma Baraz, the 91-year-old mother of meditation teacher James Baraz, describing the gratitude practice her son taught her: how to finish complaints with the phrase " . . . and my life is truly blessed." This charming video can be found on YouTube (*www.youtube.com/watch?v=FRbL46mWx9w*).

Gratitude for Small Things
(10 minutes)

The following informal practice of "counting blessings" demonstrates how gratitude can generate positive emotions (Fredrickson, 2004b). It is based on research (Emmons & McCullough, 2003; Krejtz, Nezlek, Michnicka, Holas, & Rusanowska, 2016) and adapted from an exercise developed by Dutch mindfulness teacher David Dewulf.

Instructions

- "Please write down 10 *small and insignificant* things—things you usually overlook—that make you feel grateful, even things in this room. Examples are buttons, rubber tires, warm water, a genuine smile, or eyeglasses." (*Wait until about 80% of the group has finished writing.*)
- "Now please say out loud, popcorn-style, one or two things *you're* grateful for."

Once everyone has mentioned at least one thing, teachers ask the group members how they feel after identifying and sharing what they are grateful for.

Discussion

Most participants remark that they feel happier after this practice, which provides experience-based evidence that gratitude can elicit happiness. However, some participants are likely to feel *worse* if they criticize themselves for not feeling happy. In that case, teachers can point out that others may have the same reaction, and can encourage a self-compassionate response.

Participants should be invited to continue the Gratitude for Small Things practice every day, perhaps at the end of the day while lying in bed before they fall asleep. They can note 10 small things that happened during the day that they feel grateful for, one thing per finger.

Self-Appreciation
(10 minutes)

Self-appreciation is the third way of cultivating happiness presented in Session 8. The first two—savoring and gratitude—provide a foundation for self-appreciation. Appreciating our good qualities means that we have the capacity to savor them, and we need gratitude toward those who have helped us in order to appreciate our strengths without feeling vulnerable and alone. The following teaching points set the stage for participants to appreciate their good qualities.

Teachers can start by asking, "Did anyone notice in the gratitude exercise that they forgot to include personal qualities in their gratitude list?" We can be grateful for many things in our lives, large and small, but we are rarely grateful for positive qualities in ourselves. We tend to criticize ourselves and focus on our inadequacies and take our good qualities for granted. This gives us a skewed perspective of who we are. As an example, a teacher can ask, "Is there anyone in the room who finds it difficult to receive a compliment?" Ordinarily, when we receive a compliment, it bounces right off us, but when we receive the slightest negative feedback, we fixate on it. It may feel uncomfortable even to *think* about what's good about ourselves.

Teachers can then ask, "Why is it so hard to celebrate, or be grateful, for our good qualities?" Students are likely to offer up a variety of suggestions:

- "We don't want to alienate our friends by seeming to brag."
- "Good qualities are not problems that need to be fixed."
- "We're afraid of falling off our pedestal."
- "It may cause jealousy."
- "It makes us feel more alone."

If we apply the three components of self-compassion to our positive qualities, we can be more self-appreciative. First, we need to be *mindful* of our good qualities rather than taking them for granted. Second, we need to be *kind* to ourselves by expressing our appreciation. Finally, we need to remember *common humanity* so we don't feel separate from or superior to others.

Common humanity is especially important in the practice of self-appreciation. Our good qualities did not arise out of thin air, or exclusively by personal effort. Rather, they were formed with the help of many other people, as well as by favorable conditions in our lives. When we contemplate the many factors that contributed to our good qualities, we may feel less alone and be more willing to accept them. Furthermore, when we appreciate our own beauty, we do so *not* because we're better than others, but because every human being has wonderful qualities in addition to not-so-wonderful qualities. We're only human. As the saying goes, "I may not be perfect, but parts of me are excellent!" Finally, self-appreciation is not selfish; it provides the emotional buoyancy and self-confidence we all need in order to give to others.

Teachers may wish to read an excerpt from Marianne Williamson's (1996) *A Return to Love* (beginning with "Our greatest fear is not that we are inadequate," p. 190), just before or at the end of the following practice, which highlights the importance of self-appreciation.

 ## Appreciating Our Good Qualities
(20 minutes)

This informal practice is an exploration of qualities that we appreciate about ourselves. Participants will also notice how much easier self-appreciation becomes when we acknowledge influences in our lives that have created and helped to support our good qualities.

Instructions

- "Please close your eyes, and let your awareness drop into your body."
- "Take a moment to think about three or four things you appreciate about yourself. (*Pause*) The first few things that come up may be somewhat superficial. See if you can open to what you *really*, deep down, like about yourself. You won't have to share this with anyone else, so please be honest." (*Long pause*)
- "If you experience any uneasiness in this practice, please make some space for whatever you're feeling, and let yourself be just as you are. Remember that you aren't saying you *always* show these good qualities, or that you're better than others. You're simply acknowledging that this, too, is true."
- "Now, please focus on *one quality in particular* that you appreciate."
- "Consider if there are any people who helped you develop this good quality—maybe friends, parents, teachers, even authors of books who had a positive impact on your life? And as you think of each positive influence, please send them some appreciation as well."
- "When we honor ourselves, we also honor those who have helped nurture us." (*Long pause*)
- "Let yourself savor, just for this moment, feeling good about yourself—let it soak in."

Inquiry

Since self-appreciation is a new practice for many participants, and it can be emotionally activating, it is often a comfort to have a period of inquiry so that participants can recognize the common humanity in their experiences.

> BEN: Okay, I will say this out loud right now . . . I'm a music student, and I have a beautiful voice. I am a strong tenor. (Gosh, that's hard to say out loud!) I have been blessed with a beautiful tenor voice. (*Pause*)
>
> TEACHER: Thank you for saying that, Ben! As you mentioned it, I was wondering: Was it easier for you to say, "I have been *blessed* with a beautiful tenor voice," or "I *have* a beautiful voice"?
>
> BEN: Yes, *blessed* was easier, perhaps because then it's not all about me.

TEACHER: That makes sense. I'm also wondering, Ben: In this exercise, were you able to acknowledge the people who helped you get where you are?

BEN: There are so many. A common thread was that I love music and work hard, but I come from a musical family, and so many people have helped me.

TEACHER: How did it feel when you expanded the circle of appreciation?

BEN: I felt very happy when I thought about these people—grateful, blessed—like I want to pass the kindness forward.

TEACHER: I'm sure you will get a chance to do that, Ben. In the meantime, how does it feel to acknowledge your beautiful voice right here in our group?

BEN: (*Long, audible exhale*) Pretty darn good! (*Smiling*)

TEACHER: Thanks, Ben.

Like most participants, Ben struggled a bit with self-appreciation when it made him feel separate from others. The teacher used inquiry to illuminate an aspect of this practice for the whole group—how gratitude toward others makes it easier to savor our own good qualities.

Some group members have much more difficulty with this practice. Here is an example of a participant who struggled.

MISSY: This was very tough for me. I come from a strict religious background. It was like I could never do anything right. I remember once when I was proud of getting the leading role in a school play, my mother told me not to get puffed up about it. That was the pattern in my whole childhood.

TEACHER: I can understand how your background might make this practice more challenging, Missy. Thanks for making that connection. Were you nonetheless able to identify one or two good qualities?

MISSY: Yes, but I started to feel queasy when I said them to myself, like something bad would happen. I think I have a lot of fear about this.

TEACHER: And how do you feel right now, talking about it?

MISSY: Same way.

TEACHER: Is there a place in your body, Missy, where you feel the fear the most?

MISSY: Yeah, my stomach . . . queasiness . . . butterflies . . .

TEACHER: Got it. Do you think you could put your hand over your stomach right now, to calm it, as you might for a child who feels afraid?

MISSY: (*Puts her hand over her stomach.*)

TEACHER: And perhaps we can all do this together (*glancing at the group*) because appreciating our good qualities can make anyone of us feel a bit queasy. (*Long pause; class members sit quietly together with their hands over their stomachs.*)

MISSY: (*Gentle tears start falling.*) Thank you, everybody.

TEACHER: We can't expect the fear to go away overnight, but do you think you can comfort yourself a little, going forward, when it comes up?

MISSY: I think so, as long as I recognize the fear and don't just space out.

TEACHER: I know you can, Missy, because you really do deserve to shine, just like that Marianne Williamson poem says—the world needs your light.

MISSY: I think it will take a while to let this sink in. I'll try, though.

TEACHER: Please do, Missy. And thank you for being so bold to speak up about the fear. This practice might have been particularly difficult for you, but you were really speaking for all of us.

MISSY: Thank you.

Appreciating Our Good Qualities is considered one of the challenging practices in the MSC program (see Chapter 6) because it poses the possibility of backdraft. Sometimes giving ourselves kindness violates an invisible contract with early caregivers, and fear arises as we anticipate rejection or criticism. Backdraft is more easily managed in the later sessions of the MSC program, due to the supportive atmosphere in the room and the self-compassion skills that participants have developed over the previous weeks. In the inquiry with Missy, the teacher capitalized on those resources (finding emotion in the body, soothing touch) and group support (common humanity). The teacher concluded the inquiry by valuing Missy (using the teacher–student relationship to facilitate *self*-appreciation) and by inviting Missy to continue using her resources outside the classroom.

Teachers may wish to close this inquiry by reading the poem "Love after Love," by Derek Walcott (1986). This poem is about greeting and welcoming the part of ourselves that loves us, knows us, and enriches our lives.

Break
(15 minutes)

Besides using the break for general refreshment, participants tend to use this final opportunity to connect or to express gratitude to one another and to the teachers.

Soft Landing
(2 minutes)

In the relaxed spirit of the final session, teachers ask participants to bring their awareness into the present moment any way they like—softly "landing their planes" in the easiest and most enjoyable way they know.

Tips for Maintaining a Practice
(12 minutes)

Participants are encouraged to continue to practice up to 30 minutes per day in any combination of formal and informal practices. Since the benefits of self-compassion training are related to how much we practice, we offer tips for how to maintain an ongoing practice. Beginning with the question "What have you discovered that helps you practice more regularly?", teachers can engage participants in an open-ended conversation about what has worked for them during the course. Many of the following points will be made by course participants, or can be added to the discussion (see also Chapter 7 for practice suggestions):

- "Make your practice as easy and pleasant as possible—self-reinforcing."
- "Start small—short practices can make a big difference."
- "Practice during daily life, when you need it the most."
- "Be compassionate when your practice lapses, and just start again."
- "Let go of any unnecessary effort."
- "Pick a consistent time to practice each day."
- "Identify obstacles to practice, and envision your way around them."
- "Use guided meditations, read books, or keep a journal."
- "Go on a retreat."
- "Stay connected—practice in community."

Mindfulness and self-compassion practice is a lifelong endeavor. For all of us, our best teacher is our authentic experience, and the most appropriate practices are the ones we find ourselves most committed to.

Practicing in Community

Participants often express an interest in continuing to meet after the MSC course ends. Toward that end, some teachers host weekly or monthly practice groups for all their students; they may encourage participants to start their own groups (sometimes providing reading material and consultation); or they may organize reunions 6–12 months down the road. Group members can also stay connected through email, Facebook, WhatsApp, or other online platforms. The Center for MSC also offers a variety of online options for continued practice (see the "Online Resources" section of Appendix C). Participants who are interested in taking their practice to a deeper level are encouraged to go on a retreat, especially one with an explicit focus on cultivating loving-kindness, compassion, and self-compassion.

Some participants express an interest in continuing to meet simply because they are not ready to say good-bye, but they are also not ready to commit to further training. For those participants, teachers can affirm the value of having learned self-compassion together, the inevitable sadness of leaving and saying good-bye, and the importance of keeping self-compassion alive in their lives.

What Would I Like to Remember?
(25 minutes)

The purposes of this exercise are to help participants (1) remember the most important lessons from the course; (2) identify which MSC practices were most meaningful or enjoyable; and (3) inspire one another by sharing insights from the MSC journey.

Instructions

- "The MSC program is nearly over, and you have learned a wide variety of principles and practices for cultivating self-compassion. You may feel overwhelmed by the sheer volume of new learning. Furthermore, learning is context-dependent, and this is the last day we will be learning together with this group in this particular place. Therefore, as a bridge to the rest of our lives, let's take a moment to reflect on what we would like to remember."

Heart Question

- "Please take out a pen and paper."
- "Please close your eyes for a moment. Then, scanning the terrain of your heart, asking yourself this question: 'What touched me, moved me, or shifted inside me during this course?'" (*Allow an adequate amount of time for writing.*)

Practice Question

- "Next, please write down any *practices* that were easiest, most enjoyable, or meaningful to you, and that you might wish to remember and practice after the program is over. You have been exposed to a variety of meditations, exercises, and informal practices in the MSC program. The question is: 'What worked for me?'" (*Long pause*)
- "We hope you will continue to practice mindfulness and self-compassion when the course ends. Feel free to customize the practices. If you customize, just remember to *keep it simple* and *keep it warm*."

Small-Group Discussion

- "Now please form groups of three to four persons, and informally share with one another—for about 5 minutes each—what you'd most like to remember from this course."

It is usually not necessary to lead inquiry or a discussion after the small-group sharing, but it can be done if there is sufficient time to do so. Students will have another opportunity to share brief reflections about the course at the end of the session.

Closing
(25 minutes)

Forgiveness

If teachers noticed any tension or interpersonal conflict during the course, they can begin the group closing by offering the same "intention to forgive" that was introduced in Session 1. However, this offering might make the closing unnecessarily solemn. Also, some participants might not be ready to forgive. Therefore, only if it feels just right, teachers can say on behalf of themselves and all of the participants:

- "Please forgive *me* for any hurt that I may have unconsciously caused you during this course." (*Asking for forgiveness*)
- "May we all forgive *ourselves* for any hurt that we may have unconsciously caused someone else." (*Forgiving ourselves*)
- "And may we forgive *others,* or at least be open to the *possibility* of forgiveness, for any hurt that others may have caused us, probably unconsciously, during this course." (*Giving forgiveness*)

Sharing

A heartwarming group activity should be used to bring the course to a close. If participants were invited last week to bring something to today's session (e.g., a reflection, poem, story, song), now would be the time to share it. Depending on the size of the group, teachers may want to limit the time of each sharing.

Three-Word Shares

Another option is to ask participants to think of a few words that capture *something* of their experience in the MSC program—something touching, funny, profound, or otherwise memorable. In large groups (over 20 participants), everyone can stand up, clear the room of furniture, form a circle (standing shoulder to shoulder), and offer three words each.

Compassion Bowl

Alternatively, participants can be invited to take two small pieces of paper apiece and write on separate pieces:

- A compassionate wish for *oneself:* "May I . . . "
- A compassionate wish for *others:* "May all beings . . . "

Then teachers can place a bowl on the floor, perhaps near a bouquet of flowers, and ask the group members to form a circle around the bowl, again standing shoulder to shoulder. Each person (starting with the teachers) then walks up to the bowl, states a wish for oneself, deposits this slip of paper in the bowl, states a wish for others, and deposits this slip. Participants are also welcome to place their wishes silently into the bowl. Another option is to pass the bowl around the group, rather than putting the bowl in the center of the circle.

Dedication

At the end of the circle exercise, teachers can thank participants for their participation in the course, perhaps adding some words of encouragement and inspiration. They should also thank each other (if there are co-teachers) and their assistants. Then teachers can invite participants to look around the group and do the following:

- Recognize that this group will never meet in quite the same form again.
- Appreciate that we have been supported and nourished by the presence of each person in the room—our learning would not have happened without each person present.
- Offer gratitude to the many unseen persons who have made it possible for us to meet each week for this purpose, such as family, friends, those who support us financially, and many others.
- Recognize that it is a privilege to learn together in this way.
- Close by dedicating the fruits of our efforts to the benefit of *all beings*, not forgetting to include ourselves in the circle of our compassion.

Everyone in the group can then hold hands and raise them up, declaring, "We did it!" Another option is to have a group bow: Members all lift their hands in the air, then place them on the shoulders of the people beside them, and bow together.

Some groups like to have a group photo taken. This can be shared online with the group.

PART IV

Integrating Self-Compassion into Psychotherapy

Whatever your difficulties—a devastated heart, financial loss,
feeling assaulted by the conflicts around you, or a seemingly hopeless
illness—you can always remember that you are free in every moment
to set the compass of your heart to your highest intentions.
                                          —JACK KORNFIELD (2014, p. 66)

Because self-compassion can have such a powerful, beneficial effect, psychotherapists inevitably ask, "How can I integrate self-compassion into psychotherapy?" Research certainly supports this endeavor (see Chapter 3). For example, self-compassion is a key underlying mechanism of action in psychotherapy (Schanche et al., 2011); lack of self-compassion is implicated in a variety of clinical conditions (Døssing et al., 2015; Hoge et al., 2013; Krieger et al., 2013; Werner et al., 2012); early childhood experiences play an important role in the development of self-compassion (Kearney & Hicks, 2016; Pepping et al., 2015); and self-compassion seems to be helpful for psychotherapists to prevent caregiver fatigue (Beaumont et al., 2016b; Olson et al., 2015).

Chapter 19 explores the three main ways that self-compassion can be integrated into psychotherapy: (1) how *therapists* relate to themselves, (2) how *therapists* relate to their *clients,* and (3) how *clients* relate to themselves. Chapter 20 addresses special issues in this integration, such as the importance of combining wisdom with compassion in therapy, working compassionately with "parts" of ourselves, self-compassion as a process of re-parenting, ways of safely addressing trauma with self-compassion, and self-compassion as an antidote to shame in psychotherapy.

These chapters have been written expressly for therapists. Our colleague Christine Brähler, clinical psychologist and MSC teacher trainer, has been instrumental in the development of the ideas in this section (see Brähler & Neff, in press). Although we focus on self-compassion in psychotherapy, we hope that individuals in other helping professions such as physicians, nurses, social workers, coaches, educators, or members of the clergy can identify similar principles and processes at work in their own professional domains. For further training in self-compassion and psychotherapy, please inquire with the Center for Mindful Self-Compassion (*https://centerformsc.org*) or the Compassionate Mind Foundation (*https://compassionatemind.co.uk*).

Chapter 19

Mindful Self-Compassion
and Psychotherapy

Don't turn your head.
Keep looking at the bandaged place.
That's where the Light enters you.
—RUMI (in Barks, 1990, p. 97)

Self-compassion is not new to psychotherapy; it has been an important part of the history of psychotherapy for over a century, under the umbrella of *self-acceptance*. William James, Sigmund Freud, and B. F. Skinner all considered self-acceptance to be psychologically beneficial (Williams & Lynn, 2010). Carl Rogers (1951) and other humanistic therapists elevated self-acceptance to the status of a core change process in psychotherapy. Interestingly, both Freud (1914/1958b) and Rogers considered self-acceptance to be a *precursor* to acceptance of others, and this perspective became a focus of empirical investigation well into the 1980s. In the 1990s, clinical research shifted away from acceptance of the self and embraced acceptance of *moment-to-moment experience,* with the introduction of Buddhist-inspired mindfulness and acceptance-based treatments such as dialectical behavior therapy (DBT), acceptance and commitment therapy (ACT), and mindfulness-based cognitive therapy (MBCT). Recently, the pendulum has begun to swing back to include acceptance of both the experiencer (compassion) and the moment-to-moment experience (mindfulness). The exciting new development since compassion was explicitly integrated into cognitive therapy by Paul Gilbert (2000), and self-compassion was operationalized for research by Kristin Neff (2003a, 2003b), is that clinical scientists and practitioners are assembling a solid research base (see Chapter 4) and a range of practical skills for cultivating self-acceptance and self-compassion in psychotherapy.

Self-compassion fits within the emerging model of mindfulness-, acceptance-, and compassion-based psychotherapy (Germer & Siegel,

2012; Germer, Siegel, & Fulton, 2013; Gilbert & Proctor, 2006; Hayes et al., 2012). Within this model, some therapists focus more on mindfulness, others on acceptance, and still others on compassion as the primary mechanism of change in treatment. For example, clinicians practicing mindfulness-based therapies (Segal et al., 2013; Shapiro & Carlson, 2009; Siegel, 2010) tend to emphasize the role of attention and awareness in how we create and alleviate emotional suffering. Those practicing acceptance-based therapies (Hayes et al., 2012; Roemer, Orsillo, & Salters-Pedneault, 2008) highlight the role of nonresistance and nonavoidance of moment-to-moment experience, and they are less likely to prescribe formal meditation for their clients. And those practicing compassion-based therapies (Desmond, 2016; Gilbert, 2009; Kirby, 2017; Tirch, Schoendorff, & Silberstein, 2014) focus on care and affiliation, rather than attention and awareness, as the core mechanism for managing difficult emotions. Nonetheless, our conceptual understandings of mindfulness, acceptance, and compassion have so much overlap that self-compassion-based therapists are likely to feel at home with colleagues working in any of these modalities.

Self-compassion makes sense to most therapists. Don't most therapists hope that an authentic, empathically attuned, therapeutic relationship will eventually rub off on their clients as a friendly, internal relationship that clients can have with themselves? If you are a therapist, imagine that a client came to your office a few years ago, suffering from anxiety or depression, and became deeply self-compassionate during the course of therapy. That means that the client learned to recognize and validate her pain as it arose; that she developed an inner sense that she was not alone, even during tough times; and that her inner dialogue became mostly kind and respectful. Additionally, the client learned skills for comforting and soothing herself, as well as for protecting, providing, and motivating herself, when life became difficult. Under those circumstances, it's likely that you, her therapist, would have concluded that this client no longer required therapy because she had developed the resources to meet the inevitable challenges of life on her own.

The Line between MSC and Psychotherapy

Teachers of MSC, especially those who are also psychotherapists, are carefully instructed during MSC teacher training how *not* to turn MSC into therapy—how to simply *meet* emotional distress with mindfulness and self-compassion, rather than trying to uncover and heal old wounds. There are multiple reasons for making this distinction, including the fact that the majority of MSC teachers are not clinicians and that participants don't sign up for MSC as a type of group therapy. Even if they did, however, a clinician would not have sufficient time in an 8-week skills training program to provide the personal attention that each individual may need for deeper therapeutic work. Hence, MSC participants who wish to explore their personal lives more intensively are encouraged to seek individual counseling or psychotherapy.

What is the line between psychotherapy and a resource-building program like MSC? Consider the following inquiry after the Working with Difficult Emotions practice in Session 6, accompanied by reflections on the MSC teacher's decision-making process:

NOOR: I chose a situation in my life that makes me really angry. As I was feeling the anger, an incident came to mind that happened many years ago that I just can't forget. I keep asking myself, "Why did he do this to me?" I feel pretty stuck right now and don't know what to do.

[Teacher process: Participants were instructed in this practice to recall a current, mild-to-moderately difficult situation in their lives. Nonetheless, the practice appears to have triggered a traumatic memory in Noor. A psychotherapist might ask Noor if she would be willing to share, or *begin* to share, what happened to her. An MSC teacher, such as this one, would be more likely to steer Noor back to the Working with Difficult Emotions practice itself, expecting that what was taught in this practice would provide at least some of the emotional support that Noor might need.]

TEACHER: I can see that the anger evoked a very painful memory. May I ask you a question?

NOOR: Yes (*cautiously*).

TEACHER: Was there some place in your body where you could feel the anger more than other places?

NOOR: Well, it started in my stomach as a kind of tightness, but then moved up to my chest. I actually got through the whole practice, but I still feel tightness in my chest.

TEACHER: Is it still anger that you are feeling in your chest, or a different feeling?

[Teacher process: The teacher suspected that the emotion had changed when it moved in Noor's body—perhaps shifting to a softer emotion— and that Noor might be resisting the new emotion.]

NOOR: (*Pause*) It's . . . sadness, I think . . . confusion, sadness . . . something like that.

[Teacher process: At this point, a psychotherapist might wait to hear what Noor would say next—perhaps inquiring after a while, "May I ask what you are thinking right now?", to learn more about Noor's possible trauma. The MSC teacher chose not to invite personal details from Noor's life, which might open her to more distress or uncomfortably expose her in the group. Instead, the teacher focused on a self-compassionate *response* to her distress—the next step in the practice. By returning Noor to the process rather than the content of what she just experienced, the teacher also provided the class with a second look at the practice.]

TEACHER: I wonder how it would feel if you let the chest region of your body soften a bit, just allowing the confusion or sadness to be there?

(*Pause; Noor begins to tear up.*)

[Teacher process: A psychotherapist might be curious what thoughts or memories were evoked as Noor began to cry. However, the MSC teacher kept the conversation focused on sensations and emotions arising in the moment.]

NOOR: A bit better . . . more relaxed.

TEACHER: May I ask you another question?

NOOR: Yes.

TEACHER: I wonder what you might you say to a dear friend who was treated by someone the same way you were?

[Teacher process: The teacher decided to move on to the next part of the practice—soothing with compassionate words—to deepen Noor's experience of comforting herself, and to keep group members reflecting on their own experiences of the practice.]

NOOR: Probably nothing . . . I'd just hold her. (*Pausing, then speaking emphatically*) I'd also say, "It wasn't your fault. It was *not* your fault. He had *no right* to do that." (*Pause, then some more tears*) It just wasn't fair. This shouldn't have happened to me.

TEACHER: (*Nodding, with a long sympathetic pause*) I wonder what is it like to hear these words just now?

[Teacher process: Again, a therapist might have explored *what* wasn't fair, and validated that it wasn't fair, as well as agreeing with Noor that she was not to blame. The MSC teacher, in contrast, allowed herself just to sit for a while with Noor's pain and be moved by it.]

NOOR: It feels like a big relief . . . I've been waiting to hear words like that for years. I don't think I have cried about this for a very long time . . . I've been so angry.

TEACHER: You have probably *needed* to be angry, and now you can cry. It sounds like the pain runs pretty deep.

[Teacher process: The teacher validated Noor's ability both to contain her vulnerable emotions and to open to them, which reflects the non-fixing agenda of MSC—"being with" whatever is arising in a participant. A psychotherapist, especially a mindfulness-based therapist, might do the same.]

NOOR: Yes, it does.

TEACHER: And you said you would hold your friend. Is that something you could do for yourself now? Maybe give yourself some soothing and supportive touch? (*Pause; Noor puts both hands over her heart and rocks a little back and forth. She starts nodding her head and a small smile appears on her face.*)

TEACHER: And how are you feeling now?

[Teacher process: Since Noor was able to evoke compassion for herself in the words she would say to a friend and also in soothing touch, the teacher felt it was time to end the inquiry, but she felt she needed to ask to be sure.]

NOOR: I feel okay—a little relieved, but I think I still have a lot of crying to do. (*Smiling shyly*)

TEACHER: Probably so. Is there anything you may need going forward, maybe to comfort yourself or to feel safe?

NOOR: Oh, I'm just grateful for being able to cry, to tell you the truth. I think it's because I feel comfortable in this group, and also that I'm learning self-compassion.

TEACHER: Well, let's check in together at the end of the class, if you don't mind, just to review together how you might take care of yourself in the coming week. Can we do that?

[Teacher process: The teacher did not know the extent of Noor's trauma, so she wanted to make sure that Noor would be safe. Therapists have the benefit of a more complete psychological history on each of their clients. The MSC teacher also wanted to encourage Noor to use the skills she had learned in MSC, thereby placing responsibility for Noor's safety in her own hands. A psychotherapist might apply a similar approach, although the therapy context would allow both therapist and client to rely more fully on their relationship to support the client during difficult times.]

NOOR: I'd like that, thanks.

TEACHER: Thank you!

This inquiry illustrates the choices an MSC teacher might make to support a student without intentionally opening old wounds. Psychotherapists are likely to have noticed missed opportunities that could have helped Noor heal her past trauma. However, within the constraints of MSC, Noor probably still managed to learn important skills that would enable her to address her traumatic past and engage it safely and effectively. She had learned the resources of mindfulness and self-compassion.

Adding Therapy to Resource-Building

When we practice self-compassion, it is usually sufficient to identify our emotional pain in a *general* way—simply aware that we're struggling *while* we're struggling—before responding with self-kindness. Sometimes, however, we need to be more *specific* about what's bothering us; we need to pinpoint emotional pain that lurks invisibly in the background of our lives. Psychotherapy can go a long way toward uncovering hidden pain and meeting it with compassion. Consider the following therapy experience that one of us (Chris) had while he was still a graduate student (Germer, 2015):

> This is a mystery story, one that began several decades ago, with a single tear. The tear wasn't mine, nor did it come from any of my clients. Instead, it rolled down the cheek of my first therapist as I impassively told him the story of my father's leaving in the middle of my high school athletic awards banquet. Proudly, I'd returned from the stage after receiving my first varsity letter for soccer only to find my father's chair vacant. My mother tried to excuse his behavior, but I knew my father had simply been bored and had left. I'd grown used to my father's inaccessibility and absence, a style of parenting all too common in his Mad Men generation, but my feelings this time were amplified by the shame of needing to find a ride home for my mother and myself.
>
> I'd tried to downplay the impact of this experience with my therapist, so when I glimpsed that tear trickling down his cheek, my first thought was "Whoa, this guy must have some serious father issues of his own." But then something shifted inside me as I suddenly sensed that he was crying not for himself, but for me, for the anger and sadness I hadn't allowed myself to feel in a long time. Soon I began to sob until the tears were gradually replaced by a sense of deep peace and connection. My therapist and I didn't talk much afterward about what that tear was about, but as I walked home, the warm summer night felt different, like a loving embrace.
>
> Of all the hours I spent with my therapist, that one moment of wordless communion, feeling so completely understood and cared for, is the one that stayed with me long after just about everything else we said faded from memory. For many years, I had no language to describe what had happened or how it seemed to awaken something I'd never before known inside myself, altering the most immediate sense of what it meant to be me. And for years afterward, when I'd find myself lost or adrift, I'd return to that moment and feel a sense of kindness toward myself,

however vague it was, which gave me hope for myself and for the profession I was beginning to learn about.

This experience, early in my career as a therapist, taught me (Chris) how carefully we can hide our suffering, even from ourselves, and sometimes we need a therapeutic relationship to get to the bottom of it. The experience also taught me how a moment of genuine compassion from a therapist can plant the seed of self-compassion.

Psychotherapy is also a helpful vehicle for learning self-compassion when emotional pain is too intense or complex to manage alone. Most clinical conditions fit into this category, such as panic disorder, major depression, or substance abuse. Even people suffering from psychosis can benefit from learning self-compassion (Brähler et al., 2013; Gumley, Braehler, Laithwaite, MacBeth, & Gilbert, 2010), especially by learning to downregulate fear with self-soothing techniques. Psychotherapy provides an opportunity to work with a skilled professional who can provide support and expertise over (hopefully) a longer period of time than MSC to resolve intractable emotional difficulties.

What follows is a wide-angle view of how mindfulness and self-compassion can be taught to clients—namely, by how therapists relate to themselves (presence), by how they relate to their clients (the therapy relationship), and by how clients relate to themselves (home practice).

Therapists Relating to Themselves

Radical Acceptance

Radical acceptance refers to an attitude of non-judging and non-fixing (see Chapter 9). It is the foundation of change—an ineffable quality of mind that accepts who we are, as well as our need to change. Radical acceptance is a way of being with *all* of it.

In order to radically accept our clients, we first need to radically accept *ourselves*. This is easier said than done. Consider, for example, how you may feel when your treatment plan isn't working, or you leave a fragile client to go on vacation, or you have just had an argument with your partner about money and now you have to counsel a couple on financial concerns. You may feel hopeless, helpless, confused, or ashamed, and also self-critical for failing to live up to your standards as a person and a professional. Sometimes being a therapist can feel like one insult after another. Therapists need a lot of self-compassion.

Presence

Presence is about being with moment-to-moment experience in a clear, open, and direct way, often without thoughts or words. Presence also has an interpersonal aspect. *Therapeutic presence* (Geller, 2017) is a way of doing therapy in which the therapist is "first (a) open and *receptive* to clients' experience, attuning to their verbal and nonverbal expressions. You then (b) *attune inwardly* to your resonance with clients' in-the-moment experience, which serves as a guide to (c) *extend and promote contact*" (p. 19). This aspect of therapy is often underrated, but when we reflect on what we most hope to find in a psychotherapist, it's probably presence.

In therapy sessions, there are many good reasons why we may *not* be present as therapists. For example, in order to understand what our clients are saying, we need to make personal associations to what is being said, and we may get lost in our own stories. Another source of distraction is our responding to empathic pain by going into our heads to solve the clients' problems, rather than staying with the felt sense of the clients in our bodies. However, when we *recognize* that the mind has wandered, which is always a moment to be celebrated, we can return to presence.

Self-compassion can help us *return* to therapeutic presence (Bibeau, Dionne, & Leblanc, 2016). For example, when we feel anxious during therapy, our perceptual field narrows and we focus on reducing the threat, usually a threat to our personal well-being. This is the opposite of mindfulness, or presence. In contrast, compassion is based on the physiology of care, which activates oxytocin and the endorphins (see Chapter 10). Taking a moment of self-compassion when we feel threatened by difficult emotions will soothe and comfort the nervous system and allow us to experience more fully what we're thinking and feeling, even when it's challenging.

As we know, self-compassion is inherently beneficial, for both therapists and clients. Being in the *company* of a compassionate person, such as a therapist, can have additional rewards. Research has shown that human beings are hardwired to feel the emotional states of others in their own bodies (Bernhardt & Singer, 2012; Decety & Cacioppo, 2011; Nummenmaa et al., 2008; Singer & Lamm, 2009). This means that, under the right conditions, mental states can be trained just by therapists sitting in the same room as clients (Davidson & McEwen, 2012; Gonzalez-Liencres, Shamay-Tsoory, & Brüne, 2013; Lamm, Batson, & Decety, 2007). Therefore, the first task of compassion-based therapists is to cultivate their own compassionate presence.

Therapists Relating to Their Clients

Most of the emotional pain in our lives was created in the context of relationships and can be alleviated in relationships, especially in a *compassionate* relationship. Just consider how much better it feels when our anger is honored rather than suppressed, vulnerability is embraced rather than shamed, and trauma is validated rather than ignored.

Curiously, the term *compassion* has been relatively absent from the clinical outcome literature. We can assume that compassion has not been absent from psychotherapy; rather, it has been implied in our definition of *empathy*. Carl Rogers (1980) defined *empathy* as "the therapist's sensitive ability and willingness to understand the client's thoughts, feelings and struggles from the client's point of view. [It is] this ability to see completely through the client's eyes, to adopt his frame of reference" (p. 85). Research shows that empathy is a key ingredient in effective therapeutic relationships (Elliott, Bohart, Watson, & Greenberg, 2011; Lambert & Barley, 2001; Norcross & Wampold, 2011).

Compassion has been defined as "a multidimensional process comprised of four key components: (1) an *awareness* of suffering (cognitive/empathic awareness), (2) *sympathetic concern* related to being emotionally moved by suffering (affective component), (3) a *wish* to see the relief of that suffering (intention), and (4) a *responsiveness* or readiness to help relieve that suffering (motivational)" (Jinpa, quoted in Jazaieri et al., 2013, p. 23). In this definition of compassion, *awareness* and *concern* refer to empathy, and the *wish* and *responsiveness* to alleviate suffering are special attributes of compassion. Since the starting point of psychotherapy has always been an effort to alleviate suffering, we can assume that compassion has been implicitly included in the clinical construct of empathy.

For much of the history of psychotherapy, the *relationship* between client and therapist has been the primary treatment modality, especially in psychodynamic psychotherapy. The assumption behind psychodynamic psychotherapy is that invisible patterns of thinking, feeling, and behaving reveal themselves in how we humans relate to others—particularly in a therapeutic context, where a clinician avoids intruding on the reality of a client, and instead creates a safe container for the client's inner experience to unfold. Insight into these invisible patterns, and interacting with a therapist in healthy new ways, can create a corrective emotional experience (Alexander & French, 1946/1980).

Modern neuroscience is beginning to provide tantalizing clues for how therapeutic relationships work (Fuchs, 2004; Grawe, 2017; Siegel, 2006). Our brains are not only hardwired to *feel* what others are feeling, but, due to experience-based neuroplasticity, they are also *changed* by those with whom we interact. Lou Cozolino (2017) eloquently explains:

> Over the last century, psychotherapists have demonstrated that many of the brain's shortcomings can be counterbalanced by the application of skillfully applied techniques in the context of a caring relationship. Thus, in our ability to link, attune, and regulate each other's brains, evolution has also provided us a way to heal one another. Because we know that relationships are capable of building and rebuilding neural structures, psychotherapy can now be understood as a neurobiological intervention with a deep cultural history. In psychotherapy, we are tapping the same

principles and process available in every relationship that allow us to connect to and heal another brain. (p. 361)

Therefore, similar neurobiological processes are probably engaged during the interactions between clients and their therapists as between MSC participants and their teachers.

Similarities between Therapy and MSC Inquiry

Therapists often wonder how they might bring the subtle relational qualities of the MSC inquiry process (see Chapter 9) into the therapeutic relationship. To do so, a good starting point is to consider the three R's of inquiry—*radical acceptance, resonance,* and *resource-building.*

Radical acceptance already frames the therapeutic enterprise, as noted previously. When clients know they are accepted and not being judged, they begin to explore their experience in a fresh, open manner and make changes in their lives based on a genuine understanding of why they suffer and what they can do about it. Radical acceptance has informed psychoanalysis from its earliest origins, when "evenly suspended" or "evenly hovering" attention was considered the ideal attitude of an analyst (Freud, 1912/1958a); without it, Freud stated, the therapist "is in danger of never finding out anything but what he already knows" (1912/1958, pp. 111–112). Carl Rogers (1962) expanded this notion (and warmed it up) by suggesting that what he called "unconditional positive regard" is the key ingredient in effective therapy: "By this I mean that the counselor prizes the client in a total, rather than a conditional way. He does not accept certain feelings in the client and disapprove others" (p. 181). The actual term *radical acceptance* was first coined by Marsha Linehan (1993) to refer to the attitude that therapists need to adopt toward their clients with borderline personality disorder in order to keep them engaged and working in therapy, and as a path to emotional well-being. "Radical acceptance . . . is without discrimination. In other words, one does not choose parts of reality to accept and parts to reject. . . . The notion of radical acceptance is that of 'total allowance now'" (Robins et al., 2004, pp. 40–41).

Radical acceptance is an ideal state of mind that therapists continually slip in and out of. Radical acceptance refers to acceptance *of this moment,* even as a therapist and client work toward a more meaningful, healthier, or happier life for the client. Moments of radical acceptance not only allow clients to stop struggling and relax; they also help therapists to temporarily give up the internal tension that springs out of the wish for clients to be other than they are at a particular point in time. An argument can be made that when therapies (or schools of therapy) are reduced to improvement strategies and lose the quality of radical acceptance, their effectiveness begins to slip away.

Resonance refers to empathic attunement between the therapist and client—the state of "feeling felt" (Siegel, 2010, p. 136). The "single tear" therapy experience described earlier in this chapter is an example of a therapist resonating with a client. In a state of resonance, the voice of another person feels like one's own. The experience of resonance helps the client to internalize the conversation with the therapist and connect with his own more benign, compassionate voice.

Finally, *resource-building* has always been part of psychotherapy, insofar as therapists have needed to balance the focus on psychological deficits with an appreciation of the client's strengths and resources. An *explicit* effort to cultivate strengths and resources in therapy began in earnest with the positive psychology movement (Seligman, 2002), and again with the advent of mindfulness-based psychotherapy. The benefit of a resource-building approach to therapy extends to clinicians themselves because therapists are more likely to remain hopeful about their clients if they keep their clients' strengths and capabilities in the forefront of their minds. No matter how hard life may become for our clients, there is always hope as long as our clients can change their *relationship* to what's bothering them. Chief among the resources that can shift the relationship to seemingly unbearable circumstances are the resources of mindfulness and self-compassion.

There are additional aspects of MSC inquiry that can be meaningfully integrated into the therapy relationship, such as the *compassionate listening* process. Compassionate listening is taught to MSC students as an informal practice of the same name in Session 5 (Chapter 14), and to teacher trainees during MSC teacher training as a foundational skill for conducting inquiry. Compassionate listening is *embodied* listening— understanding the student through one's own body sensations as well as through one's ears and the eyes. In the process of compassionate listening, an MSC teacher is attentive to salient moments, or visceral *pings*, that may reflect either a moment of pain hidden among the speaker's words or evidence of a resource such as compassion, courage, or wisdom. When it is the teacher's turn to speak, finding language for the pings keeps the conversation at a deeper level—out of the mind and in the body. Such an encounter may be experienced by a student as a direct transmission of *loving-kindness* when the teacher admires a student's strengths, or as a moment of *compassion* when psychological pain is validated and tenderly embraced. The same process of embodied listening, and finding language for the visceral pings, can be applied to psychotherapy to maintain a sense of presence—*therapeutic presence* (Geller & Greenberg, 2012)—even during conversation.

Finally, the attitude of *mutuality* and *interdependence* found in MSC inquiry transfers nicely to psychotherapy. In this view, all beneficial insights arise out of a unique interpersonal field that consists of "you" and "I," but

in which the field is greater than the sum of the parts. This approach is similar to the intersubjective metatheory of modern psychoanalysis (Atwood
& Stolorow, 2014). The client and the therapist are experts on their own
lives, but neither person holds a monopoly on the truth. Both MSC inquiry
and the therapeutic conversation seem to flow most easily when they are
collaborative ventures characterized by curiosity, humility, and awareness
of everyone's limitations.

Differences between Therapy and MSC Inquiry

There are key differences between MSC inquiry and psychotherapy. The
main difference is that the purpose of psychotherapy is to *alleviate* or *cure*
a disorder, whereas the purpose of MSC inquiry is to *hold* suffering in a
mindful and compassionate way. The intention to eliminate or cure a problem in therapy can subtly introduce striving for a particular outcome and
pull both the therapist and client out of their present-moment experience.
Therefore, the challenge for mindfulness- and compassion-based psychotherapists is not to give up the idea of cure, but rather to focus on *how* the
goal is achieved—namely, by continuing to suffuse the conversation with a
mindful and compassionate attitude. When that happens, psychotherapists
and clients have the best of both worlds: They can go deeper and explore
the hidden details of the clients' lives, while also enjoying the benefits of
therapeutic presence.

Another difference between MSC inquiry and psychotherapy is the role
of *interpretation*. In MSC inquiry, a teacher only asks "what" is occurring
in a student's experience, whereas a therapist can also ask "why" something happened. For example, a person who was abused as a child is likely
to blame herself for what happened and develop the belief that she is a "bad
person." In MSC, a student would hopefully develop a more compassionate
attitude toward himself in general, but in therapy the client could explore
why the negative core belief arose in the first place and establish a more
intimate relationship with the wounded inner child. Perhaps the child was
traumatized and explicitly told by an abusive caregiver that she deserved
the treatment she received, or perhaps the child was neglected rather than
abused and didn't hear these messages, but concluded that she must *be* bad
because she *felt* so bad. Psychotherapy is an opportunity to reinterpret the
patterns of a client's life and create a new, personal narrative.

The *context* of asking questions in MSC is also different from that of
psychotherapy. In MSC, inquiry usually follows a group practice or exercise and is anchored in a student's direct experience of the preceding practice. In other words, the options for what is discussed during inquiry are
limited. In psychotherapy clients tend to talk about whatever seems most
relevant at the time, and therapists usually know a lot more about their
clients' lives so they can also follow the conversation.

Working with Empathic Distress

It is as natural for a clinician to become distracted during a therapy hour as it is for the mind to wander during meditation. Becoming distracted is not a problem per se, as long as the clinician can return to therapeutic presence. Sometimes therapists are simply too overwhelmed by the suffering of their clients—they become overidentified with it—to sustain an emotional connection with their clients or with themselves. This is a natural consequence of listening to the suffering of others, hour after hour. People unfamiliar with psychotherapy often wonder how it is even possible to do this kind of work. The answer lies in the difference between empathy and compassion, and the power of compassion to alleviate empathic distress (see also Chapter 17).

Empathy Fatigue versus Compassion Fatigue

As mentioned earlier, empathy is the capacity to *see* and *feel* the experience of others as our own. The definition of empathy does not discriminate between joy and suffering; we feel everything. But when others are suffering, we experience *empathic distress.* Compassion may *begin* with empathic distress, but compassion adds an element of goodwill—the *wish* and *effort* to alleviate the suffering.

The element of goodwill in compassion seems to mitigate the negative impact of empathic distress. Tania Singer and colleagues (Klimecki, Leiberg, Lamm, & Singer, 2012; Singer & Klimecki, 2014) have identified nonoverlapping neural networks for empathic distress and for compassion. Empathic distress activated areas associated with empathy and negative affect (the anterior insula and the anterior middle cingulate cortex), and compassion activated brain areas associated with positive affect and affiliation (the medial orbitofrontal cortex and the ventral striatum). Singer (personal communication, November 16, 2017) explains that although these brain networks are nonoverlapping when empathic distress and compassion are fully present, a moment of empathic distress is a necessary precursor for compassion to arise.

The reason therapists sometimes feel enlivened while listening to painful stories is that they are actually experiencing compassion, and compassion is a positive, energizing emotion. However, even the most loving caregivers have their limits. When they experience too much empathic distress and start to resist it, they are likely to become distracted, irritated, anxious, detached, or fatigued. The common term for this syndrome is *compassion fatigue,* but it might be better understood as *empathy fatigue* (Klimecki & Singer, 2012; see Chapter 17).

Self-Compassion for Empathic Distress

As therapists, how do we return to therapeutic presence when we are caught in empathic distress? The key is to activate compassion, starting with compassion for ourselves. A practice for doing this, Compassion with Equanimity, is taught in Session 7 (see Chapter 17). To start, when we realize that we are feeling distant and disconnected from a client—when the mind has wandered—we can return to presence by feeling the body breathing in, allowing each in-breath to be for ourselves, one in-breath after another. When we feel reconnected with ourselves, we can begin to feel the out-breath and offer the ease of each out-breath to the client. Eventually, we let the body breathe "in for me and out for you," staying in connection with the client through the natural ebb and flow of our breathing.

Usually a few breaths are all we require to return to therapeutic presence, and then we can let our breathing slip into the background of awareness and resume listening to the client. When we need to gain additional perspective or distance from what is happening in the therapy room, we can also whisper equanimity phrases to ourselves, such as "I am not the cause of this person's suffering, nor is it entirely in my power to make it go away." Together, self-compassion and equanimity reduce the tendency to overidentify with our clients' emotional pain while remaining emotionally engaged.

The shift to a compassionate state of mind is a shift from feeling threatened to a state of care. A core conceptual feature of compassion-focused therapy (Gilbert, 2009) is the three-circle model of motivation—threat, drive, and care—with each motivation having its own physiology. Being with ourselves in a compassionate manner (yin self-compassion) appears to activate the physiology of care. Therefore, when we feel emotionally overwhelmed in the consultation room, the easiest way to activate the care state is by *giving care to ourselves,* and once we feel calmed and soothed, we are in the right state of mind and can extend care to our clients. Consider the following example:

> Priscilla suffered from severe depression, and sometimes it was only the thought of suicide that helped her endure her painful life. To prove her point, Priscilla announced shortly before she left our session that she had lined up all her medicines on the night stand beside her bed, and it was a relief to know that she could "end it" whenever she needed to. Upon hearing this news, my first reaction was dread because it became clear to me that my client had both a plan and the means to end her life. Instinctively, I started thinking about how I might prevent the suicide (commit her to a hospital, wrangle a promise from Priscilla that she would not do it, engage her friends and other caregivers in a safety plan). Although these safety strategies are essential and often life-saving, I eventually realized that Priscilla was still talking, and I had not heard another word she said. Furthermore, I knew that it was important to stay in connection with Priscilla—that knowing there is one other person in the world who is aware how bad we feel can sometimes keep a person alive through a long, dark night.

To reconnect with Priscilla, I started breathing in for myself, validating how frightened I felt, reminding myself that therapy is hard work, and telling myself that I am ultimately not capable of protecting people from self-harm when they are determined to do so. I kept breathing in for myself, again and again, until I could actually hear what Priscilla was saying. Then I started breathing out for Priscilla, one breath after another. Then back and forth, in for me and out for Priscilla.

As I breathed, my focus quietly shifted from self-absorbed dread to admiration for Priscilla's capacity to endure so much despair. From the bottom of my heart, I said to Priscilla, "You amaze me . . . I don't know how you manage with all you are up against. I know that it feels hopeless sometimes, but you might be one of the strongest people I know. How *do* you do it?" In reply, Priscilla described the comfort she got from her dog, from giving food to homeless people, and from prayer. As she spoke, her mood improved, and we discussed what she might do the next time she was in the depths of despair and wanted to take her life. Just before Priscilla left the session, we gave each other a brief glance that spoke of genuine, mutual gratitude and appreciation. I knew she would be okay.

This brief vignette illustrates how feeling afraid makes a therapist disconnect from herself and from the client, and how a moment of self-compassion can begin the process of returning to therapeutic presence.

Clients Relating to Themselves

The last way that self-compassion can be integrated into psychotherapy is to create exercises and practices, or *interventions,* that clients can practice at home to cultivate self-compassion. This makes sense because we know that the human brain is plastic and changes through experience, including mental experience such as meditation (Kang et al., 2015; Lazar et al., 2005; Valk et al., 2017). Without home practice, clients might only enjoy the benefit of compassion for 1 hour per week while in the company of their therapists. With home practice, the therapy relationship becomes portable, and clients can enjoy compassion for many hours each week.

How to Approach Interventions

When therapists first discover the transformative power of self-compassion, they may be tempted to rush out and teach home practices to all their clients. This effort is well intentioned but not always helpful because clients are likely to interpret such attempts as dismissive of their struggles and the complexity of their lives. For example, it is all too common these days that a client arrives in therapy with an anxiety disorder and is told in the first session, "You should learn mindfulness meditation." In that scenario, the client arrives for therapy with one problem (anxiety) and leaves with two problems (anxiety, plus lack of mindfulness). A therapist doesn't need to add self-compassion to a client's list of perceived inadequacies. Teaching mindfulness and self-compassion practices is an important part of effective treatment, but a better way to start is for the therapist to listen carefully to what the client is saying and to reach a deep understanding of the client's dilemma. In other words, the best approach is radical acceptance.

The relational qualities of radical acceptance, resonance, presence, non-fixing, humility, and mutuality discussed earlier in this chapter are no less relevant when, as therapists, we consider teaching mindfulness and self-compassion exercises to our clients. As a kind of clinical self-discipline to reduce striving and maintain emotional resonance with our clients, it may help to give up the notion that we are actually "teaching" self-compassion, and look at it more as a process of "removing obstacles" or "unfolding the clients' resources." Another way of reducing unnecessary therapeutic striving is to avoid using the words *mindfulness* and *self-compassion* altogether, unless a client brings them up in conversation. Then the therapist and client can focus on the actual business of relating mindfully and compassionately to the client's experience. And when we keep interventions "experience-near" like that, they can be seamlessly integrated into the therapeutic relationship.

A clinical example might be Ruth, who came to therapy for help with bitter arguments she was having with her partner. These arguments were leaving Ruth increasingly angry and resentful. Her therapist thought that learning the Self-Compassion Break in Relationships (Session 7) would help Ruth disengage from such a quarrel by helping her step away from the argument, and also by shifting her frame of mind from anger to caregiving, starting with caring for herself. Rather than teaching this practice on the spot, however, the therapist decided to start by exploring Ruth's anger a little more. In that discussion, Ruth discovered that an underlying sense of loneliness, as well as desperation about losing her partner and feeling even more alone, fueled her side of these arguments. Ruth let out a sigh of relief when this insight dawned on her, whereupon the therapist wondered aloud what might happen if Ruth remembered, the next time she was in a fight with her partner, that she was not only angry but also lonely and afraid. Ruth thought it might shift her frame of mind if she just said to herself, "Loneliness . . . loneliness." The therapist added that if it felt right at the time, Ruth could also squeeze her own hand as an expression of sympathy and support.

Ruth went home and actually managed to do this small component of the practice. In the next session, she reported how doing this had made her lose her appetite for fighting. Without mentioning the Self-Compassion Break in Relationships itself, the therapist then invited Ruth to consider other elements of it, such as "This is painful" (mindfulness), "This is what loneliness feels like" (common humanity), and compassionate words such as "I love you. I am here for you." Ruth preferred, however, to stick with what she had already learned: She was hoping to reinforce the habit of feeling what lay beneath her anger, and she was also curious about the whole learning process.

Interestingly, Ruth probably would not have made this discovery if the therapist had not taken time during therapy to explore Ruth's actual experience. The rule of thumb for designing interventions is that we want to teach self-compassion *through* our clients' lived experience, not to teach our clients *about* self-compassion.

Just as self-compassion practitioners go through stages of progress (as described in Chapter 13), compassion-based therapists also go through stages of progress. Initially, therapists urgently want to prove themselves as effective therapists, and they take great pleasure when their clients improve. This is the *striving* stage, and it can get in the way of actual progress because when obstacles arise, therapists are likely to blame themselves or their clients for lack of improvement. That becomes the second stage—*disillusionment:* "What did I do wrong?" or "Why is my client sabotaging treatment?" The final stage—*radical acceptance*—comes about when a therapist opens to the fullness of a client's predicament, perhaps the slowness of change, and gets a clearer picture of the client's strengths and weaknesses. Then the therapist is in a good position to explore, with fewer preconceptions or unrealistic expectations, what may actually help the client. The three stages of development as a therapist reflect a subtle shift in therapeutic intention from "fixing" the client to "being with" the client in a compassionate way; a shift in motivation from drive to care (Gilbert, 2009).

Types of Interventions

There are 27 meditations and informal practices in the MSC program, all described in this book. Any of these practices can also be customized (indeed, *should* be customized) for the needs of individual clients. Seven of these 27 practices are formal meditations, and clients who have an inclination to meditate can access guided recordings of most of these meditations on this book's companion website (see the box at the end of the table of contents).

Short practices are especially appropriate for therapy clients, or for anyone who is not particularly interested in formal meditation. Any of the 20 *informal* practices taught in MSC can be integrated into a client's life to cultivate mindfulness and self-compassion. Additionally, each of the 14 class exercises in the MSC program contain components that can be practiced informally by clients. For example, in the Meeting Unmet Needs exercise (Session 7), participants (1) validate their experience of anger, (2) explore soft emotions that may lie behind anger, (3) identify unmet needs, and (4) learn to give themselves, verbally and/or behaviorally, what they may have been missing for a long time. Any of these elements can be applied in daily life.

The MSC curriculum also contains a brief Soft Landing in each session, immediately following the break. The Soft Landing is an opportunity to condense anything learned in the MSC course into 1–2 minutes. For example, after learning Affectionate Breathing in Session 2, a student might shorten the meditation into 2 minutes by simply savoring the internal rocking motion of the breath. After learning the Compassionate Body Scan during the retreat, a student might simply touch a part of the body that is in pain and offer that body part a word of kindness. Therapists can collaborate with their clients to develop very brief interventions, based on the principles and practices of the MSC program, that correspond to the needs, interests, and life circumstances of their clients.

Psychotherapy, especially cognitive-behavioral therapy, offers a wealth of techniques that can also be reconfigured as compassion-based interventions. For example, exposure therapy could become "compassionate exposure therapy" when clients are taught to self-soothe as they place themselves in a feared situation, or behavioral activation could include a Compassionate Letter (Session 4) to enhance motivation. The *purpose* of an intervention subtly shifts when it becomes a compassion practice. Rather than merely augmenting desensitization or behavioral activation with compassion, compassion interventions work best when the motivation behind them shifts as well. The immediate focus of a compassion intervention is to simply hold our suffering with compassion, and symptom reduction is allowed to emerge as a *side effect* of compassion. The long-term goal of alleviating emotional pain still remains the same, but the *means* by which we achieve symptom reduction is radical acceptance and compassion for what is.

The possibilities for self-compassion home practice are endless. Compassion-focused therapy (Gilbert, 2009, 2012) contains a wealth of interventions for therapy clients (see *https://compassionatemind.co.uk/ resources/audio*). These include exercises for (1) *developing an inner compassionate self*—imagining oneself as a compassionate person; (2) *compassion flowing out to others*—savoring our own compassion and extending it outward; (3) *compassion flowing into the self*—visualizing an ideal compassionate being and relating to oneself from that perspective; and (4) *compassion toward oneself*—relating to challenging parts of oneself from the perspective of our own compassionate self.

Another resource for treatment interventions is *The Mindful Self-Compassion Workbook,* which can be used by clients as an adjunct to therapy (Neff & Germer, 2018) (see also Appendices B and C). Although the MSC curriculum is probably most effective in a group format, due to the power of common humanity, some therapists use the workbook in a structured way with clients who have a personal commitment to learning self-compassion.

POINTS TO REMEMBER

* Self-compassion is an underlying mechanism of action in psychotherapy.

* MSC is therapeutic, but it is not therapy. In psychotherapy, clients have an opportunity to explore their personal lives more fully and over time, uncovering hidden wounds and making them available for a transformative, compassionate response.

* Self-compassion can be integrated into psychotherapy at three levels: (1) how therapists relate to themselves (compassionate presence), (2) how therapists relate to their clients (compassionate relationship), and (3) how clients relate to themselves (interventions/home practice).

* A therapist's *presence* (i.e., loving, connected presence) is the first step. A personal self-compassion practice can help therapists stay present while doing therapy. Presence can have a positive impact on clients through the mechanism of empathic attunement.

* The therapy *relationship* can be supported by the three R's of MSC inquiry (radical acceptance, resonance, and resource-building). A challenge in therapy is to simultaneously maintain radical acceptance and not to give up the idea of cure. Therapy has the added benefit of allowing a client to co-create a new, personal narrative with a therapist.

* Many therapists have a natural capacity for empathizing with pain, which can lead to empathy fatigue and burnout. Compassion, especially *self*-compassion, can offer therapists a buffer against empathy fatigue.

* Home practice, or *interventions,* should emerge naturally from the therapeutic dialogue and be customized, in collaboration with clients, to seamlessly integrate into clients' lives.

Chapter 20

Special Issues in Therapy

Although the world is full of suffering,
it is full also of the overcoming of it.
—HELEN KELLER (1903/2015, p. 5)

The issues addressed in this chapter are likely to arise in the context of any MSC course and have been mentioned earlier in this book. They are also common topics in psychotherapy: acting wisely in the world, working with parts of ourselves, attachment and re-parenting, and healing trauma and shame. This chapter explores ways in which self-compassion training can inform psychotherapy, as well as insights that these clinical issues can provide to MSC teachers and practitioners who are not therapists.

Compassion and Wisdom

Participants in MSC classes often ask, "From the standpoint of compassion, what should I *do* about [such and such] problem?" These questions cannot be answered by MSC teachers because teachers rarely know enough about a participant's life circumstances to do so. Therapists know a lot more about their clients' lives, but therapists still avoid giving advice because they can't know the best plan of action for another person, at another time, under another set of circumstances. The best any of us—participants, teachers, clients, and therapists—can do when the time comes is to decide for ourselves what action to take by blending as much wisdom and compassion as we can muster.

There are many definitions of *wisdom* (Siegel & Germer, 2012). One definition might be (1) understanding the complexity of a situation and (2) seeing our way through it. We rarely ever know enough about the short- and long-term consequences of our behavior to know *for sure* how

378

to proceed, but trying to understand the complexity of a situation is a good initial step toward making wise decisions.

Wisdom and compassion are "like a bird's two wings" (Ricard, in Luisi, 2008, p. 94). That means that to be fully wise, we also need to be compassionate, and to be truly compassionate, we need to be wise. Consider the following clinical example of compassion *without* wisdom:

> Early in my (Chris's) career as a clinical psychologist, I had a client, Anna, who suffered from borderline personality disorder. I was by nature a warm-hearted therapist and believed in the power of kindness, even then. What I could not understand was why this client got worse and worse in therapy. We initially met once a week for therapy and, feeling safe, Anna began to recount her early childhood trauma. Over the next few months, Anna because increasingly agitated—to the extent that it interfered with her functioning at work. I thought that Anna might need more support and offered to meet with her twice a week, which Anna eagerly accepted. Eventually, old suicidal ideation resurfaced as Anna ruminated more and more about her traumatic past. When she became a real danger to herself, Anna agreed to go into the hospital. A wise clinician at the hospital suggested that our psychotherapy was the cause of Anna's deteriorating mental condition and advised us to discontinue treatment, which we managed to do. Anna was transferred to a more experienced clinician.

This clinical error occurred before Marsha Linehan (1993) developed DBT and showed us how to help clients regulate their *own* emotions, rather than relying on the therapeutic relationship to do all the work. I recall hearing Linehan say years later, "What good is compassion if it doesn't actually *help*?" Our compassion needs to be tempered with wisdom.

Clinical wisdom includes a thorough understanding of psychopathology (in Anna's case, complex trauma), the therapy relationship (especially transference), and a healthy dose of common sense. Wisdom is also necessary to *maintain* a compassionate attitude in therapy. For example, when we understand that sometimes the only way a client with early childhood trauma can function in daily life is by projecting shame into a therapist (projective identification), our reaction is different. Clinical wisdom allows us to see the pain behind the poison and to respond with compassion, rather than react habitually with fear and anger.

Wisdom is commonly associated with perspective taking. Neuroimaging research by Tania Singer and colleagues (see Valk et al., 2017, including supplementary materials) showed that compassion and perspective-taking activate different networks in the brain. They also discovered in their 9-month study that their mindfulness/presence and compassion/affect training modules didn't necessarily lead to enhanced perspective-taking, but that a module specifically designed to enhance perspective-taking (especially "theory of mind") was more successful (Hildebrandt et al., 2017). This study suggests that different types of training have different outcomes, and that a single practice like compassion is not sufficient to achieve all goals.

For clients who want to become more self-compassionate, getting perspective on their psychological patterns through psychotherapy can help. For any of us, when we step back and develop an understanding of the causes and conditions of our struggles, we are more likely to see our actions as innocent attempts to cope with difficult circumstances and have compassion for ourselves.

Working Compassionately with Parts of Ourselves

As therapists, when we work with clients, we discover that the human personality has different parts, or selves. For example, one part may want to stop drinking, and another part may want to drink to oblivion. Or one part may have panic attacks, and another part may be strong and reliable when a crisis occurs in the family. Typically, different parts express themselves under different circumstances. Harry Stack Sullivan (1950/1964) once remarked, "For all I know, every human being has as many personalities as he has interpersonal relations" (p. 221).

Insight into these different selves also arises during meditation. The Buddhist monk Thanissaro Bhikku (2013) wrote:

> One of the first things you learn about the mind as you get started in meditation is that it has many minds. . . . Some of your "yous" are in harmony, others are incompatible, and still others are totally unrelated to one another. Each of these "yous" is a member of the committee of the mind. Each committee member is like a politician, with its own supporters and strategies for satisfying their desires . . . the mind's committee is less like a communion of saints planning a charity event, and more like a corrupt city council, with the balance of power constantly shifting between different factions, and many deals being made in back rooms. (p. 9)

Students of meditation may discover that they have different parts even *before* they meditate. A typical argument between parts can occur each morning: One part probably just wants to drink a cup of coffee and hear the morning news, and another part wants to meditate and experience the benefits of regular meditation. A special function of psychotherapy (and also of contemplative practice) is that it enables us to understand our different parts better so that we don't find ourselves inexplicably at cross-purposes with ourselves. Research also shows that learning more about our parts enhances our capacity to understand others (Böckler, Herrmann, Trautwein, Holmes, & Singer, 2017).

Internal family systems (IFS), a model of psychotherapy developed by Richard Schwartz (1995; Schwartz & Falconer, 2017), separates our parts into different categories, which Schwartz calls "protectors" (or "managers" and "firefighters") and "exiles." An exile is usually a child part—locked away, stuck in time, and bearing burdens of shame, fear, or a sense of worthlessness. Protectors keep exiles safe from harm and protect the person from the pain of exiles. Examples of a protector/manager are the "inner critic," a "people pleaser," or an "intellectual," and the function of a manager is to make the person behave properly. A protector/firefighter is often angry and tries to drown or bury difficult feelings with troublesome behaviors such as addiction or numbing. All parts have good intentions, although they are often stuck in time.

One way of conceptualizing self-compassion is to have compassion for *all* our parts, no matter what their nature or role may be. The *depth* to which we explore our parts is a difference between MSC and psychotherapy, and, generally speaking, we do not engage exile parts in the context of MSC. Rather, we might try to *understand* a protector, such as the inner critic (see Session 4), and we can *acknowledge* that an exile part may be holding pain, but teachers cannot expect to provide a safe enough container in the context of an MSC class for parts to open up and share the burdens they are carrying. That is the work of psychotherapy.

Parts do come out in MSC, however. For example, an old trauma may have been activated by an MSC exercise, and a participant could be feeling a lingering lump in the throat after the exercise ended. During inquiry, the teacher could invite the student to place a hand gently on her throat as an expression of compassion for the struggle being waged in that part of the body. If the participant remains unsettled, the teacher can gently invite the participant to talk inwardly and compassionately to the lump in the throat as if it were a part of herself. And if it feels safe enough to do so, the teacher could even invite the participant to *listen* to what that part has to say—but for no longer than 10–20 seconds, to limit the depth of engagement. In IFS therapy, however, clients can unpack the story that each part (including exiles) has to tell and meet it with compassion. Therapists who work with parts psychology notice that their clients increase their capacity to meet challenging parts with compassion when they have a self-compassion practice. In other words, IFS and MSC are increasingly seen as complementary systems of compassionate care.

Attachment and Re-Parenting

As described in Chapter 11 (Session 2), *backdraft* refers to the pain—often very old pain—that may arise when we begin to give ourselves kindness and compassion. Backdraft can emerge as negative beliefs ("I'm worthless"), repressed emotions (shame, dread, grief), or body memories (aches, pains). It refers to the principle that when we receive unconditional love, we discover the conditions under which we were *un*loved.

Most therapists have heard the expression "Sometimes it needs to get worse before it gets better." When therapists know why this phenomenon occurs, they can make therapy safer for vulnerable clients, especially those who struggle with early childhood abuse and neglect. An example of poorly managed backdraft has been given earlier in the vignette about Anna: Her trauma emerged in proportion to the amount of warmth and kindness she received in therapy. Therefore, to keep therapy safe, clients usually need to "warm up slowly."

Fortunately, backdraft is a temporary state. Backdraft usually consists of memories reexperienced in the present, rather than an ongoing problem. Ironically, we only experience backdraft *because* we feel safe enough to relax our defenses and open to old wounds. Mindfulness and self-compassion provide a sense of inner safety, and when old wounds reemerge, we can relate to them in a new, more mindful, and more compassionate manner than we experienced in the past. Backdraft is an intrinsic part of the process whereby self-compassion transforms emotional suffering.

Self-compassion training can be understood as a way of *re-parenting* ourselves. As children, we instinctively reached out to our primary caregivers for comfort and solace when we were emotionally distraught. However, due to our caregivers' limitations or the circumstances of caregiving, these efforts did not always have the expected outcome. Each frustrating or painful interaction eventually became woven into a pattern that was internalized during childhood as an attachment style (Mikulincer, Shaver, & Pereg, 2003). As adults, when we give ourselves the compassion we hoped to receive as children, our attachment wounds are often laid bare. When we *meet* these wounds with the kindness and understanding that we hoped to receive as children, we can establish a more secure base within ourselves (Ainsworth & Marvin, 1995; Bowlby, 1988; Fay, 2017; Holmes, 2001; Mikulincer & Shaver, 2017). This is the experience of feeling strong and confident that self-compassion practitioners often describe.

We usually need to *receive* compassion from others before we can bring compassion to ourselves. This is why MSC teachers focus on creating a "culture of kindness" in the classroom, and why so much attention is given to maintaining a compassionate attitude during the inquiry process. These sources of compassion may still not be enough for some individuals, especially those in severe emotional distress. In that case, a more personal relationship with a psychotherapist is a useful option for cultivating self-compassion.

The same re-parenting process described above occurs in any compassionate psychotherapy. Old wounds emerge in the context of a safe, compassionate relationship; the therapist and client respond to the wounds in a more benign, understanding manner; and gradually the conversation with the clinician is internalized by the client as his own compassionate voice. It may take years for this process to occur, however. Unfortunately, until the client has established a secure inner base to work with difficult emotions, the client may not have the inner strength to manage traumatic memories that can emerge in the relative safety of the consultation room. (This was the case with Anna.) That is when self-compassion practice, especially *behavioral* self-compassion (see Chapter 11), can be an important adjunct to psychotherapy. Over time, mental training such as cultivating a compassionate inner voice allows clients to take the therapeutic relationship with them wherever they go; it makes therapy portable.

Working with Trauma

Traumatic memories are likely to emerge during self-compassion training. In the United States, the prevalence of exposure to a traumatic event (e.g., fire, physical or sexual assault, war zone combat, disaster) is 89.7%, with multiple exposures being the norm; and the prevalence of PTSD is 8.3% (Kilpatrick et al., 2013). Therefore, MSC teachers need to know how to manage trauma that may emerge during the training, and also when to refer trauma survivors for psychotherapy.

Self-compassion training can be both a trigger and a solution for unresolved trauma. Recent research shows that how individuals *interpret* and *regulate* traumatic experiences predicts whether they will develop PTSD (Barlow et al., 2017). Self-compassion is an important resource for emotion regulation (see Chapter 2). For example, levels of trait self-compassion were found to be a stronger predictor of PTSD than levels of combat exposure (Hiraoka et al., 2015). Self-compassion was negatively related to PTSD symptom severity and emotion dysregulation in a clinical population of women with severe and repeated interpersonal trauma (Scoglio et al., 2018). Barlow and colleagues (2017) found that self-compassion is inversely associated with negative trauma appraisals (such as shame) and emotion regulation difficulties. A study of cognitive therapy for PTSD showed that self-kindness increased, and self-judgment decreased, over the course of therapy (Hoffart et al., 2015). Other research demonstrated that self-compassion practice can reduce trauma-related guilt and PTSD (Held & Owens, 2015; Kearney et al., 2013).

The three symptom clusters traditionally associated with PTSD are (1) arousal, (2) avoidance, and (3) intrusions. Interestingly, these three categories closely correspond to the stress response (fight–flight–freeze) and to the reactions to internal stress (self-criticism, isolation, and rumination) mentioned earlier (see Table 20.1). Together, they point toward self-compassion as a healthy response to trauma. Self-kindness can have a calming effect on autonomic hyperarousal; common humanity is an antidote to hiding in shame; and mindfulness allows a traumatized person to disentangle from intrusive memories and feelings. In a study of undergraduate students who

TABLE 20.1. Components of the Stress Response, PTSD, and Self-Compassion

Stress response	Stress response turned inward	PTSD symptoms	Self-compassion
Fight	Self-criticism	Arousal	Self-kindness
Flight	Isolation	Avoidance	Common humanity
Freeze	Rumination	Intrusions	Mindfulness

Note. From Germer and Neff (2015, p. 46). Copyright © 2015 The Guilford Press. Reprinted by permission.

met criteria for PTSD (mostly with adulthood traumas such as accidents or deaths), Thompson and Waltz (2008) found that the avoidance cluster of symptoms was negatively correlated with self-compassion. Self-compassion seems to protect against the development of PTSD, primarily by decreasing avoidance of emotional discomfort and facilitating desensitization.

In work with traumatized clients, especially those with early childhood trauma who have internalized their abuse (i.e., they feel they deserved it) and developed insecure attachments to caregivers, the therapeutic relationship is a key vehicle for recovery (Briere, 1992; Cloitre, Cohen, & Koenen, 2006). Some traumatized clients learned as children that "being perfect" was an effective strategy for avoiding trauma, but working too hard at self-compassion can be a prescription for excessive backdraft. Therefore, therapists may need to encourage their traumatized clients to become "slow learners" to benefit from therapy and remain safe. Trauma survivors may also need to be told to slow down their retelling of traumatic events, in order to absorb the experience of speaking with a compassionate therapist (Mendelsohn et al., 2011).

The capacity to return to safety is essential for compassion-based trauma treatment. Just as MSC teachers do for participants, therapists can teach their clients about the zones of safety (see Chapter 6, Figure 6.2), and can collaborate with the clients to help them remain in either the safe or challenged zone and stay out of the overwhelmed zone. The metaphor of opening and closing used in MSC is also applicable to psychotherapy (see Chapter 10). To move toward safety, clients need to have permission to close—that is, to disengage from whatever they are thinking about or doing that is activating their distress.

What should therapists and MSC teachers keep in mind when working with traumatized individuals who want a home practice? The overarching question that trauma survivors should ask themselves is "What do I need?" If a trauma survivor cannot answer that question, it can be made more specific: "What do I need . . . *to feel safe?*" or "What do I need . . . *to comfort and soothe myself?*" The easiest question is "How do I care for myself already?" The focus should be on practicing *behavioral* self-compassion—doing pleasant, ordinary activities as compassionate responses to suffering, such as listening to music, taking a nap, or getting some exercise. When a trauma survivor wants to engage in *mental* training, such as meditation, it is generally advisable to keep the practices short (perhaps no more than 10–15 minutes per day). The dosage of mental training is the key factor for regulating backdraft. In general, *informal* home practices are safest, such as the Self-Compassion Break taught in Session 1 (Chapter 10) or the Sense and Savor Walk taught during the retreat (Chapter 15).

Therapists and their clients should pay attention to whether doing the practices is *actually* self-compassionate—how the practice "lands" for each individual. An MSC participant once told us, with tears streaming down his face, that he typically dissociated from his body a few times a day. During the MSC course, for the first time in his life, he managed to stay in his body by putting a hand over his heart and gently rubbing his chest. That simple gesture was soothing for him (i.e., genuinely self-compassionate). Another trauma survivor, however, was triggered by the same practice. His name was Luke, and he was a therapy client who had been severely abused as a child. When Luke simply had the *thought* that he could comfort himself with a hand over his heart, voices in his head became extremely loud and told him he was "garbage" and "didn't deserve to live." With that feedback, Luke's therapist dropped the idea of home practice altogether and focused instead on keeping the therapy relationship safe and supportive.

When should MSC teachers refer their students for psychotherapy? Careful screening of MSC applicants (as described in Chapter 5) can significantly reduce the need for a therapy referral. Nevertheless, if it appears that participation in MSC is diminishing a student's ability to function (e.g., increased anxiety, depression, or poor concentration), despite recommendations to reduce the length or type of practice, then the teacher and student should have a conversation about the advisability of the student's discontinuing the course, going to psychotherapy, or both. Students who experience adverse effects during training are probably more likely to skip sessions or withdraw emotionally, rather than inform their teachers of their difficulties, so teachers should regularly ask students to share *all* types of experiences—negative as well as positive ones. For a review of meditation-related challenges that may appear during contemplative training, see Lindahl and colleagues (2017).

Self-Compassion as an Antidote to Shame

Shame is ubiquitous in psychotherapy. It is usually present from the moment clients walk through the door, perhaps feeling that they are defective and can't fix themselves without paying for help. Shame also has many masks. It can hide behind self-criticism, hostility, narcissism, or suicidality, or can lurk quietly beneath the surface of awareness as self-consciousness, embarrassment, or self-consciousness. Shame is often the glue that makes other difficult emotions so sticky, such as anxiety, grief, or anger. Shame affects therapists and clients alike (Alonso & Rutan, 1988; Hahn, 2000). It is therefore useful to identify shame and see it for what it is (Dearing & Tangney, 2011; DeYoung, 2011; Tangney & Dearing, 2002; see Chapter 16).

A formal definition of *shame* is "a complex combination of emotions, physiological responses and imagery associated with the real or imagined rupture of relational ties" (Hahn, 2000, p. 10). Judith Herman (2011), an expert in the treatment of trauma, wrote the following about shame:

> Shame is a relatively wordless state, in which speech and thought are inhibited. It is also an acutely self-conscious state; the person wishes to "sink through the floor" or "crawl in a hole and die." Shame is always implicitly a relational experience. According to Lewis (1987), one of the early pioneers in the study of shame, shame is "one's own vicarious experience of the other's scorn . . . the self-in-the-eyes-of-the-other is the focus of awareness in shame" (p. 15). . . . Thus, shame represents a complex form of mental representation in which the person imagines the mind of another. (p. 263)

Therefore, shame is constructed in the context of relationships. It is often quite arbitrary, such as when people belong to a minority that is invisible or devalued in a particular culture, or when caregivers are unable to give their children the attention required to develop a healthy sense of self.

Shame is a key component of PTSD. For example, in the aftermath of a crime, shame was the strongest predictor of PTSD 6 months later (Andrews, Brewin, Rose, & Kirk, 2000).

Shame is especially associated with PTSD from early childhood trauma. Talbot (1996) describes the process in which children are helpless to control what happens to them, are deprived of the self-confidence that comes with mastery, and have no opportunity to develop a healthy sense of self though an emotionally attuned, compassionate response from others. In that context, children are likely to conclude that they deserved what happened to them and are essentially worthless. As described in Chapter 16, the cognitive component of shame is usually a negative core belief such as "I'm worthless," "I'm defective." "I'm stupid," or "I'm unlovable."

Self-compassion is uniquely helpful as an antidote to shame (Gilbert & Procter, 2006; Johnson & O'Brien, 2013). This is because the self-worth derived from self-compassion is not contingent upon external evaluation (see Chapter 3). Rather, self-worth from self-compassion arises from the sense of feeling supported and loved, particularly when things go wrong. By activating the resource of self-compassion, we can move from "I am worthless" to "I *feel* worthless" to "I am *worthwhile*."

The first step toward meeting shame with self-compassion is *psychoeducation*—in other words, "de-shaming" shame. In psychotherapy, identifying shame for a client can be an eye-opening experience. For example, in my (Chris's) struggle with public speaking anxiety, identifying my anxiety as a shame disorder made it much easier to accept my anxiety, feel less self-conscious, and focus on the task at hand—making a speech.

Through the lens of self-compassion, shame is positively reframed in a way that has important implications for psychotherapy. This approach does not deny that the consequences of unrecognized shame can be cruel and unforgiving, such as violence, substance abuse, depression, and suicide. However, when we look deeply into shame (see also Chapter 16), we are likely to discover the following paradoxes:

- Shame feels *blameworthy,* but it is an *innocent* emotion.
- Shame makes us feel *isolated,* but it *connects* us to the rest of humanity.
- Shame feels *permanent,* but it is a *temporary* state—like all emotions.

These paradoxes correspond roughly to the three components of self-compassion—self-kindness, common humanity, and mindfulness. They also provide a roadmap for working with shame in psychotherapy. For example, the notion that shame is an innocent emotion stems from the observation that behind the rupture in relational ties that constitutes shame is the wish to be connected to others in a loving, compassionate manner. This wish is also a necessity for physical survival since infancy. When adults are caught in shame, they can say, "I just want[ed] to be loved!," and the shame is likely to subside enough to allow them to begin addressing what actually happened. Similarly, recognizing that shame is a universal emotion, and that we all feel unfit for social connection from time to time, frees us from the terrible isolation induced by shame. Finally, remembering that shame is just an emotion, with a beginning and an end, helps us disconnect our identification with shame and let it go.

A particularly poignant example of discovering the innocent wish to be loved behind shame occurred with Luke, the client mentioned above. At one point in therapy when Luke related (yet again) that he felt like garbage because his voices were telling him so, his therapist asked, "Even though you *feel* like garbage, I wonder if you have always *wished* to be loved, even though you weren't?" Luke nodded gently. Then the therapist added, "So you are saying that even though you still believe what the voices are telling you, there has always been a part of you that wanted to be loved, and never stopped wanting to be loved despite all you went through?" With tears in his eyes now, Luke softly responded, "Yes." Even though Luke *felt* he didn't deserve to be loved, he became determined to let in the love and compassion around him, as a first step toward self-compassion. He had survived as a child, and he would not give up on his deepest wish now.

The Healing Balm of Self-Compassion

Because self-compassion is essentially the process of holding pain with love, it has a unique and powerful ability to heal our wounds. Without needing to get rid of the pain or make it go away, self-compassion allows us to be with our pain in a courageous way. It uses the power of warmth and kindness to help us remain strong in the midst of struggle, allowing us to feel connected to others in the human experience of suffering. Pain is a part of life. Whether it occurs in minor, everyday ways or becomes entrenched as a clinical disorder, pain hurts. This is why we all need compassion as the wise and loving response to any moment of suffering—for our students, for our clients, for our friends, for strangers, but most of all for ourselves.

POINTS TO REMEMBER

* When we are deciding what to actions to take in our lives, compassion needs to be tempered with wisdom. *Wisdom,* including clinical wisdom, refers to understanding the complexity of a situation and choosing the most beneficial action. Wisdom is closely associated with perspective-taking.

* The personality consists of numerous parts, or selves. Both psychotherapy and MSC provide an opportunity to discover different parts and bring compassion to them, but psychotherapy provides a container for deeper parts work, especially for alleviating the burdens of wounded childhood parts.

* Self-compassion training is an opportunity to re-parent ourselves—to establish a secure inner base. Re-parenting can also occur through a therapeutic relationship. Self-compassion practice can mimic the therapy relationship, making therapy more portable.

* Due to the high prevalence of trauma in society, self-compassion training is likely to trigger old traumas. The capacity to return to safety is important in both self-compassion training and psychotherapy. Excessive zeal in self-compassion training can lead to excessive backdraft. Self-compassion is an important factor that prevents trauma from developing into PTSD.

* Self-compassion is an antidote to shame, the most difficult human emotion. A compassion-based perspective on shame suggests that shame is an innocent emotion, arising from the wish to be loved. Shame is ubiquitous in psychotherapy, and this positive approach to shame has important implications for psychotherapy.

* Self-compassion gives us the power to hold any moment of suffering with love.

Appendices

Appendix A

Ethical Guidelines

As a teacher of MSC, I am aware of my responsibility to my course participants. For this reason, I observe the following ethical guidelines:

1. *Transparency and openness.* In advance of the course, I will accurately inform all participants about the content, form, duration, and costs of the course. I will also be forthright about my own qualifications and training to teach MSC.

2. *Embracing diversity.* MSC is a learning environment that is inclusive of all. I will respect the differences between people (both visible and invisible) and will attempt to teach without biases based on differences of any kind, to the best of my ability. I will honor the unique challenges that each individual faces as we learn together to embrace our common humanity.

3. *Financial integrity.* Although I recognize that I am entitled to be fairly compensated for my time teaching MSC, my primary goal is to be of service to others, and I agree always to balance my own economic needs and those of my participants when making financial decisions such as reducing fees and granting scholarships for those in need.

4. *Respecting the integrity of the program.* Being a member of this teacher organization, I will ground my teaching in what I learned during MSC teacher training and subsequent training opportunities. I respect the integrity of the MSC curriculum, and when using the MSC trademark, I will maintain a minimum of 85% adherence to the curriculum or receive approval from the Center for Mindful Self-Compassion.

5. *Acknowledging the limitations of the program.* I am aware that MSC is not a substitute for medical or mental health treatment and I will endeavor to assure that my public communications (e.g., advertising, writing, speaking) make this clear to all prospective and current participants.

Note. Adapted with permission from the Ethical Guidelines of the German MBSR-MBCT Association (MBSR/MBCT Verband, *www.mbsr-verband.de*).

6. *Ongoing learning and personal practice.* In order to remain qualified to teach, I will stay abreast of developments in the fields of mindfulness and self-compassion and will participate in the professional community of MSC teachers. I am also aware that an ongoing personal practice of mindfulness, compassion, and self-compassion is a foundation of effective teaching.

7. *Responsibility for my relationship to participants.* I understand that to teach self-compassion, I have to be compassionate toward my students. I will take responsibility for this relationship without seeking further material or immaterial rewards and, above all else, will hold the emotional and psychological safety of my MSC participants as paramount. For this reason, I will maintain a professional teacher–student relationship with every participant while teaching an MSC course.

8. *Respect toward other teachers and programs.* I understand that being a compassionate teacher includes my behavior toward other teachers as well as toward other mindfulness- and compassion-based programs. This includes adopting a respectful and appreciative attitude—recognizing our shared goals of bringing mindfulness and compassion to the world—and not speaking in a disparaging way about other teachers or programs. I will attempt to address any existing or potential conflicts directly, in a constructive and compassionate manner.

9. *Ideological neutrality.* When teaching MSC, I will refrain from political, ideological, or religious indoctrination. I may, of course, discuss the background of MSC, or my own practice, if asked.

Appendix B

Companion Reading

While participating in an MSC course, students are encouraged to read *The Mindful Self-Compassion Workbook* (Neff & Germer, 2018), which closely follows the content and structure of MSC as described in the present book.

As students follow the course, they can also read *Self-Compassion: The Proven Power of Being Kind to Yourself* (Neff, 2011a) or *The Mindful Path to Self-Compassion* (Germer, 2009). The following outlines identify the chapters in these books that correspond to related sessions in the MSC program.

Self-Compassion: The Proven Power of Being Kind to Yourself

Session 1—Chapters 1 and 2
Session 2—Chapter 5
Session 3—Chapters 3 and 4
Session 4—Chapter 8
Session 5—Chapter 12
Session 6—Chapter 6
Session 7—Chapter 9
Session 8—Chapter 13

The Mindful Path to Self-Compassion

Session 1—Chapter 1
Session 2—Chapter 2
Session 3—Chapters 4 and 6
Session 4—Chapter 5
Session 5—Appendix B
Session 6—Chapter 3
Session 7—Chapter 7
Session 8—Chapters 8 and 9

Appendix C

Resources

Books

Baraz, J. (2012). *Awakening joy*. Berkeley, CA: Parallax Press.

Bluth, K. (2017). *The self-compassion workbook for teens*. Oakland, CA: New Harbinger.

Brach, T. (2003). *Radical acceptance: Embracing your life with the heart of a Buddha*. New York: Bantam Books.

Brown, B. (2010). *The gifts of imperfection*. Center City, MI: Hazelden.

Chödrön, P. (1997). *When things fall apart: Heart advice for difficult times*. Boston: Shambhala.

Cozolino, L. (2017). *The neuroscience of psychotherapy: Healing the social brain* (3rd ed.). New York: Norton.

Dalai Lama. (1995). *The power of compassion*. New York: HarperCollins.

Davidson, R., & Begley, S. (2012). *The emotional life of your brain*. New York: Plume.

Dearing, R. L., & Tangney, J. P. (Eds.). (2011). *Shame in the therapy hour*. Washington, DC: American Psychological Association.

Desmond, T. (2016). *Self-compassion in psychotherapy*. New York: Norton.

Desmond, T. (2017). *The self-compassion skills workbook*. New York: Norton.

Doty, J. (2016). *Into the magic shop*. New York: Avery.

Engel, B. (2010). *It wasn't your fault*. Oakland, CA: New Harbinger.

Epstein, M. (2013). *The trauma of everyday life*. New York: Penguin.

Feldman, C. (2017). *Boundless heart*. Boston: Shambhala.

Geller, S. M., & Greenberg, L. S. (2012). *Therapeutic presence: A mindful approach to effective therapy*. Washington, DC: American Psychological Association.

Germer, C. (2009). *The mindful path to self-compassion*. New York: Guilford Press.

Germer, C., & Siegel, R. (Eds.). (2012). *Wisdom and compassion in psychotherapy*. New York: Guilford Press.

Germer, C., Siegel, R., & Fulton, P. (Eds.). (2013). *Mindfulness and psychotherapy* (2nd ed.). New York: Guilford Press.

Gilbert, P. (2009). *The compassionate mind*. Oakland, CA: New Harbinger.

Gilbert, P. (Ed.). (2017). *Compassion: Concepts, research and applications.* London: Routledge.

Hanh, T. N. (1976). *The miracle of mindfulness.* Boston: Beacon Press.

Hanh, T. N. (1998). *Teaching on love.* Berkeley, CA: Parallax Press.

Hanson, R. (2009). *The Buddha's brain.* Oakland, CA: New Harbinger.

Hanson, R. (2013). *Hardwiring happiness.* New York: Harmony Books.

Hayes, S. (2005). *Get out of your mind and into your life.* Oakland, CA: New Harbinger.

Jinpa, T. (2015). *A fearless heart.* New York: Avery.

Kabat-Zinn, J. (1990). *Full catastrophe living.* New York: Dell.

Keltner, D. (2009). *Born to be good.* New York: Norton.

Kolts, R. (2016). *CFT made simple.* Oakland, CA: New Harbinger.

Kornfield, J. (1993a). *A path with heart.* New York: Bantam Books.

Kornfield, J. (1993b). *No time like the present.* New York: Atria Books.

Lieberman, M. D. (2013). *Social: Why our brains are wired to connect.* New York: Crown.

Linehan, M. M. (2015). *DBT skills training manual* (2nd ed.). New York: Guilford Press.

Makransky, J. (2007). *Awakening through love.* Somerville, MA: Wisdom.

Neff, K. (2011). *Self-compassion: The proven power of being kind to yourself.* New York: Morrow.

Neff, K. (2013). *Self-compassion: Step by step.* Louisville, CO: Sounds True.

Rosenberg, M. (2003). *Nonviolent communication: A language of life.* Encinitas, CA: Puddledancer Press.

Salzberg, S. (1995). *Lovingkindness: The revolutionary art of happiness.* Boston: Shambhala.

Salzberg, S. (2017). *Real love: The art of mindful connection.* New York: Flatiron Books.

Schwartz, R. C. (1995). *Internal family systems therapy.* New York: Guilford Press.

Schwartz, R. C., & Falconer, R. (2017). *Many minds, one self.* Oak Park, IL: Center for Self Leadership.

Seppälä, E., Simon-Thomas, E., Brown, S. L., Worline, M. C., Cameron, C. D., & Doty, J. R. (Eds.). (2017). *The Oxford handbook of compassion science.* New York: Oxford University Press.

Siegel, D. J. (2010). *Mindsight.* New York: Bantam Books.

Teasdale, J., Williams, J. M., & Segal, Z. (2014). *The mindful way workbook.* New York: Guilford Press.

Tirch, D., Schoendorff, B., & Silberstein, L. (2014). *The ACT practitioner's guide to the science of compassion: Tools for fostering psychological flexibility.* Oakland, CA: New Harbinger.

Treleaven, D. (2018). *Trauma-sensitive mindfulness.* New York: Norton.

van den Brink, E., & Koster, R. (2015). *Mindfulness-based compassionate living.* New York: Routledge.

Welford, M. (2013). *The power of self-compassion: Using compassion-focused therapy to end self-criticism and build self-confidence.* Oakland, CA: New Harbinger.

Worline, M., & Dutton, J. (2017). *Awakening compassion at work.* Oakland, CA: Berrett-Koehler.

Online Resources

Center for Mindful Self-Compassion

- Website: *https://centerformsc.org*
  - Audio and video recordings of MSC practices
  - Live online MSC courses
  - Resources to support continuing study and practice
  - Information about upcoming retreats, workshops, and other activities related to self-compassion
  - A searchable database of MSC teachers and programs worldwide
- Social media
  - Facebook page: *www.facebook.com/centerformsc*
  - Twitter: *@centerformsc*

Authors' Websites

- Christopher Germer, PhD: *https://chrisgermer.com*
  - Exercises and guided meditations
  - Videos
- Kristin Neff, PhD: *https://self-compassion.org*
  - A self-compassion test (the Self-Compassion Scale, or SCS)
  - Exercises and guided meditations
  - Videos
  - PDFs of self-compassion research

Related Websites

- Acceptance and Commitment Therapy, Association for Contextual Behavioral Science
  www.contextualscience.org/act
- Center for Compassion and Altruism Research and Education, Stanford Medicine
  http://ccare.stanford.edu
- Center for Healthy Minds, University of Wisconsin–Madison
  www.centerhealthyminds.org
- Center for Mindfulness and Compassion, Cambridge Health Alliance, Harvard Medical School Teaching Hospital
  www.chacmc.org
- Center for Mindfulness in Medicine, Health Care, and Society, University of Massachusetts Medical School
  www.umassmed.edu/cfm
- Cognitively-Based Compassion Training, Emory University, Emory–Tibet Partnership
  www.tibet.emory.edu/cognitively-based-compassion-training

- Compassion Cultivation Training, Compassion Institute
  www.compassioninstitute.com
- Compassion Focused Therapy, Compassionate Mind Foundation
  https://.compassionatemind.co.uk
- Greater Good Magazine, Greater Good Science Center at University
  of California, Berkeley
  www.greatergood.berkeley.edu
- Institute for Meditation and Psychotherapy
  www.meditationandpsychotherapy.org
- Internal Family Systems, Center for Self Leadership
  https://selfleadership.org
- Mindfulness-Based Compassionate Living
  www.compassionateliving.info
- Mindfulness-Based Cognitive Therapy
  www.mbct.com

References

Adams, C. E., & Leary, M. R. (2007). Promoting self-compassionate attitudes toward eating among restrictive and guilty eaters. *Journal of Social and Clinical Psychology, 26,* 1120–1144.

Adolphs, R. (2009). The social brain: Neural basis of social knowledge. *Annual Review of Psychology, 60,* 693–716.

Ainsworth, M., & Marvin, R. S. (1995). On the shaping of attachment theory and research: An interview with Mary D. S. Ainsworth (Fall 1994). *Monographs of the Society for Research in Child Development, 60*(2–3), 2–21. Retrieved June 17, 2017, from *www.jstor.org/stable/1166167.*

Akhtar, S., & Barlow, J. (2018). Forgiveness therapy for the promotion of mental well-being: A systematic review and meta-analysis. *Trauma, Violence, and Abuse, 19*(1), 107–122.

Albertson, E. R., Neff, K. D., & Dill-Shackleford, K. E. (2015). Self-compassion and body dissatisfaction in women: A randomized controlled trial of a brief meditation intervention. *Mindfulness, 6*(3), 444–454.

Alexander, F., & French, T. M. (1980). *Psychoanalytic therapy: Principles and application.* Lincoln: University of Nebraska Press. (Original work published 1946)

Allen, A., Barton, J., & Stevenson, O. (2015). Presenting a self-compassionate image after an interpersonal transgression. *Self and Identity, 14*(1), 33–50.

Allen, A., Goldwasser, E. R., & Leary, M. R. (2012). Self-compassion and well-being among older adults. *Self and Identity, 11*(4), 428–453.

Allen, A., & Leary, M. R. (2010). Self-compassion, stress, and coping. *Social and Personality Psychology Compass, 4*(2), 107–118.

Allen, A., & Leary, M. R. (2014). A self-compassionate response to aging. *The Gerontologist, 54*(2), 190–200.

Allen, M., Bromley, A., Kuyken, W., & Sonnenberg, S. J. (2009). Participants' experiences of mindfulness-based cognitive therapy: "It changed me in just about every way possible." *Behavioural and Cognitive Psychotherapy, 37*(4), 413–430.

Alonso, A., & Rutan, J. S. (1988). Shame and guilt in psychotherapy supervision. *Psychotherapy: Theory, Research, Practice, Training, 25*(4), 576–581.

Anderson, J. C. (2012, May 15). Maya Angelou opens women's health and wellness center, calls disparities "embarrassing." *HuffPost*. Retrieved January 23, 2019, from *www.huffingtonpost.com/2012/05/15/maya-angelou-opens-womens-health-center-calls-disparities-embarrassing_n_1517418.html?ref=black-voices*.

Andrews, B., Brewin, C. R., Rose, S., & Kirk, M. (2000). Predicting PTSD symptoms in victims of violent crime: The role of shame, anger, and childhood abuse. *Journal of Abnormal Psychology, 109*(1), 69–73.

Arao, B., & Clemens, K. (2013). From safe spaces to brave spaces. In B. Arao & K. Clemens (Eds.), *The art of effective facilitation: Reflections from social justice educators.* (pp. 135–150). Sterling, VA: Stylus.

Arch, J. J., Brown, K. W., Dean, D. J., Landy, L. N., Brown, K. D., & Laudenslager, M. L. (2014). Self-compassion training modulates alpha-amylase, heart rate variability, and subjective responses to social evaluative threat in women. *Psychoneuroendocrinology, 42*, 49–58.

Arimitsu, K., & Hofmann, S. G. (2015). Effects of compassionate thinking on negative emotions. *Cognition and Emotion, 31*(1), 160–167.

Armstrong, K. (2010). *Twelve steps to a compassionate life.* New York: Knopf.

Astin, J. (2013). This constant lover. In J. Astin, *This is always enough.* Scotts Valley, CA: CreateSpace Independent Publishing Platform.

Atkinson, D. M., Rodman, J. L., Thuras, P. D., Shiroma, P. R., & Lim, K. O. (2017). Examining burnout, depression, and self-compassion in Veterans Affairs mental health staff. *Journal of Alternative and Complementary Medicine, 23*(7), 551–557.

Atwood, G. E., & Stolorow, R. D. (2014). *Structures of subjectivity: Explorations in psychoanalytic phenomenology and contextualism.* London: Routledge.

Avalos, L., Tylka, T. L., & Wood-Barcalow, N. (2005). The Body Appreciation Scale: Development and psychometric evaluation. *Body Image, 2*(3), 285–297.

Baer, R. A. (2010). Self-compassion as a mechanism of change in mindfulness- and acceptance-based treatments. In R. A. Baer (Ed.), *Assessing mindfulness and acceptance processes in clients* (pp. 135–154). Oakland, CA: New Harbinger.

Baer, R. A., Lykins, E. L. B., & Peters, J. R. (2012). Mindfulness and self-compassion as predictors of psychological wellbeing in long-term meditators and match nonmeditators. *Journal of Positive Psychology, 7*(3), 230–238.

Baker, L. R., & McNulty, J. K. (2011). Self-compassion and relationship maintenance: The moderating roles of conscientiousness and gender. *Journal of Personality and Social Psychology, 100*, 853–873.

Barks, C. (1990). Childhood friends. In *Delicious laughter: Rambunctious teaching stories from the mathnawi of Jelaluddin Rumi.* Athens, GA: Maypop Books.

Barlow, M. R., Turow, R. E. G., & Gerhart, J. (2017). Trauma appraisals, emotion regulation difficulties, and self-compassion predict posttraumatic stress symptoms following childhood abuse. *Child Abuse and Neglect, 65*, 37–47.

Barnard, L., & Curry, J. (2011). Self-compassion: Conceptualizations, correlates, and interventions. *Review of General Psychology, 15*(4), 289–303.

Bartels-Velthuis, A. A., Schroevers, M. J., van der Ploeg, K., Koster, F., Fleer, J.,

& van den Brink, E. (2016). A mindfulness-based compassionate living training in a heterogeneous sample of psychiatric outpatients: A feasibility study. *Mindfulness, 7*(4), 809–818.

Beaumont, E., Durkin, M., Hollins Martin, C. J., & Carson, J. (2016a). Compassion for others, self-compassion, quality of life and mental well-being measures and their association with compassion fatigue and burnout in student midwives: A quantitative survey. *Midwifery, 34,* 239–244.

Beaumont, E., Durkin, M., Hollins Martin, C. J., & Carson, J. (2016b). Measuring relationships between self-compassion, compassion fatigue, burnout and well-being in student counsellors and student cognitive behavioural psychotherapists: A quantitative survey. *Counselling and Psychotherapy Research, 16*(1), 15–23.

Beaumont, E., Galpin, A., & Jenkins, P. (2012). Being kinder to myself: A prospective comparative study, exploring post-trauma therapy outcome measures, for two groups of clients, receiving either cognitive behaviour therapy or cognitive behaviour therapy and compassionate mind training. *Counseling Psychology Review, 27*(1), 31–43.

Beaumont, E., Irons, C., Rayner, G., & Dagnall, N. (2016). Does compassion-focused therapy training for health care educators and providers increase self-compassion and reduce self-persecution and self-criticism? *Journal of Continuing Education in the Health Professions, 36*(1), 4–10.

Bennett, D. S., Sullivan, M. W., & Lewis, M. (2010). Neglected children, shame-proneness, and depressive symptoms. *Child Maltreatment, 15*(4), 305–314.

Bernhardt, B. C., & Singer, T. (2012). The neural basis of empathy. *Annual Review of Neuroscience, 35,* 1–23.

Berry, W. (2012). The silence. In W. Berry, *New collected poems* (p. 127). Berkeley, CA: Counterpoint Press.

Bessenoff, G. R., & Snow, D. (2006). Absorbing society's influence: Body image self-discrepancy and internalized shame. *Sex Roles, 54*(9–10), 727–731.

Bhikku, T. (2013). With each and every breath: A guide to meditation. Retrieved January 1, 2018, from *www.dhammatalks.org/Archive/Writings/withEachAndEveryBreath_v160221.pdf.*

Bibeau, M., Dionne, F., & Leblanc, J. (2016). Can compassion meditation contribute to the development of psychotherapists' empathy?: A review. *Mindfulness, 7*(1), 255–263.

Biber, D. D., & Ellis, R. (2017). The effect of self-compassion on the self-regulation of health behaviors: A systematic review. *Journal of Health Psychology.* [Epub ahead of print]

Birnie, K., Speca, M., & Carlson, L. E. (2010). Exploring self-compassion and empathy in the context of mindfulness-based stress reduction (MBSR). *Stress and Health, 26,* 359–371.

Bishop, S. R., Lau, M., Shapiro, S., Carlson, L., Anderson, N. D., Carmody, J., et al. (2004). Mindfulness: A proposed operational definition. *Clinical Psychology: Science and Practice, 11,* 191–206.

Blatt, S. J. (1995). Representational structures in psychopathology. In D. Cicchetti & S. Toth (Eds.), *Rochester Symposium on Developmental Psychopathology: Vol. 6. Emotion, cognition, and representation* (pp. 1–34). Rochester, NY: University of Rochester Press.

Bloom, P. (2017). Empathy and its discontents. *Trends in Cognitive Sciences, 21*(1), 24–31.

Blum, L. (1980). Compassion. In A. O. Rorty (Ed.), *Explaining emotions* (pp. 507–517). Berkeley: University of California Press.

Bluth, K., & Blanton, P. W. (2015). The influence of self-compassion on emotional well-being among early and older adolescent males and females. *Journal of Positive Psychology, 10*(3), 219–230.

Bluth, K., Campo, R. A., Futch, W. S., & Gaylord, S. A. (2016). Age and gender differences in the associations of self-compassion and emotional well-being in a large adolescent sample. *Journal of Youth and Adolescence, 46*(4), 840–853.

Bluth, K., & Eisenlohr-Moul, T. A. (2017). Response to a mindful self-compassion intervention in teens: A within-person association of mindfulness, self-compassion, and emotional well-being outcomes. *Journal of Adolescence, 57,* 108–118.

Bluth, K., Gaylord, S. A., Campo, R. A., Mullarkey, M. C., & Hobbs, L. (2016). Making friends with yourself: A mixed methods pilot study of a mindful self-compassion program for adolescents. *Mindfulness, 7*(2), 479–492.

Böckler, A., Herrmann, L., Trautwein, F. M., Holmes, T., & Singer, T. (2017). Know thy selves: Learning to understand oneself increases the ability to understand others. *Journal of Cognitive Enhancement, 1*(2), 197–209.

Boellinghaus, I., Jones, F. W., & Hutton, J. (2014). The role of mindfulness and loving-kindness meditation in cultivating self-compassion and other-focused concern in health care professionals. *Mindfulness, 5*(2), 129–138.

Bowlby, J. (1988). *A secure base: Parent–child attachment and healthy human development.* New York: Basic Books.

Boykin, D. M., Himmerich, S. J., Pinciotti, C. M., Miller, L. M., Miron, L. R., & Orcutt, H. K. (2018). Barriers to self-compassion for female survivors of childhood maltreatment: The roles of fear of self-compassion and psychological inflexibility. *Child Abuse and Neglect, 76,* 216–224.

Brach, T. (2003). *Radical acceptance: Embracing your life with the heart of a Buddha.* New York: Bantam Books.

Brähler, C. (2015). *Selbstmitgefühl entwickeln.* Munich: Scorpio Verlag.

Brähler, C., Gumley, A., Harper, J., Wallace, S., Norrie, J., & Gilbert, P. (2013). Exploring change processes in compassion focused therapy in psychosis: Results of a feasibility randomized controlled trial. *British Journal of Clinical Psychology, 52*(2), 199–214.

Brähler, C., & Neff, K. (in press). Self-compassion in PTSD. In M. T. Tull & N. Kimbrel (Eds.), *Emotion in posttraumatic stress disorder.* New York: Elsevier.

Brandsma, R. (2017). *The mindfulness teaching guide.* Oakland, CA: New Harbinger.

Braun, T. D., Park, C. L., & Gorin, A. (2016). Self-compassion, body image, and disordered eating: A review of the literature. *Body Image, 17,* 117–131.

Breen, W. E., Kashdan, T. B., Lenser, M. L., & Fincham, F. D. (2010). Gratitude and forgiveness: Convergence and divergence on self-report and informant ratings. *Personality and Individual Differences, 49*(8), 932–937.

Breines, J. G., & Chen, S. (2012). Self-compassion increases self-improvement motivation. *Personality and Social Psychology Bulletin, 38*(9), 1133–1143.

Breines, J. G., & Chen, S. (2013). Activating the inner caregiver: The role of support-giving schemas in increasing state self-compassion. *Journal of Experimental Social Psychology, 49*(1), 58–64.

Breines, J. G., McInnis, C. M., Kuras, Y. I., Thoma, M. V., Gianferante, D., Hanlin, L., et al. (2015). Self-compassionate young adults show lower salivary alpha-amylase responses to repeated psychosocial stress. *Self and Identity, 14*(4), 390–402.

Breines, J. G., Thoma, M. V., Gianferante, D., Hanlin, L., Chen, X., & Rohleder, N. (2014). Self-compassion as a predictor of interleukin-6 response to acute psychosocial stress. *Brain, Behavior, and Immunity, 37*, 109–114.

Breines, J., Toole, A., Tu, C., & Chen, S. (2014). Self-compassion, body image, and self-reported disordered eating. *Self and Identity, 13*(4), 432–448.

Brewer, J. A., Garrison, K. A., & Whitfield-Gabrieli, S. (2013). What about the "self" is processed in the posterior cingulate cortex? *Frontiers in Human Neuroscience, 7*, 647.

Brewer, J. A., Mallik, S., Babuscio, T. A., Nich, C., Johnson, H. E., Deleone, C. M., et al. (2011). Mindfulness training for smoking cessation: Results from a randomized controlled trial. *Drug and Alcohol Dependence, 119*(1–2), 72–80.

Briere, J. (1992). *Child abuse trauma: Theory and treatment of the lasting effects.* Newbury Park, CA: SAGE.

Brion, J. M., Leary, M. R., & Drabkin, A. S. (2014). Self-compassion and reactions to serious illness: The case of HIV. *Journal of Health Psychology, 19*(2), 218–229.

Brito-Pons, G., Campos, D., & Cebolla, A. (2018). Implicit or explicit compassion?: Effects of compassion cultivation training and comparison with mindfulness-based stress reduction. *Mindfulness, 9*(5), 1494–1508.

Brooks, M., Kay-Lambkin, F., Bowman, J., & Childs, S. (2012). Self-compassion amongst clients with problematic alcohol use. *Mindfulness, 3*(4), 308–317.

Brown, L., Huffman, J. C., & Bryant, C. (2018). Self-compassionate aging: A systematic review. *The Gerontologist.* [Epub ahead of print]

Bryant, F., & Veroff, J. (2007). *Savoring: A new model of positive experience.* Mahwah, NJ: Erlbaum.

Buckner, R. L., Andrews-Hanna, J. R., & Schacter, D. L. (2008). The brain's default network. *Annals of the New York Academy of Sciences, 1124*(1), 1–38.

Burt, C. H., Lei, M. K., & Simons, R. L. (2017). Racial discrimination, racial socialization, and crime: Understanding mechanisms of resilience. *Social Problems, 64*(3), 414–438.

Calkins, S. D. (1994). Origins and outcomes of individual differences in emotion regulation. *Monographs of the Society for Research in Child Development, 59*(2–3), 53–72.

Campo, R. A., Bluth, K., Santacroce, S. J., Knapik, S., Tan, J., Gold, S., et al. (2017). A mindful self-compassion videoconference intervention for nationally recruited posttreatment young adult cancer survivors: Feasibility, acceptability, and psychosocial outcomes. *Supportive Care in Cancer, 25*(6), 1759–1768.

Campos, D., Cebolla, A., Quero, S., Bretón-López, J., Botella, C., Soler, J., et al. (2016). Meditation and happiness: Mindfulness and self-compassion may mediate the meditation–happiness relationship. *Personality and Individual Differences, 93*, 80–85.

Cassell, E. J. (2002). Compassion. In C. R. Snyder & S. J. Lopez (Eds.), *Handbook of positive psychology* (pp. 434–445). New York: Oxford University Press.

Chang, E. C., Yu, T., Najarian, A. S. M., Wright, K. M., Chen, W., Chang, O. D., et al. (2016). Understanding the association between negative life events and suicidal risk in college students: Examining self-compassion as a potential mediator. *Journal of Clinical Psychology, 73*(6), 745–755.

Chesterton, G. K. (2015). *Orthodoxy.* Scotts Valley, CA: CreateSpace Independent Publishing Platform. (Original work published 1908)

Chiesa, A., & Serretti, A. (2009). Mindfulness-based stress reduction for stress management in healthy people: A review and meta-analysis. *Journal of Alternative and Complementary Medicine, 15,* 593–600.

Chittister, J. (2000). *Illuminated life: Monastic wisdom for seekers of light.* Maryknoll, NY: Orbis Books.

Chödrön, P. (2001). *The wisdom of no escape and the path of loving-kindness.* Boston: Shambhala. (Original work published 1991)

Christensen, A., Doss, B., & Jacobson, N. (2014). *Reconcilable differences* (2nd ed.). New York: Guilford Press.

Claesson, K., & Sohlberg, S. (2002). Internalized shame and early interactions characterized by indifference, abandonment and rejection: Replicated findings. *Clinical Psychology and Psychotherapy, 9*(4), 277–284.

Cleare, S., Gumley, A., Cleare, C. J., & O'Connor, R. C. (2018). An investigation of the factor structure of the Self-Compassion Scale. *Mindfulness, 9*(2), 618–628.

Cloitre, M., Cohen, L. R., & Koenen, K. C. (2006). *Treating survivors of childhood abuse: Psychotherapy for the interrupted life.* New York: Guilford Press.

Collett, N., Pugh, K., Waite, F., & Freeman, D. (2016). Negative cognitions about the self in patients with persecutory delusions: An empirical study of self-compassion, self-stigma, schematic beliefs, self-esteem, fear of madness, and suicidal ideation. *Psychiatry Research, 239,* 79–84.

Collins, B. (2014). Aimless love. In B. Collins, *Aimless love: New and selected poems* (pp. 9–10). New York: Random House.

Compson, J. (2014). Meditation, trauma and suffering in silence: Raising questions about how meditation is taught and practiced in Western contexts in the light of a contemporary trauma resiliency model. *Contemporary Buddhism, 15*(2), 274–297.

Cornell, A. (2013). *Focusing in clinical practice: The essence of change.* New York: Norton.

Costa, J., Marôco, J., Pinto-Gouveia, J., Ferreira, C., & Castilho, P. (2015). Validation of the psychometric properties of the Self-Compassion Scale: Testing the factorial validity and factorial invariance of the measure among borderline personality disorder, anxiety disorder, eating disorder and general populations. *Clinical Psychology and Psychotherapy, 23*(5), 460–468.

Costa, J., & Pinto-Gouveia, J. (2011). Acceptance of pain, self-compassion and psychopathology: Using the Chronic Pain Acceptance Questionnaire to identify patients subgroups. *Clinical Psychology and Psychotherapy, 18,* 292–302.

Cousins, N. (1991). *The celebration of life: A dialogue on hope, spirit, and the immortality of the soul.* New York: Bantam Books. (Original work published 1974)

Covello, V. T., & Yoshimura, Y. (2009). *The Japanese art of stone appreciation: Suiseki and its use with bonsai.* North Clarendon, VT: Tuttle.

Covey, S. R. (2013). *The 7 habits of highly effective people: Powerful lessons in personal change.* New York: Simon & Schuster.

Cozolino, L. (2017). *The neuroscience of psychotherapy: Healing the social brain* (3rd ed.). New York: Norton.

Crane, R. S., Eames, C., Kuyken, W., Hastings, R. P., Williams, J. M. G., Bartley, T., et al. (2013). Development and validation of the Mindfulness-Based Interventions—Teaching Assessment Criteria (MBI: TAC). *Assessment, 20*(6), 681–688.

Creswell, J. D. (2015). Biological pathways linking mindfulness with health. In K. W. Brown, J. D. Creswell, & R. M. Ryan (Eds.), *Handbook of mindfulness: Theory, research, and practice* (pp. 426–440). New York: Guilford Press.

Creswell, J. D., Way, B. M., Eisenberger, N. I., & Lieberman, M. D. (2007). Neural correlates of dispositional mindfulness during affect labeling. *Psychosomatic Medicine, 69*(6), 560–565.

Crews, D., & Crawford, M. (2015). Exploring the role of being out on a queer person's self-compassion. *Journal of Gay and Lesbian Social Services, 27*(2), 172–186.

Crews, D. A., Stolz-Newton, M., & Grant, N. S. (2016). The use of yoga to build self-compassion as a healing method for survivors of sexual violence. *Journal of Religion and Spirituality in Social Work: Social Thought, 35*(3), 139–156.

Crocker, J., & Canevello, A. (2008). Creating and undermining social support in communal relationships: The role of compassionate and self-image goals. *Journal of Personality and Social Psychology, 95,* 555–575.

Crocker, J., Luhtanen, R. K., Cooper, M. L., & Bouvrette, S. (2003). Contingencies of self-worth in college students: Theory and measurement. *Journal of Personality and Social Psychology, 85,* 894–908.

Crocker, J., & Park, L. E. (2004). The costly pursuit of self-esteem. *Psychological Bulletin, 130,* 392–414.

Dahm, K., Meyer, E. C., Neff, K. D., Kimbrel, N. A., Gulliver, S. B., & Morissette, S. B (2015). Mindfulness, self-compassion, posttraumatic stress disorder symptoms, and functional disability in U.S. Iraq and Afghanistan war veterans. *Journal of Traumatic Stress, 28*(5), 460–464.

Dalai Lama. (2003). *Lighting the path: The Dalai Lama teaches on wisdom and compassion.* South Melbourne, Australia: Thomas C. Lothian.

Dalai Lama. (2012a). *Kindness, clarity, and insight.* Boston: Snow Lion. (Original work published 1984)

Dalai Lama. (2012b). Training the mind: Verse 7. Retrieved February 1, 2019, from *www.dalailama.com/teachings/training-the-mind/training-the-mind-verse-7.*

Damasio, A. R. (2004). Emotions and feelings: A neurobiological perspective. In A. S. R. Manstead, N. Frijda, & A. Fischer (Eds.), *Studies in emotion and social interaction: Feelings and emotions: The Amsterdam symposium* (pp. 49–57). Cambridge, UK: Cambridge University Press.

Davidson, R. J., & McEwen, B. S. (2012). Social influences on neuroplasticity: Stress and interventions to promote well-being. *Nature Neuroscience, 15*(5), 689–695.

Davis, D. M., & Hayes, J. A. (2011). What are the benefits of mindfulness?: A practice review of psychotherapy-related research. *Psychotherapy, 48*(2), 198–208.

Daye, C. A., Webb, J. B., & Jafari, N. (2014). Exploring self-compassion as a refuge against recalling the body-related shaming of caregiver eating messages on dimensions of objectified body consciousness in college women. *Body Image, 11*(4), 547–556.

Dearing, R. L., & Tangney, J. P. (Eds.). (2011). *Shame in the therapy hour.* Washington, DC: American Psychological Association.

Decety, J., & Cacioppo, J. T. (Eds.). (2011). *The Oxford handbook of social neuroscience.* New York: Oxford University Press.

Decety, J., & Lamm, C. (2006). Human empathy through the lens of social neuroscience. *Scientific World Journal, 6*, 1146–1163.

Deci, E. L., & Ryan, R. M. (1995). Human autonomy: The basis for true self-esteem. In M. H. Kernis (Ed.), *Efficacy, agency, and self-esteem* (pp. 31–49). New York: Plenum Press.

Delaney, M. C. (2018). Caring for the caregivers: Evaluation of the effect of an eight-week pilot mindful self-compassion (MSC) training program on nurses' compassion fatigue and resilience. *PLOS ONE, 13*(11), e0207261.

Denkova, E., Dolcos, S., & Dolcos, F. (2014). Neural correlates of "distracting" from emotion during autobiographical recollection. *Social Cognitive and Affective Neuroscience, 10*(2), 219–230.

Desbordes, G., Negi, L. T., Pace, T. W., Wallace, B. A., Raison, C. L., & Schwartz, E. L. (2012). Effects of mindful-attention and compassion meditation training on amygdala response to emotional stimuli in an ordinary, non-meditative state. *Frontiers in Human Neuroscience, 6*, 292.

Desmond, T. (2016). *Self-compassion in psychotherapy.* New York: Norton.

DeYoung, P. (2011). *Understanding and treating chronic shame: A relational, neurobiological approach.* New York: Routledge.

Diac, A. E., Constantinescu, N., Sefter, I. I., Rașia, E. L., & Târgoveçu, E. (2017). Self-compassion, well-being and chocolate addiction. *Romanian Journal of Cognitive Behavioral Therapy and Hypnosis, 4*(1–2).

Dickens, L. R. (2017). Using gratitude to promote positive change: A series of meta-analyses investigating the effectiveness of gratitude interventions. *Basic and Applied Social Psychology, 39*(4), 193–208.

Dickinson, E. (1872). Dickinson/Higginson correspondence: Late 1872. Dickinson Electronic Archives, Institute for Advanced Technology in the Humanities (IATH), University of Virginia. Retrieved July 21, 2004, from *http://jefferson.village.virginia.edu/cgi-bin/AT-Dickinsonsearch.cgi.*

Diedrich, A., Burger, J., Kirchner, M., & Berking, M. (2016). Adaptive emotion regulation mediates the relationship between self-compassion and depression in individuals with unipolar depression. *Psychology and Psychotherapy: Theory, Research and Practice, 90*(3), 247–263.

Diedrich, A., Grant, M., Hofmann, S. G., Hiller, W., & Berking, M. (2014). Self-compassion as an emotion regulation strategy in major depressive disorder. *Behaviour Research and Therapy, 58*, 43–51.

Diedrich, A., Hofmann, S. G., Cuijpers, P., & Berking, M. (2016). Self-compassion enhances the efficacy of explicit cognitive reappraisal as an emotion regulation strategy in individuals with major depressive disorder. *Behaviour Research and Therapy, 82,* 1–10.

Dodds, S. E., Pace, T. W., Bell, M. L., Fiero, M., Negi, L. T., Raison, C. L., et al. (2015). Feasibility of cognitively-based compassion training (CBCT) for breast cancer survivors: A randomized, wait-list controlled pilot study. *Supportive Care in Cancer, 23*(12), 3599–3608.

Dolcos, S., & Albarracin, D. (2014). The inner speech of behavioral regulation: Intentions and task performance strengthen when you talk to yourself as a you. *European Journal of Social Psychology, 44*(6), 636–642.

Døssing, M., Nilsson, K. K., Svejstrup, S. R., Sørensen, V. V., Straarup, K. N., & Hansen, T. B. (2015). Low self-compassion in patients with bipolar disorder. *Comprehensive Psychiatry, 60,* 53–58.

Dowd, A. J., & Jung, M. E. (2017). Self-compassion directly and indirectly predicts dietary adherence and quality of life among adults with celiac disease. *Appetite, 113,* 293–300.

Dozois, D. J., & Beck, A. T. (2008). Cognitive schemas, beliefs and assumptions. *Risk Factors in Depression, 1,* 121–143.

Duarte, C., Ferreira, C., Trindade, I. A., & Pinto-Gouveia, J. (2015). Body image and college women's quality of life: The importance of being self-compassionate. *Journal of Health Psychology, 20*(6), 754–764.

Duarte, J., McEwan, K., Barnes, C., Gilbert, P., & Maratos, F. A. (2015). Do therapeutic imagery practices affect physiological and emotional indicators of threat in high self-critics? *Psychology and Psychotherapy: Theory, Research and Practice, 88*(3), 270–284.

Duckworth, A. (2016). *Grit: The power of passion and perseverance.* New York: Simon & Schuster.

Dugo, J. M., & Beck, A. P. (1997). Significance and complexity of early phases in the development of the co-therapy relationship. *Group Dynamics: Theory, Research, and Practice, 1*(4), 294–305.

Dundas, I., Binder, P. E., Hansen, T. G., & Stige, S. H. (2017). Does a short self-compassion intervention for students increase healthy self-regulation?: A randomized control trial. *Scandinavian Journal of Psychology, 58*(5), 443–450.

Dunne, S., Sheffield, D., & Chilcot, J. (2018). Brief report: Self-compassion, physical health and the mediating role of health-promoting behaviours. *Journal of Health Psychology, 23*(7), 993–999.

Durkin, M., Beaumont, E., Hollins Martin, C. J., & Carson, J. (2016). A pilot study exploring the relationship between self-compassion, self-judgement, self-kindness, compassion, professional quality of life and wellbeing among UK community nurses. *Nurse Education Today, 46,* 109–114.

Dweck, C. S. (1986). Motivational processes affecting learning. *American Psychologist, 41,* 1040–1048.

Egan, H., Mantzios, M., & Jackson, C. (2017). Health practitioners and the directive towards compassionate healthcare in the UK: Exploring the need to educate health practitioners on how to be self-compassionate and mindful alongside mandating compassion towards patients. *Health Professions Education, 3*(2), 61–63.

Ehret, A. M., Joormann, J., & Berking, M. (2018). Self-compassion is more effective than acceptance and reappraisal in decreasing depressed mood in currently and formerly depressed individuals. *Journal of Affective Disorders, 226,* 220–226.

Eicher, A. E., Davis, L. W., & Lysaker, P. H. (2013). Self-compassion: A novel link with symptoms in schizophrenia? *Journal of Nervous and Mental Disease, 201*(5), 1–5.

Elliott, R., Bohart, A. C., Watson, J. C., & Greenberg, L. S. (2011). Empathy. *Psychotherapy, 48*(1), 43–49.

Elwafi, H. M., Witkiewitz, K., Mallik, S., Thornhill, T. A., IV, & Brewer, J. A. (2013). Mindfulness training for smoking cessation: Moderation of the relationship between craving and cigarette use. *Drug and Alcohol Dependence, 130*(1–3), 222–229.

Emerson, R. W. (1883). Spiritual laws. In R. W. Emerson, *Works of Ralph Waldo Emerson* (pp. 30–37). London: Routledge. (Original work published 1841)

Emmons, R. A., & McCullough, M. E. (2003). Counting blessings versus burdens: An experimental investigation of gratitude and subjective well-being in daily life. *Journal of Personality and Social Psychology, 84*(2), 377.

Emmons, R. A., & McCullough, M. (Eds.). (2004). *The psychology of gratitude.* New York: Oxford University Press.

Enright, R. D., & Fitzgibbons, R. P. (2000). *Helping clients forgive: An empirical guide for resolving anger and restoring hope.* Washington, DC: American Psychological Association.

Evans, S., Wyka, K., Blaha, K. T., & Allen, E. S. (2018). Self-compassion mediates improvement in well-being in a mindfulness-based stress reduction program in a community-based sample. *Mindfulness, 9*(4), 1280–1287.

Ewert, C., Gaube, B., & Geisler, F. C. M. (2018). Dispositional self-compassion impacts immediate and delayed reactions to social evaluation. *Personality and Individual Differences, 125,* 91–96.

Falconer, C. J., Slater, M., Rovira, A., King, J. A., Gilbert, P., Antley, A., et al. (2014). Embodying compassion: A virtual reality paradigm for overcoming excessive self-criticism. *PLOS ONE, 9*(11), e111933.

Faulds, D. (2002). Allow. In D. Faulds, *Go in and in: Poems from the heart of yoga.* Berkeley, CA: Peaceable Kingdom Press.

Fay, D. (2017). *Attachment-based yoga and meditation for trauma recovery: Simple, safe, and effective practices for therapy.* New York: Norton.

Fein, S., & Spencer, S. J. (1997). Prejudice as self-image maintenance: Affirming the self through derogating others. *Journal of Personality and Social Psychology, 73,* 31–44.

Ferguson, L. J., Kowalski, K. C., Mack, D. E., & Sabiston, C. M. (2015). Self-compassion and eudaimonic well-being during emotionally difficult times in sport. *Journal of Happiness Studies, 16*(5), 1263–1280.

Ferrari, M., Dal Cin, M., & Steele, M. (2017). Self-compassion is associated with optimum self-care behaviour, medical outcomes and psychological well-being in a cross-sectional sample of adults with diabetes. *Diabetic Medicine, 34*(11), 1546–1553.

Ferreira, C., Pinto-Gouveia, J., & Duarte, C. (2013). Self-compassion in the face of shame and body image dissatisfaction: Implications for eating disorders. *Eating Behaviors, 14*(2), 207–210.

Finlay-Jones, A., Kane, R., & Rees, C. (2017). Self-compassion online: A pilot study of an Internet-based self-compassion cultivation program for psychology trainees. *Journal of Clinical Psychology, 73*(7), 797–816.

Finlay-Jones, A. L., Rees, C. S., & Kane, R. T. (2015). Self-compassion, emotion regulation and stress among Australian psychologists: Testing an emotion regulation model of self-compassion using structural equation modeling. *PLOS ONE, 10*(7), e0133481.

Finlay-Jones, A., Xie, Q., Huang, X., Ma, X., & Guo, X. (2018). A pilot study of the 8-week Mindful Self-Compassion training program in a Chinese community sample. *Mindfulness, 9*(3), 993–1002.

Fredrickson, B. L. (2004a). The broaden-and-build theory of positive emotions. *Philosophical Transactions of the Royal Society of London, Series B, Biological Sciences, 359*, 1367–1378.

Fredrickson, B. L. (2004b). Gratitude, like other positive emotions, broadens and builds. In R. Emmons & M. McCullough (Eds.), *The psychology of gratitude* (pp. 145–166). New York: Oxford University Press.

Fredrickson, B. L., Cohn, M. A., Coffey, K. A., Pek, J., & Finkel, S. M. (2008). Open hearts build lives: Positive emotions, induced through loving-kindness meditation, build consequential personal resources. *Journal of Personality and Social Psychology, 95*(5), 1045–1062.

Fresnics, A., & Borders, A. (2016). Angry rumination mediates the unique associations between self-compassion and anger and aggression. *Mindfulness, 8*(3), 554–564.

Freud, S. (1958a). Recommendations to physicians on practicing psycho-analysis. In J. Strachey (Ed. & Trans.), *The standard edition of the complete psychological works of Sigmund Freud* (Vol. 12, pp. 109–120). London: Hogarth Press. (Original work published 1912)

Freud, S. (1958b). Remembering, repeating and working-through (further recommendations on the technique of psycho-analysis II). In J. Strachey (Ed. & Trans.), *The standard edition of the complete psychological works of Sigmund Freud* (Vol. 12, pp. 145–156). London: Hogarth Press. (Original work published 1914)

Friis, A. M., Johnson, M. H., Cutfield, R. G., & Consedine, N. S. (2015). Does kindness matter?: Self-compassion buffers the negative impact of diabetes-distress on HbA1c. *Diabetic Medicine, 32*(12), 1634–1640.

Friis, A. M., Johnson, M. H., Cutfield, R. G., & Consedine, N. S. (2016). Kindness matters: A randomized controlled trial of a Mindful Self-Compassion intervention improves depression, distress, and HbA1c among patients with diabetes. *Diabetes Care, 39*(11), 1963–1971.

Fuchs, T. (2004). Neurobiology and psychotherapy: An emerging dialogue. *Current Opinion in Psychiatry, 17*(6), 479–485.

Füstös, J., Gramann, K., Herbert, B. M., & Pollatos, O. (2013). On the embodiment of emotion regulation: Interoceptive awareness facilitates reappraisal. *Social Cognitive and Affective Neuroscience, 8*(8), 911–917.

Galhardo, A., Cunha, M., Pinto-Gouveia, J., & Matos, M. (2013). The mediator role of emotion regulation processes on infertility-related stress. *Journal of Clinical Psychology in Medical Settings, 20*(4), 497–507.

Galili-Weinstock, L., Chen, R., Atzil-Slonim, D., Bar-Kalifa, E., Peri, T., & Rafaeli, E. (2018). The association between self-compassion and treatment outcomes: Session-level and treatment-level effects. *Journal of Clinical Psychology, 74*(6), 849–866.

Galla, B. M. (2016). Within-person changes in mindfulness and self-compassion predict enhanced emotional well-being in healthy, but stressed adolescents. *Journal of Adolescence, 49,* 204–217.

Gallant, M. P. (2014). Social networks, social support, and health-related behavior. In L. R. Martin & M. R. DiMatteo (Eds.), *The Oxford handbook of health communication, behavior change, and treatment adherence* (pp. 305–322). New York: Oxford University Press.

Gallese, V., Eagle, M. N., & Migone, P. (2007). Intentional attunement: Mirror neurons and the neural underpinnings of interpersonal relations. *Journal of the American Psychoanalytic Association, 55*(1), 131–175.

Gard, T., Brach, N., Hölzel, B. K., Noggle, J. J., Conboy, L. A., & Lazar, S. W. (2012). Effects of a yoga-based intervention for young adults on quality of life and perceived stress: The potential mediating roles of mindfulness and self-compassion. *Journal of Positive Psychology, 7*(3), 165–175.

Garland, E. L., Fredrickson, B., Kring, A. M., Johnson, D. P., Meyer, P. S., & Penn, D. L. (2010). Upward spirals of positive emotions counter downward spirals of negativity: Insights from the broaden-and-build theory and affective neuroscience on the treatment of emotion dysfunctions and deficits in psychopathology. *Clinical Psychology Review, 30*(7), 849–864.

Geller, S. M. (2017). *A practical guide to cultivating therapeutic presence.* Washington, DC: American Psychological Association.

Geller, S. M., & Greenberg, L. S. (2012). *Therapeutic presence: A mindful approach to effective therapy.* Washington, DC: American Psychological Association.

Gendlin, E. T. (1990). The small steps of the therapy process: How they come and how to help them come. In G. Lietaer, J. Rombauts, & R. Van Balen (Eds.), *Client-centered and experiential psychotherapy in the nineties* (pp. 205–224). Leuven, Belgium: Leuven University Press.

Gerber, Z., Tolmacz, R., & Doron, Y. (2015). Self-compassion and forms of concern for others. *Personality and Individual Differences, 86,* 394–400.

Germer, C. (2009). *The mindful path to self-compassion.* New York: Guilford Press.

Germer, C. (2013). Mindfulness: What is it? What does it matter? In C. Germer, R. Siegel, & P. Fulton (Eds.), *Mindfulness and psychotherapy* (2nd ed., pp. 3–35). New York: Guilford Press.

Germer, C. (2015, September–October). Inside the heart of healing: When moment-to-moment awareness isn't enough. *Psychotherapy Networker,* Article No. 3. Retrieved January 23, 2019, from *www.psychotherapynetworker.org/magazine/article/3/inside-the-heart-of-healing.*

Germer, C., & Barnhofer, T. (2017). Mindfulness and compassion: Similarities and differences. In P. Gilbert (Ed.), *Compassion: Concepts, research and applications* (pp. 69–86). London: Routledge.

Germer, C., & Neff, K. (2013). Self-compassion in clinical practice. *Journal of Clinical Psychology, 69*(8), 856–867.

Germer, C., & Neff, K. (2015). Cultivating self-compassion in trauma survivors. In V. Follette, J. Briere, D. Rozelle, J. Hopper, & D. Rome (Eds.),

Mindfulness-oriented interventions for trauma: Integrating contemplative practices (pp. 43–58). New York: Guilford Press.

Germer, C., & Siegel, R. (Eds.). (2012). *Wisdom and compassion in psychotherapy.* New York: Guilford Press.

Germer, C., Siegel, R., & Fulton, P. (Eds.). (2013). *Mindfulness and psychotherapy* (2nd ed.). New York: Guilford Press.

Gharraee, B., Tajrishi, K. Z., Farani, A. R., Bolhari, J., & Farahani, H. (2018). A randomized controlled trial of compassion focused therapy for social anxiety disorder. *Iranian Journal of Psychiatry and Behavioral Sciences, 12*(4).

Gilbert, P. (2000). Social mentalities: Internal "social" conflicts and the role of inner warmth and compassion in cognitive therapy. In P. Gilbert & K. G. Bailey (Eds.), *Genes on the couch: Explorations in evolutionary psychotherapy* (pp. 118–150). Hove, UK: Psychology Press.

Gilbert, P. (Ed.). (2005). *Compassion: Conceptualisations, research and use in psychotherapy.* London: Routledge.

Gilbert, P. (2009). *The compassionate mind: A new approach to life's challenges.* Oakland, CA: New Harbinger.

Gilbert, P. (2012). Depression: Suffering in the flow of life. In C. Germer & R. Siegel (Eds.), *Wisdom and compassion in psychotherapy* (pp. 249–264). New York: Guilford Press.

Gilbert, P., & Andrews, B. (Eds.). (1998). *Shame: Interpersonal behavior, psychopathology, and culture.* New York: Oxford University Press.

Gilbert, P., Catarino, F., Duarte, C., Matos, M., Kolts, R., Stubbs, J., et al. (2017). The development of compassionate engagement and action scales for self and others. *Journal of Compassionate Health Care, 4.* Retrieved March 27, 2019, from *https://jcompassionatehc.biomedcentral.com/articles/10.1186/s40639-017-0033-3.*

Gilbert, P., & Choden. (2014). *Mindful compassion.* Oakland, CA: New Harbinger.

Gilbert, P., Clarke, M., Hempel, S., Miles, J. N., & Irons, C. (2004). Criticizing and reassuring oneself: An exploration of forms, styles and reasons in female students. *British Journal of Clinical Psychology, 43*(1), 31–50.

Gilbert, P., & Irons, C. (2009). Shame, self-criticism, and self-compassion in adolescence. In N. Allen & L. Sheeber (Eds.), *Adolescent emotional development and the emergence of depressive disorders* (pp. 195–214). Cambridge, UK: Cambridge University Press.

Gilbert, P., McEwan, K., Matos, M., & Rivis, A. (2011). Fears of compassion: Development of three self-report measures. *Psychology and Psychotherapy: Theory, Research and Practice, 84,* 239–255.

Gilbert, P., & Procter, S. (2006). Compassionate mind training for people with high shame and self-criticism: Overview and pilot study of a group therapy approach. *Clinical Psychology and Psychotherapy, 13,* 353–379.

Gillanders, D. T., Sinclair, A. K., MacLean, M., & Jardine, K. (2015). Illness cognitions, cognitive fusion, avoidance and self-compassion as predictors of distress and quality of life in a heterogeneous sample of adults, after cancer. *Journal of Contextual Behavioral Science, 4*(4), 300–311.

Goetz, J. L., Keltner, D., & Simon-Thomas, E. (2010). Compassion: An evolutionary analysis and empirical review. *Psychological Bulletin, 136*(3), 351–374.

Gonzalez-Hernandez, E., Romero, R., Campos, D., Burichka, D., Diego-Pedro, R., Baños, R., et al. (2018). Cognitively-based compassion training (CBCT) in breast cancer survivors: A randomized clinical trial study. *Integrative Cancer Therapies, 17*(3), 684–696.

Gonzalez-Liencres, C., Shamay-Tsoory, S. G., & Brüne, M. (2013). Towards a neuroscience of empathy: Ontogeny, phylogeny, brain mechanisms, context and psychopathology. *Neuroscience and Biobehavioral Reviews, 37*(8), 1537–1548.

Goodman, J. H., Guarino, A., Chenausky, K., Klein, L., Prager, J., Petersen, R., et al. (2014). CALM Pregnancy: Results of a pilot study of mindfulness-based cognitive therapy for perinatal anxiety. *Archives of Women's Mental Health, 17*(5), 373–387.

Grawe, K. (2017). *Neuropsychotherapy: How the neurosciences inform effective psychotherapy.* London: Routledge.

Greenberg, J., Datta, T., Shapero, B. G., Sevinc, G., Mischoulon, D., & Lazar, S. W. (2018). Compassionate hearts protect against wandering minds: Self-compassion moderates the effect of mind-wandering on depression. *Spirituality in Clinical Practice, 5*(3), 155–169.

Greenberg, L. S. (1983). Toward a task analysis of conflict resolution in Gestalt therapy. *Psychotherapy: Theory, Research and Practice, 20*(2), 190–201.

Greenberg, L., & Iwakabe, S. (2011). Emotion-focused therapy and shame. In R. L. Dearing & J. P. Tangney (Eds.), *Shame in the therapy hour* (pp. 69–90). Washington, DC: American Psychological Association.

Greene, D. C., & Britton, P. J. (2015). Predicting adult LGBTQ happiness: Impact of childhood affirmation, self-compassion, and personal mastery. *Journal of LGBT Issues in Counseling, 9*(3), 158–179.

Greeson, J. M., Juberg, M. K., Maytan, M., James, K., & Rogers, H. (2014). A randomized controlled trial of Koru: A mindfulness program for college students and other emerging adults. *Journal of American College Health, 62*(4), 222–233.

Grossman, P., Niemann, L., Schmidt, S., & Walach, H. (2004). Mindfulness-based stress reduction and health benefits: A meta-analysis. *Journal of Psychosomatic Research, 57*(1), 35–43.

Gumley, A., Braehler, C., Laithwaite, H., MacBeth, A., & Gilbert, P. (2010). A compassion focused model of recovery after psychosis. *International Journal of Cognitive Therapy, 3*(2), 186–201.

Gunnell, K. E., Mosewich, A. D., McEwen, C. E., Eklund, R. C., & Crocker, P. R. (2017). Don't be so hard on yourself!: Changes in self-compassion during the first year of university are associated with changes in well-being. *Personality and Individual Differences, 107*, 43–48.

Gusnard, D. A., & Raichle, M. E. (2001). Searching for a baseline: Functional imaging and the resting human brain. *Nature Reviews Neuroscience, 2*(10), 685–694.

Hafiz. (1999). With that moon language. In Hafiz, *The gift: Poems by Hafiz, the great Sufi master* (D. Ladinsky, Trans.). Melbourne, Australia: Penguin Books.

Hahn, W. K. (2000). Shame: Countertransference identifications in individual psychotherapy. *Psychotherapy, 37*(1), 10–21.

Halifax, J. (2012a, May 12). *Compassion and challenges to compassion: The art of living and dying.* Paper presented at the Meditation and Psychotherapy conference, Harvard Medical School, Boston, MA.

Halifax, J. (2012b, September 19). Practicing G.R.A.C.E.: How to bring compassion into your interaction with others. *The Blog, Huffington Post.* Retrieved May 31, 2017, from *https://www.huffpost.com/entry/compassion_n_1885877.*

Hall, C. W., Row, K. A., Wuensch, K. L., & Godley, K. R. (2013). The role of self-compassion in physical and psychological well-being. *Journal of Psychology, 147*(4), 311–323.

Hanh, T. N. (2014). *No mud, no lotus: The art of transforming suffering.* Berkeley, CA: Parallax Press.

Hanson, R. (2013). *Hardwiring happiness: The new brain science of contentment, calm, and confidence.* New York: Harmony Books.

Harter, S. (1999). *The construction of the self: A developmental perspective.* New York: Guilford Press.

Harwood, E. M., & Kocovski, N. L. (2017). Self-compassion induction reduces anticipatory anxiety among socially anxious students. *Mindfulness, 8*(6), 1544–1551.

Hasenkamp, W., & Barsalou, L. W. (2012). Effects of meditation experience on functional connectivity of distributed brain networks. *Frontiers in Human Neuroscience, 6,* 38.

Hatfield, E., Cacioppo, J. T., & Rapson, R. L. (1993). Emotional contagion. *Current Directions in Psychological Science, 2*(3), 96–100.

Hayes, S. C., Strosahl, K. D., & Wilson, K. G. (2012). *Acceptance and commitment therapy: The process and practice of mindful change* (2nd ed.). New York: Guilford Press.

Hayter, M. R., & Dorstyn, D. S. (2013). Resilience, self-esteem and self-compassion in adults with spina bifida. *Spinal Cord, 52*(2), 167–171.

Heath, P. J., Brenner, R. E., Vogel, D. L., Lannin, D. G., & Strass, H. A. (2017). Masculinity and barriers to seeking counseling: The buffering role of self-compassion. *Journal of Counseling Psychology, 64*(1), 94–103.

Heatherton, T. F., & Polivy, J. (1990). Chronic dieting and eating disorders: A spiral model. In J. H. Crowther, D. L. Tennenbaum, S. E. Hobfoll, & M. A. P. Stephens (Eds.), *The etiology of bulimia nervosa: The individual and familial context* (pp. 133–155). Washington, DC: Hemisphere.

Heffernan, M., Griffin, M., McNulty, S., & Fitzpatrick, J. J. (2010). Self-compassion and emotional intelligence in nurses. *International Journal of Nursing Practice, 16,* 366–373.

Heine, S. J., Lehman, D. R., Markus, H. R., & Kitayama, S. (1999). Is there a universal need for positive self-regard? *Psychological Review, 106,* 766–794.

Held, P., & Owens, G. P. (2015). Effects of self-compassion workbook training on trauma-related guilt in a sample of homeless veterans: A pilot study. *Journal of Clinical Psychology, 71,* 513–526.

Herman, J. L. (2011). Posttraumatic stress disorder as a shame disorder. In R. L. Dearing & J. P. Tangney (Eds.), *Shame in the therapy hour* (pp. 261–275). Washington, DC: American Psychological Association.

Herriot, H., Wrosch, C., & Gouin, J. P. (2018). Self-compassion, chronic age-related stressors, and diurnal cortisol secretion in older adulthood. *Journal of Behavioral Medicine, 41*(6), 850–862.

Hertenstein, M. J., Keltner, D., App, B., Bulleit, B. A., & Jaskolka, A. R. (2006). Touch communicates distinct emotions. *Emotion, 6*(3), 528–533.

Hildebrandt, L., McCall, C., & Singer, T. (2017). Differential effects of attention-, compassion-, and socio-cognitively based mental practices on self-reports of mindfulness and compassion. *Mindfulness, 8*(6), 1488–1512.

Hiraoka, R., Meyer, E. C., Kimbrel, N. A., DeBeer, B. B., Gulliver, S. B., & Morissette, S. B. (2015). Self-compassion as a prospective predictor of PTSD symptom severity among trauma-exposed US Iraq and Afghanistan war veterans. *Journal of Traumatic Stress, 28*(2), 127–133.

Hoagland, T. (2011). The word. *The writer's almanac with Garrison Keillor.* Retrieved on June 16, 2017, from *http://writersalmanac.publicradio.org/index.php?date=2011/09/10.*

Hobbs, L., & Bluth, K. (2016). *Making friends with yourself: A Mindful Self-Compassion program for teens and young adults.* Unpublished training manual.

Hoffart, A., Øktedalen, T., & Langkaas, T. F. (2015). Self-compassion influences PTSD symptoms in the process of change in trauma-focused cognitive-behavioral therapies: A study of within-person processes. *Frontiers in Psychology, 6,* 1273.

Hofmann, S. G., Grossman, P., & Hinton, D. E. (2011). Loving-kindness and compassion meditation: Potential for psychological interventions. *Clinical Psychology Review, 31,* 1126–1132.

Hofmann, S. G., Sawyer, A. T., Witt, A. A., & Oh, D. (2010). The effect of mindfulness-based therapy on anxiety and depression: A meta-analytic review. *Journal of Consulting and Clinical Psychology, 78,* 169–183.

Hoge, E. A., Hölzel, B. K., Marques, L., Metcalf, C. A., Brach, N., Lazar, S. W., et al. (2013). Mindfulness and self-compassion in generalized anxiety disorder: Examining predictors of disability. *Evidence-Based Complementary and Alternative Medicine, 2013,* 576258.

Hollis-Walker, L., & Colosimo, K. (2011). Mindfulness, self-compassion, and happiness in non-meditators: A theoretical and empirical examination. *Personality and Individual Differences, 50,* 222–227.

Holmes, J. (2001). *The search for the secure base.* London: Routledge.

Hölzel, B. K., Lazar, S. W., Gard, T., Schuman-Olivier, Z., Vago, D. R., & Ott, U. (2011). How does mindfulness meditation work?: Proposing mechanisms of action from a conceptual and neural perspective. *Perspectives on Psychological Science, 6*(6), 537–559.

Homan, K. J., & Sirois, F. M. (2017). Self-compassion and physical health: Exploring the roles of perceived stress and health-promoting behaviors. *Health Psychology Open, 4*(2), 2055102917729542.

Homan, K. J., & Tylka, T. L. (2015). Self-compassion moderates body comparison and appearance self-worth's inverse relationships with body appreciation. *Body Image, 15,* 1–7.

Hope, N., Koestner, R., & Milyavskaya, M. (2014). The role of self-compassion in goal pursuit and well-being among university freshmen. *Self and Identity, 13*(5), 579–593.

Horney, K. (1950). *Neurosis and human growth: The struggle toward self-realization.* New York: Norton.

Howell, A. J., Dopko, R. L., Turowski, J. B., & Buro, K. (2011). The disposition to apologize. *Personality and Individual Differences, 51*(4), 509–514.

Hurd, B. (2008). *Stirring the mud: On swamps, bogs, and human imagination.* Athens: University of Georgia Press.

Isgett, S. F., Algoe, S. B., Boulton, A. J., Way, B. M., & Fredrickson, B. L. (2016). Common variant in OXTR predicts growth in positive emotions from loving-kindness training. *Psychoneuroendocrinology, 73*, 244–251.

Jackowska, M., Brown, J., Ronaldson, A., & Steptoe, A. (2016). The impact of a brief gratitude intervention on subjective well-being, biology and sleep. *Journal of Health Psychology, 21*(10), 2207–2217.

James, K., & Rimes, K. A. (2018). Mindfulness-based cognitive therapy versus pure cognitive behavioural self-help for perfectionism: A pilot randomised study. *Mindfulness, 9*(3), 801–814.

Jazaieri, H., Jinpa, G. T., McGonigal, K., Rosenberg, E. L., Finkelstein, J., Simon-Thomas, E., et al. (2013). Enhancing compassion: A randomized controlled trial of a compassion cultivation training program. *Journal of Happiness Studies, 14*(4), 1113–1126.

Jazaieri, H., Lee, I. A., McGonigal, K., Jinpa, T., Doty, J. R., Gross, J. J., & Goldin, P. R. (2016). A wandering mind is a less caring mind: Daily experience sampling during compassion meditation training. *Journal of Positive Psychology, 11*(1), 37–50.

Jazaieri, H., McGonigal, K., Jinpa, T., Doty, J. R., Gross, J. J., & Goldin, P. R. (2014). A randomized controlled trial of compassion cultivation training: Effects on mindfulness, affect, and emotion regulation. *Motivation and Emotion, 38*(1), 23–35.

Jazaieri, H., McGonigal, K., Lee, I. A., Jinpa, T., Doty, J. R., Gross, J. J., et al. (2018). Altering the trajectory of affect and affect regulation: The impact of compassion training. *Mindfulness, 9*(1), 283–293.

Jiang, Y., You, J., Hou, Y., Du, C., Lin, M. P., Zheng, X., et al. (2016). Buffering the effects of peer victimization on adolescent non-suicidal self-injury: The role of self-compassion and family cohesion. *Journal of Adolescence, 53*, 107–115.

Jinpa, T. (2016). *A fearless heart: How the courage to be compassionate can change your life.* New York: Avery.

Joeng, J. R., Turner, S. L., Kim, E. Y., Choi, S. A., Lee, Y. J., & Kim, J. K. (2017). Insecure attachment and emotional distress: Fear of self-compassion and self-compassion as mediators. *Personality and Individual Differences, 112*, 6–11.

Johnson, E. A., & O'Brien, K. A. (2013). Self-compassion soothes the savage EGO-threat system: Effects on negative affect, shame, rumination, and depressive symptoms. *Journal of Social and Clinical Psychology, 32*(9), 939–963.

Jones, E. (1955). *The life and work of Sigmund Freud: Vol. 2. Years of maturity, 1901–1919.* London: Hogarth Press.

Jung, C. G. (2014a). *Collected works of C. G. Jung: Vol. 11. Psychology and religion: West and East.* Princeton, NJ: Princeton University Press. (Original work published 1958)

Jung, C. G. (2014b). *Memories, dreams, reflections.* New York: Vintage Books. (Original work published 1963)

Kabat-Zinn, J. (1990). *Full catastrophe living: Using the wisdom of your body and mind to face stress, pain, and illness.* New York: Dell.

Kabat-Zinn, J. (1994). *Wherever you go, there you are: Mindfulness meditation in everyday life.* New York: Hyperion.

Kabat-Zinn, J. (2003). Mindfulness-based interventions in context: Past, present, and future. *Clinical Psychology: Science and Practice, 10*(2), 144–156.

Kabat-Zinn, J. (2005). *Coming to our senses.* New York: Hyperion.

Kahneman, D. (2011, October 23). Don't blink!: The hazards of confidence. *New York Times.* Retrieved December 26, 2018, from *www.nytimes.com/2011/10/23/magazine/dont-blink-the-hazards-of-confidence.html.*

Kang, Y., Gray, J. R., & Dovidio, J. F. (2015). The head and the heart: Effects of understanding and experiencing lovingkindness on attitudes toward the self and others. *Mindfulness, 6*(5), 1063–1070.

Kant, I. (2016). Critique of pure reason (J. M. D. Meiklejohn, Trans.). Retrieved from *https://ebooks.adelaide.edu.au/k/kant/immanuel/k16p/index.html.* (Original work published 1781)

Kearney, D. J., Malte, C. A., McManus, C., Martinez, M. E., Felleman, B., & Simpson, T. L. (2013). Loving-kindness meditation for posttraumatic stress disorder: A pilot study. *Journal of Traumatic Stress, 26*(4), 426–434.

Kearney, K. G., & Hicks, R. E. (2016). Early nurturing experiences, self-compassion, hyperarousal and scleroderma the way we relate to ourselves may determine disease progression. *International Journal of Psychological Studies, 8*(4), 16.

Kearney, K. G., & Hicks, R. E. (2017). Self-compassion and breast cancer in 23 cancer respondents: Is the way you relate to yourself a factor in disease onset and progress? *Psychology, 8,* 14–26.

Keller, H. (2000). *To love this life: Quotations by Helen Keller.* New York: AFB Press.

Keller, H. (2015). *Optimism: An essay.* Scotts Valley, CA: CreateSpace Independent Publishing Platform. (Original work published 1903)

Kelliher Rabon, J., Sirois, F. M., & Hirsch, J. K. (2018). Self-compassion and suicidal behavior in college students: Serial indirect effects via depression and wellness behaviors. *Journal of American College Health, 66*(2), 114–122.

Kelly, A. C., & Carter, J. C. (2014). Eating disorder subtypes differ in their rates of psychosocial improvement over treatment. *Journal of Eating Disorders, 2,* 1–10.

Kelly, A. C., & Carter, J. C. (2015). Self-compassion training for binge eating disorder: A pilot randomized controlled trial. *Psychology and Psychotherapy, 88,* 285–303.

Kelly, A. C., Carter, J. C., & Borairi, S. (2014). Are improvements in shame and self-compassion early in eating disorders treatment associated with better patient outcomes? *International Journal of Eating Disorders, 47,* 54–64.

Kelly, A. C., Carter, J. C., Zuroff, D. C., & Borairi, S. (2013). Self-compassion and fear of self-compassion interact to predict response to eating disorders treatment: A preliminary investigation. *Psychotherapy Research, 23*(3), 252–264.

Kelly, A. C., Wisniewski, L., Martin-Wagar, C., & Hoffman, E. (2017). Group-based compassion-focused therapy as an adjunct to outpatient treatment for eating disorders: A pilot randomized controlled trial. *Clinical Psychology and Psychotherapy, 24*(2), 475–487.

Kelly, A. C., Zuroff, D. C., Foa, C. L., & Gilbert, P. (2009). Who benefits from training in self-compassionate self-regulation?: A study of smoking reduction. *Journal of Social and Clinical Psychology, 29,* 727–755.

Keltner, D. (2009). *Born to be good.* New York: Norton.

Kemper, K. J., Mo, X., & Khayat, R. (2015). Are mindfulness and self-compassion associated with sleep and resilience in health professionals? *Journal of Alternative and Complementary Medicine, 21*(8), 496–503.

Keng, S., Smoski, M. J., Robins, C. J., Ekblad, A. G., & Brantley, J. G. (2012). Mechanisms of change in mindfulness-based stress reduction: Self-compassion and mindfulness as mediators of intervention outcomes. *Journal of Cognitive Psychotherapy, 26*(3), 270–280.

Kernis, M. H., Cornell, D. P., Sun, C. R., Berry, A., & Harlow, T. (1993). There's more to self-esteem than whether it is high or low: The importance of stability of self-esteem. *Journal of Personality and Social Psychology, 65,* 1190–1204.

Kernis, M. H., Paradise, A. W., Whitaker, D. J., Wheatman, S. R., & Goldman, B. N. (2000). Master of one's psychological domain?: Not likely if one's self-esteem is unstable. *Personality and Social Psychology Bulletin, 26,* 1297–1305.

Keysers, C., Kaas, J. H., & Gazzola, V. (2010). Somatosensation in social perception. *Nature Reviews Neuroscience, 11*(6), 417–428.

Killingsworth, M. A., & Gilbert, D. T. (2010). A wandering mind is an unhappy mind. *Science, 330,* 932.

Kilpatrick, D. G., Resnick, H. S., Milanak, M. E., Miller, M. W., Keyes, K. M., & Friedman, M. J. (2013). National estimates of exposure to traumatic events and PTSD prevalence using DSM-IV and DSM-5 criteria. *Journal of Traumatic Stress, 26*(5), 537–547.

Kim, J., Talbot, N. L., & Cicchetti, D. (2009). Childhood abuse and current interpersonal conflict: The role of shame. *Child Abuse and Neglect, 33*(6), 362–371.

King, M. L., Jr. (1965, June). *Remaining awake through a great revolution.* Commencement address for Oberlin College, Oberlin, OH. Retrieved January 31, 2019, from *www2.oberlin.edu/external/EOG/BlackHistoryMonth/MLK/CommAddress.html.*

King, M. L., Jr. (2014). *The papers of Martin Luther King, Jr.: Vol. 7. To save the soul of America, January 1961–August 1962* (C. Carson, Ed.). Berkeley: University of California Press.

King, S. D. (1964). *Training within the organization.* London: Tavistock.

Kirby, J. N. (2017). Compassion interventions: The programmes, the evidence, and implications for research and practice. *Psychology and Psychotherapy: Theory, Research and Practice, 90*(3), 432–455.

Kirby, J. N., Tellegen, C. L., & Steindl, S. R. (2017). A meta-analysis of compassion-based interventions: Current state of knowledge and future directions. *Behavior Therapy, 48*(6), 778–792.

Kirschner, H., Kuyken, W., Wright, K., Roberts, H., Brejcha, C., & Karl, A. (2019). Soothing your heart and feeling connected: A new experimental paradigm to study the benefits of self-compassion. *Clinical Psychological Science.* [Epub ahead of print]

Klimecki, O. M., Leiberg, S., Lamm, C., & Singer, T. (2012). Functional neural plasticity and associated changes in positive affect after compassion training. *Cerebral Cortex, 23*(7), 1552–1561.

Klimecki, O., & Singer, T. (2012). Empathic distress fatigue rather than compassion fatigue?: Integrating findings from empathy research in psychology and social neuroscience. In B. Oakley, A. Knafo, G. Mahdavan, & D. Wilson (Eds.), *Pathological altruism* (pp. 368–383). New York: Oxford University Press.

Knabb, J. (2018). *The compassion-based workbook for Christian clients: Finding freedom from shame and negative self-judgments.* New York: Routledge.

Knox, M., Neff, K., & Davidson, O. (2016, June). *Comparing compassion for self and others: Impacts on personal and interpersonal well-being.* Paper presented at the 14th annual Association for Contextual Behavioral Science World Conference, Seattle, WA.

Kolb, D. A. (2015). *Experiential learning: Experience as the source of learning and development* (2nd ed.). Upper Saddle River, NJ: Pearson Education.

Kornfield, J. (1993). *A path with heart.* New York: Bantam Books.

Kornfield, J. (2008, May 16). *Buddhist practices at the heart of psychotherapy.* Paper presented at the Meditation and Psychotherapy conference, Harvard Medical School, Boston, MA.

Kornfield, J. (2014). *A lamp in the darkness: Illuminating a path through difficulties in hard times.* Louisville, CO: Sounds True.

Kornfield, J. (2017). *Freedom of the heart: Heart wisdom, Episode 11.* Retrieved on June 29, 2017, from *https://jackkornfield.com/freedom-heart-heart-wisdom-episode-11.*

Krakovsky, M. (2017, May–June). The self-compassion solution. *Scientific American Mind,* pp. 65–70.

Kraus, M. (2017). Voice-only communication enhances empathic accuracy. *American Psychologist, 72*(7), 644–654.

Kraus, S., & Sears, S. (2009). Measuring the immeasurables: Development and initial validation of the Self–Other Four Immeasurables (SOFI) scale based on Buddhist teachings on loving kindness, compassion, joy, and equanimity. *Social Indicators Research, 92*(1), 169–181.

Kreemers, L. M., van Hooft, E. A., & van Vianen, A. E. (2018). Dealing with negative job search experiences: The beneficial role of self-compassion for job seekers' affective responses. *Journal of Vocational Behavior, 106,* 165–179.

Krejtz, I., Nezlek, J. B., Michnicka, A., Holas, P., & Rusanowska, M. (2016). Counting one's blessings can reduce the impact of daily stress. *Journal of Happiness Studies, 17*(1), 25–39.

Krieger, T., Altenstein, D., Baettig, I., Doerig, N., & Holtforth, M. (2013). Self-compassion in depression: Associations with depressive symptoms, rumination, and avoidance in depressed outpatients. *Behavior Therapy, 44*(3), 501–513.

Krieger, T., Berger, T., & Holtforth, M. G. (2016). The relationship of self-compassion and depression: Cross-lagged panel analyses in depressed patients after outpatient therapy. *Journal of Affective Disorders, 202,* 39–45.

Krieger, T., Hermann, H., Zimmermann, J., & Holtforth, M. G. (2015).

Associations of self-compassion and global self-esteem with positive and negative affect and stress reactivity in daily life: Findings from a smart phone study. *Personality and Individual Differences, 87,* 288–292.

Krieger, T., Martig, D. S., van den Brink, E., & Berger, T. (2016). Working on self-compassion online: A proof of concept and feasibility study. *Internet Interventions, 6,* 64–70.

Kross, E., Bruehlman-Senecal, E., Park, J., Burson, A., Dougherty, A., Shablack, H., et al. (2014). Self-talk as a regulatory mechanism: How you do it matters. *Journal of Personality and Social Psychology, 106*(2), 304–324.

Kuyken, W., Watkins, E., Holden, E., White, K., Taylor, R. S., Byford, S., et al. (2010). How does mindfulness-based cognitive therapy work? *Behaviour Research and Therapy, 48,* 1105–1112.

Kyeong, L. W. (2013). Self-compassion as a moderator of the relationship between academic burn-out and psychological health in Korean cyber university students. *Personality and Individual Differences, 54*(8), 899–902.

Lambert, M. J., & Barley, D. E. (2001). Research summary on the therapeutic relationship and psychotherapy outcome. *Psychotherapy: Theory, Research, Practice, Training, 38*(4), 357–361.

Lamm, C., Batson, C. D., & Decety, J. (2007). The neural substrate of human empathy: Effects of perspective-taking and cognitive appraisal. *Journal of Cognitive Neuroscience, 19*(1), 42–58.

Lamott, A. (1997, March 13). My mind is a bad neighborhood I try not to go into alone. *Salon.* Retrieved June 7, 2017, from *www.salon.com/1997/03/13/lamott970313.*

Lapsley, D. K., FitzGerald, D., Rice, K., & Jackson, S. (1989). Separation-individuation and the "new look" at the imaginary audience and personal fable: A test of an integrative model. *Journal of Adolescent Research 4,* 483–505.

Larsson, H., Andershed, H., & Lichtenstein, P. (2006). A genetic factor explains most of the variation in the psychopathic personality. *Journal of Abnormal Psychology, 115*(2), 221–230.

Lazar, S. W., Kerr, C. E., Wasserman, R. H., Gray, J. R., Greve, D. N., Treadway, M. T., et al. (2005). Meditation experience is associated with increased cortical thickness. *NeuroReport, 16*(17), 1893–1897.

Leadbeater, B. J., Kuperminc, G. P., Blatt, S. J., & Hertzog, C. (1999). A multivariate model of gender differences in adolescents' internalizing and externalizing problems. *Developmental Psychology, 35*(5), 1268–1282.

Leary, M. R. (1999). Making sense of self-esteem. *Current Directions in Psychological Science, 8,* 32–35.

Leary, M. R., Tate, E. B., Adams, C. E., Allen, A. B., & Hancock, J. (2007). Self-compassion and reactions to unpleasant self-relevant events: The implications of treating oneself kindly. *Journal of Personality and Social Psychology, 92,* 887–904.

Leaviss, J., & Uttley, L. (2015). Psychotherapeutic benefits of compassion-focused therapy: An early systematic review. *Psychological Medicine, 45*(5), 927–945.

Lee, T., Leung, M., Hou, W., Tang, J., Yin, J., So, K., et al. (2012). Distinct neural activity associated with focused-attention meditation and loving-kindness meditation. *PLOS ONE, 7*(8), e40054.

Leung, M. K., Chan, C. C., Yin, J., Lee, C. F., So, K. F., & Lee, T. M. (2013). Increased gray matter volume in the right angular and posterior parahippocampal gyri in loving-kindness meditators. *Social Cognitive and Affective Neuroscience, 8*(1), 34–39.

Lewis, H. B. (1987). Introduction: Shame, the "sleeper" in psychopathology. In H. B. Lewis (Ed.), *The role of shame in symptom formation* (pp. 1–28). Hillsdale, NJ: Erlbaum.

Lieberman, M. D. (2007). Social cognitive neuroscience: A review of core processes. *Annual Review of Psychology, 58,* 259–289.

Lieberman, M. D. (2013). *Social: Why our brains are wired to connect.* New York: Crown.

Lindahl, J. R., Fisher, N. E., Cooper, D. J., Rosen, R. K., & Britton, W. B. (2017). The varieties of contemplative experience: A mixed-methods study of meditation-related challenges in Western Buddhists. *PLOS ONE, 12*(5), e0176239.

Lindsay, E. K., & Creswell, J. D. (2014). Helping the self help others: Self-affirmation increases self-compassion and pro-social behaviors. *Frontiers in Psychology, 5,* 421.

Linehan, M. M. (1993). *Cognitive-behavioral treatment of borderline personality disorder.* New York: Guilford Press.

Lloyd, J., Muers, J., Patterson, T. G., & Marczak, M. (2018). Self-compassion, coping strategies, and caregiver burden in caregivers of people with dementia. *Clinical Gerontologist, 42*(1), 47–59.

Lockard, A. J., Hayes, J. A., Neff, K. D., & Locke, B. D. (2014). Self-compassion among college counseling center clients: An examination of clinical norms and group differences. *Journal of College Counseling, 17,* 249–259.

LoParo, D., Mack, S. A., Patterson, B., Negi, L. T., & Kaslow, N. J. (2018). The efficacy of cognitively-based compassion training for African American suicide attempters. *Mindfulness, 9*(6), 1951–1954.

Luckner, J. L., & Nadler, R. S. (1997). *Processing the experience: Strategies to enhance and generalize learning.* Dubuque, IA: Kendall/Hunt.

Luisi, P. L. (2008). The two pillars of Buddhism—consciousness and ethics. *Journal of Consciousness Studies, 15*(1), 84–107.

Luo, X., Qiao, L., & Che, X. (2018). Self-compassion modulates heart rate variability and negative affect to experimentally induced stress. *Mindfulness, 9*(5), 1522–1528.

Luoma, J. B., & Platt, M. G. (2015). Shame, self-criticism, self-stigma, and compassion in acceptance and commitment therapy. *Current Opinion in Psychology, 2,* 97–101.

Lutz, A., Slagter, H. A., Dunne, J. D., & Davidson, R. J. (2008). Attention regulation and monitoring in meditation. *Trends in Cognitive Sciences, 12*(4), 163–169.

MacBeth, A., & Gumley, A. (2012). Exploring compassion: A meta-analysis of the association between self-compassion and psychopathology. *Clinical Psychology Review, 32,* 545–552.

Mackintosh, K., Power, K., Schwannauer, M., & Chan, S. W. (2018). The relationships between self-compassion, attachment and interpersonal problems in clinical patients with mixed anxiety and depression and emotional distress. *Mindfulness, 9*(3), 961–971.

Macy, J. (2007). *World as lover, world as self.* Berkeley, CA: Parallax Press.

Magnus, C. M. R., Kowalski, K. C., & McHugh, T.-L. F. (2010). The role of self-compassion in women's self-determined motives to exercise and exercise-related outcomes. *Self and Identity, 9,* 363–382.

Magyari, T. (2016). Teaching individuals with traumatic stress. In D. McCown, D. Reibel, & M. Micozzi (Eds.), *Resources for teaching mindfulness: An international handbook* (pp. 339–358). New York: Springer.

Mak, W. W., Tong, A. C., Yip, S. Y., Lui, W. W., Chio, F. H., Chan, A. T., et al. (2018). Efficacy and moderation of mobile app–based programs for mindfulness-based training, self-compassion training, and cognitive behavioral psychoeducation on mental health: Randomized controlled noninferiority trial. *JMIR Mental Health, 5*(4), e60.

Maratos, F. A., Duarte, J., Barnes, C., McEwan, K., Sheffield, D., & Gilbert, P. (2017). The physiological and emotional effects of touch: Assessing a hand-massage intervention with high self-critics. *Psychiatry Research, 250,* 221–227.

Marsh, I. C., Chan, S. W., & MacBeth, A. (2018). Self-compassion and psychological distress in adolescents—a meta-analysis. *Mindfulness, 9*(4), 1011–1027.

Marshall, S. L., Parker, P. D., Ciarrochi, J., Sahdra, B., Jackson, C. J., & Heaven, P. C. (2015). Self-compassion protects against the negative effects of low self-esteem: A longitudinal study in a large adolescent sample. *Personality and Individual Differences, 74,* 116–121.

Marta-Simões, J., Ferreira, C., & Mendes, A. L. (2016). Exploring the effect of external shame on body appreciation among Portuguese young adults: The role of self-compassion. *Eating Behaviors, 23,* 174–179.

Marta-Simões, J., Ferreira, C., & Mendes, A. L. (2018). Self-compassion: An adaptive link between early memories and women's quality of life. *Journal of Health Psychology, 23*(7), 929–938.

Mascaro, J. S., Kelley, S., Darcher, A., Negi, L. T., Worthman, C., Miller, A., et al. (2018). Meditation buffers medical student compassion from the deleterious effects of depression. *Journal of Positive Psychology, 13*(2), 133–142.

Mascaro, J. S., Rilling, J. K., Negi, L. T., & Raison, C. L. (2013). Compassion meditation enhances empathic accuracy and related neural activity. *Social Cognitive and Affective Neuroscience, 8*(1), 48–55.

Matos, M., Duarte, J., Duarte, C., Gilbert, P., & Pinto-Gouveia, J. (2018). How one experiences and embodies compassionate mind training influences its effectiveness. *Mindfulness, 9*(4), 1224–1235.

Mayer, P. (2010). Japanese bowl. On *Heaven below* [Audio CD]. Stillwater, MN: Blueboat.

McCullough, M. E., Pargament, K. I., & Thoresen, C. E. (Eds.). (2001). *Forgiveness: Theory, research, and practice.* New York: Guilford Press.

McEwan, K., & Gilbert, P. (2016). A pilot feasibility study exploring the practising of compassionate imagery exercises in a nonclinical population. *Psychology and Psychotherapy: Theory, Research and Practice, 89*(2), 239–243.

McGehee, P., Germer, C., & Neff, K. (2017). Core values in mindful self-compassion.

In L. Montiero, J. Compson, & F. Musten (Eds.), *Practitioner's guide to ethics and mindfulness-based interventions* (pp. 279–294). New York: Springer.

Mendelsohn, M., Herman, J. L., Schatzow, E., Kallivayalil, D., Levitan, J., & Coco, M. (2011). *The trauma recovery group: A guide for practitioners.* New York: Guilford Press.

Merton, T. (1975). *My argument with the Gestapo.* New York: New Directions.

Michaels, L. (Producer), & Waters, M. (Director). (2004). *Mean girls* [Motion picture]. United States: Paramount Pictures.

Mikulincer, M., & Shaver, P. R. (2017). Adult attachment and compassion: Normative and individual difference components. In E. M. Seppälä, E. Simon-Thomas, S. L. Brown, M. C. Worline, C. D. Cameron, & J. R. Doty (Eds.), *The Oxford handbook of compassion science* (pp. 79–90). New York: Oxford University Press.

Mikulincer, M., Shaver, P. R., & Pereg, D. (2003). Attachment theory and affect regulation: The dynamics, development, and cognitive consequences of attachment-related strategies. *Motivation and Emotion, 27*(2), 77–102.

Miller, W., Matthews, D., C'de Baca, J., & Wilbourne, P. (2011). Personal values card sort. Retrieved June 18, 2017, from *www.guilford.com/add/miller2/values.pdf*.

Mills, J., & Chapman, M. (2016). Compassion and self-compassion in medicine: Self-care for the caregiver. *Australasian Medical Journal, 9*(5), 87–91.

Moffitt, R. L., Neumann, D. L., & Williamson, S. P. (2018). Comparing the efficacy of a brief self-esteem and self-compassion intervention for state body dissatisfaction and self-improvement motivation. *Body Image, 27,* 67–76.

Møller, S. A. Q., Sami, S., & Shapiro, S. L. (2019). Health benefits of (mindful) self-compassion meditation and the potential complementarity to mindfulness-based interventions: A review of randomized-controlled trials. *OBM Integrative and Complementary Medicine, 4*(1), 1–20.

Morgan, W. D. (1990). *Change in meditation: A phenomenological study of vipassana meditators' views of progress* (Order No. 0568811). ProQuest Dissertations and Theses Global (No. 303920675). Retrieved from *http://search.proquest.com.ezp-prod1.hul.harvard.edu/docview/303920675?accountid=11311.*

Morris, A. S., Silk, J. S., Steinberg, L., Myers, S. S., & Robinson, L. R. (2007). The role of the family context in the development of emotion regulation. *Social Development, 16*(2), 361–388.

Mosewich, A. D., Crocker, P. E., Kowalski, K. C., & DeLongis, A. (2013). Applying self-compassion in sport: An intervention with women athletes. *Journal of Sport and Exercise Psychology, 35*(5), 514–524.

Mosewich, A. D., Kowalski, K. C., Sabiston, C. M., Sedgwick, W. A., & Tracy, J. L. (2011). Self-compassion: A potential resource for young women athletes. *Journal of Sport and Exercise Psychology, 33,* 103–123.

Moyers, W., with Ketcham, K. (2006). *Broken: My story of addiction and redemption.* New York: Viking.

Muris, P. (2015). A protective factor against mental health problems in youths?: A critical note on the assessment of self-compassion. *Journal of Child and Family Studies, 25*(5), 1461–1465.

Nairn, R. (2009, September). [Lecture as part of foundation training in compassion]. Lecture presented at Kagyu Samye Ling Monastery, Dumfriesshire, Scotland, UK.

Nathanson, D. (Ed.). (1987). *The many faces of shame*. New York: Guilford Press.

Neely, M. E., Schallert, D. L., Mohammed, S. S., Roberts, R. M., & Chen, Y. (2009). Self-kindness when facing stress: The role of self-compassion, goal regulation, and support in college students' well-being. *Motivation and Emotion, 33,* 88–97.

Neff, K. D. (2003a). Development and validation of a scale to measure self-compassion. *Self and Identity, 2,* 223–250.

Neff, K. D. (2003b). Self-compassion: An alternative conceptualization of a healthy attitude toward oneself. *Self and Identity, 2,* 85–102.

Neff, K. D. (2011a). *Self-compassion: The proven power of being kind to yourself.* New York: Morrow.

Neff, K. D. (2011b). Self-compassion, self-esteem, and well-being. *Social and Personality Compass, 5,* 1–12.

Neff, K. D. (2015, September–October). The 5 myths of self-compassion. *Psychotherapy Networker.* Retrieved June 6, 2017, from *www.psychotherapynetworker.org/magazine/article/4/the-5-myths-of-self-compassion.*

Neff, K. D. (2016a). Does self-compassion entail reduced self-judgment, isolation, and over-identification?: A response to Muris, Otgaar, and Petrocchi. *Mindfulness, 7*(3), 791–797.

Neff, K. D. (2016b). The Self-Compassion Scale is a valid and theoretically coherent measure of self-compassion. *Mindfulness, 7*(1), 264–274.

Neff, K. D., & Beretvas, S. N. (2013). The role of self-compassion in romantic relationships. *Self and Identity, 12*(1), 78–98.

Neff, K. D., & Faso, D. J. (2014). Self-compassion and well-being in parents of children with autism. *Mindfulness, 6*(4), 938–947.

Neff, K. D., & Germer, C. (2013). A pilot study and randomized controlled trial of the Mindful Self-Compassion program. *Journal of Clinical Psychology, 69*(1), 28–44.

Neff, K. D., & Germer, C. (2018). *The Mindful Self-Compassion workbook.* New York: Guilford Press.

Neff, K. D., Hsieh, Y., & Dejitterat, K. (2005). Self-compassion, achievement goals, and coping with academic failure. *Self and Identity, 4,* 263–287.

Neff, K. D., Kirkpatrick, K., & Rude, S. S. (2007). Self-compassion and its link to adaptive psychological functioning. *Journal of Research in Personality, 41,* 139–154.

Neff, K. D., Long, P., Knox, M., Davidson, O., Kuchar, A., Costigan, A., et al. (2018). The forest and the trees: Examining the association of self-compassion and its positive and negative components with psychological functioning. *Self and Identity, 17*(6), 627–645.

Neff, K. D., & McGehee, P. (2010). Self-compassion and psychological resilience among adolescents and young adults. *Self and Identity, 9,* 225–240.

Neff, K. D., Pisitsungkagarn, K., & Hseih, Y. (2008). Self-compassion and self-construal in the United States, Thailand, and Taiwan. *Journal of Cross-Cultural Psychology, 39*(3), 267–285.

Neff, K. D., & Pommier, E. (2013). The relationship between self-compassion and other-focused concern among college undergraduates, community adults, and practicing meditators. *Self and Identity, 12*(2), 160–176.

Neff, K. D., Rude, S. S., & Kirkpatrick, K. (2007). An examination of self-compassion in relation to positive psychological functioning and personality traits. *Journal of Research in Personality, 41*, 908–916.

Neff, K., & Tirch, D. (2013). Self-compassion and ACT. In T. B. Kashdan & J. Ciarrochi (Eds.), *Mindfulness, acceptance, and positive psychology: The seven foundations of well-being* (pp. 78–106). Oakland, CA: Context Press/ New Harbinger.

Neff, K. D., Tóth-Király, I., & Colisomo, K. (2018). Self-compassion is best measured as a global construct and is overlapping with but distinct from neuroticism: A response to Pfattheicher, Geiger, Hartung, Weiss, and Schindler (2017). *European Journal of Personality, 32*(4), 371–392.

Neff, K. D., Tóth-Király, I., Yarnell, L. M., Arimitsu, K., Castilho, P., Ghorbani, N., et al. (2018). Examining the factor structure of the Self-Compassion Scale using exploratory SEM bifactor analysis in 20 diverse samples: Support for use of a total score and six subscale scores. *Psychological Assessment, 31*(1), 27–45.

Neff, K. D., & Vonk, R. (2009). Self-compassion versus global self-esteem: Two different ways of relating to oneself. *Journal of Personality, 77*, 23–50.

Neff, K. D., Whittaker, T., & Karl, A. (2017). Evaluating the factor structure of the Self-Compassion Scale in four distinct populations: Is the use of a total self-compassion score justified? *Journal of Personality Assessment, 99*(6), 596–607.

Negi, L. T. (2009, 2016). *CBCT® (cognitively-based compassion training) manual.* Unpublished manuscript, Emory University, Atlanta, GA.

Nepo, M. (2000). Being direct. In M. Nepo, *The book of awakening.* Newburyport, MA: Conari Press.

Nery-Hurwit, M., Yun, J., & Ebbeck, V. (2018). Examining the roles of self-compassion and resilience on health-related quality of life for individuals with multiple sclerosis. *Disability and Health Journal, 11*(2), 256–261.

Niebuhr, R. (1986). *The essential Reinhold Niebuhr: Selected essays and addresses.* New Haven, CT: Yale University Press.

Nolen-Hoeksema, S. (1991). Responses to depression and their effects on the duration of depressive episodes. *Journal of Abnormal Psychology, 100*, 569–582.

Nolen-Hoeksema, S., Larson, J., & Grayson, C. (1999). Explaining the gender difference in depressive symptoms. *Journal of Personality and Social Psychology, 77*, 1061–1072.

Nolen-Hoeksema, S., & Morrow, J. (1991). A prospective study of depression and posttraumatic stress symptoms after a natural disaster: The 1989 Loma Prieta earthquake. *Journal of Personality and Social Psychology, 61*(1), 115–121.

Nolen-Hoeksema, S., Wisco, B. E., & Lyubomirsky, S. (2008). Rethinking rumination. *Perspectives on Psychological Science, 3*(5), 400–424.

Norcross, J. C., & Wampold, B. E. (2011). Evidence-based therapy relationships: Research conclusions and clinical practices. *Psychotherapy, 48*(1), 98–102.

Nouwen, H. (2004). *Out of solitude: Three meditations on the Christian life.* Notre Dame, IN: Ave Maria Press.

Nummenmaa, L., Glerean, E., Hari, R., & Hietanen, J. K. (2014). Bodily maps of emotions. *Proceedings of the National Academy of Sciences of the USA, 111*(2), 646–651.

Nummenmaa, L., Hirvonen, J., Parkkola, R., & Hietanen, J. K. (2008). Is emotional contagion special?: An fMRI study on neural systems for affective and cognitive empathy. *NeuroImage, 43*(3), 571–580.

Nye, N. S. (1995). Kindness. In N. S. Nye, *Words under the words: Selected poems* (pp. 42–43). Portland, OR: Eighth Mountain Press.

O'Donohue, J. (2008). For belonging. In J. O'Donohue, *To bless the space between us: A book of blessings* (p. 44). New York: Harmony Books.

O'Donohue, J. (2011). Beannacht. In J. O'Donohue, *Echoes of memory* (pp. 8–9). New York: Harmony Books.

Odou, N., & Brinker, J. (2014). Exploring the relationship between rumination, self-compassion, and mood. *Self and Identity, 13*(4), 449–459.

Odou, N., & Brinker, J. (2015). Self-compassion, a better alternative to rumination than distraction as a response to negative mood. *Journal of Positive Psychology, 10*(5), 447–457.

Ogden, P., Minton, K., & Pain, C. (2009). *Trauma and the body: A sensorimotor approach to psychotherapy*. New York: Norton.

Olendzki, A. (2012). Wisdom in Buddhist psychology. In C. Germer & R. Siegel (Eds.), *Wisdom and compassion in psychotherapy* (pp. 121–137). New York: Guilford Press.

Oliver, M. (2004a). The journey. In M. Oliver, *New and selected poems* (Vol. 1, pp. 114–115). Boston: Beacon Press.

Oliver, M. (2004b). Wild geese. In M. Oliver, *New and selected poems* (Vol. 1, p. 110). Boston: Beacon Press.

Olson, K., Kemper, K. J., & Mahan, J. D. (2015). What factors promote resilience and protect against burnout in first-year pediatric and medicine-pediatric residents? *Journal of Evidence-Based Complementary and Alternative Medicine, 20*(3), 192–198.

Ozawa-de Silva, B., & Dodson-Lavelle, B. (2011). An education of heart and mind: Practical and theoretical issues in teaching cognitive-based compassion training to children. *Practical Matters, 4,* 1–28.

Pace, T. W., Negi, L. T., Adame, D. D., Cole, S. P., Sivilli, T. I., Brown, T. D., et al. (2009). Effect of compassion meditation on neuroendocrine, innate immune and behavioral responses to psychosocial stress. *Psychoneuroendocrinology, 34*(1), 87–98.

Pace, T. W., Negi, L. T., Dodson-Lavelle, B., Ozawa-de Silva, B., Reddy, S. D., Cole, S. P., et al. (2013). Engagement with cognitively-based compassion training is associated with reduced salivary C-reactive protein from before to after training in foster care program adolescents. *Psychoneuroendocrinology, 38*(2), 294–299.

Palmeira, L., Pinto-Gouveia, J., & Cunha, M. (2017). Exploring the efficacy of an acceptance, mindfulness and compassionate-based group intervention for women struggling with their weight (Kg-Free): A randomized controlled trial. *Appetite, 112,* 107–116.

Parrish, M. H., Inagaki, T. K., Muscatell, K. A., Haltom, K. E., Leary, M. R., & Eisenberger, N. I. (2018). Self-compassion and responses to negative social feedback: The role of fronto-amygdala circuit connectivity. *Self and Identity,* 17(6), 723–738.

Parry, S. L., & Malpus, Z. (2017). Reconnecting the mind and body: A pilot study of developing compassion for persistent pain. *Patient Experience Journal,* 4(1), 145–153.

Parzuchowski, M., Szymkow, A., Baryla, W., & Wojciszke, B. (2014). From the heart: Hand over heart as an embodiment of honesty. *Cognitive Processing,* 15(3), 237–244.

Patzak, A., Kollmayer, M., & Schober, B. (2017). Buffering impostor feelings with kindness: The mediating role of self-compassion between gender-role orientation and the impostor phenomenon. *Frontiers in Psychology, 8,* 1289.

Pepping, C. A., Davis, P. J., O'Donovan, A., & Pal, J. (2015). Individual differences in self-compassion: The role of attachment and experiences of parenting in childhood. *Self and Identity, 14*(1), 104–117.

Petrocchi, N., Ottaviani, C., & Couyoumdjian, A. (2016). Compassion at the mirror: Exposure to a mirror increases the efficacy of a self-compassion manipulation in enhancing soothing positive affect and heart rate variability. *Journal of Positive Psychology, 12*(6), 525–536.

Phelps, C. L., Paniagua, S. M., Willcockson, I. U., & Potter, J. S. (2018). The relationship between self-compassion and the risk for substance use disorder. *Drug and Alcohol Dependence, 183,* 78–81.

Pires, F. B., Lacerda, S. S., Balardin, J. B., Portes, B., Tobo, P. R., Barrichello, C. R., et al. (2018). Self-compassion is associated with less stress and depression and greater attention and brain response to affective stimuli in women managers. *BMC Women's Health, 18*(1), 195.

Pisitsungkagarn, K., Taephant, N., & Attasaranya, P. (2013). Body image satisfaction and self-esteem in Thai female adolescents: The moderating role of self-compassion. *International Journal of Adolescent Medicine and Health,* 26(3), 333–338.

Pittman, F. S., III, & Wagers, T. P. (2005). The relationship, if any, between marriage and infidelity. In F. P. Piercy, K. M. Hertlein, & J. L. Wetchler (Eds.), *Handbook of the clinical treatment of infidelity* (pp. 135–148). Binghamton, NY: Haworth Press.

Porges, S. W. (2003). The polyvagal theory: Phylogenetic contributions to social behavior. *Physiology and Behavior, 79*(3), 503–513.

Porges, S. W. (2007). The polyvagal perspective. *Biological Psychology, 74,* 116–143.

Powers, T. A., Koestner, R., & Zuroff, D. C. (2007). Self-criticism, goal motivation, and goal progress. *Journal of Social and Clinical Psychology, 26,* 826–840.

Proeve, M., Anton, R., & Kenny, M. (2018). Effects of mindfulness-based cognitive therapy on shame, self-compassion and psychological distress in anxious and depressed patients: A pilot study. *Psychology and Psychotherapy: Theory, Research and Practice, 91*(4), 434–449.

Przezdziecki, A., & Sherman, K. A. (2016). Modifying affective and cognitive responses regarding body image difficulties in breast cancer survivors using a self-compassion-based writing intervention. *Mindfulness, 7*(5), 1142–1155.

Przezdziecki, A., Sherman, K. A., Baillie, A., Taylor, A., Foley, E., & Stalgis-Bilinski,

K. (2013). My changed body: Breast cancer, body image, distress and self-compassion. *Psycho-Oncology, 22*(8), 1872–1879.

Pujji/O'Shea, J. (2007). My balm. In J. Pujji/O'Shea, *Follow yourself home.* Jacksonville, FL: Living Well.

Quoidbach, J., Berry, E. V., Hansenne, M., & Mikolajczak, M. (2010). Positive emotion regulation and well-being: Comparing the impact of eight savoring and dampening strategies. *Personality and Individual Differences, 49*(5), 368–373.

Raab, K. (2014). Mindfulness, self-compassion, and empathy among health care professionals: A review of the literature. *Journal of Health Care Chaplaincy, 20*(3), 95–108.

Raab, K., Sogge, K., Parker, N., & Flament, M. F. (2015). Mindfulness-based stress reduction and self-compassion among mental healthcare professionals: A pilot study. *Mental Health, Religion and Culture, 18*(6), 503–512.

Raes, F. (2010). Rumination and worry as mediators of the relationship between self-compassion and depression and anxiety. *Personality and Individual Differences, 48*, 757–761.

Raes, F., Pommier, E., Neff, K. D., & Van Gucht, D. (2011). Construction and factorial validation of a short form of the Self-Compassion Scale. *Clinical Psychology and Psychotherapy, 18*, 250–255.

Raque-Bogdan, T. L., Ericson, S. K., Jackson, J., Martin, H. M., & Bryan, N. A. (2011). Attachment and mental and physical health: Self-compassion and mattering as mediators. *Journal of Counseling Psychology, 58*, 272–278.

Reddy, S. D., Negi, L. T., Dodson-Lavelle, B., Ozawa-de Silva, B., Pace, T. W., Cole, S. P., et al. (2013). Cognitive-based compassion training: A promising prevention strategy for at-risk adolescents. *Journal of Child and Family Studies, 22*(2), 219–230.

Reid, R. C., Temko, J., Moghaddam, J. F., & Fong, T. W. (2014). Shame, rumination, and self-compassion in men assessed for hypersexual disorder. *Journal of Psychiatric Practice, 20*(4), 260–268.

Reilly, E. D., Rochlen, A. B., & Awad, G. H. (2014). Men's self-compassion and self-esteem: The moderating roles of shame and masculine norm adherence. *Psychology of Men and Masculinity, 15*, 22–28.

Richardson, C. M., Trusty, W. T., & George, K. A. (2018). Trainee wellness: Self-critical perfectionism, self-compassion, depression, and burnout among doctoral trainees in psychology. *Counselling Psychology Quarterly.* [Epub ahead of print]

Rimes, K. A., & Wingrove, J. (2011). Pilot study of mindfulness-based cognitive therapy for trainee clinical psychologists. *Behavioural and Cognitive Psychotherapy, 39*(2), 235–241.

Ringenbach, R. T. (2009). *A comparison between counselors who practice meditation and those who do not on compassion fatigue, compassion satisfaction, burnout and self-compassion.* Unpublished doctoral dissertation, University of Akron, Akron, OH.

Rizzolatti, G., Fadiga, L., Gallese, V., & Fogassi, L. (1996). Premotor cortex and the recognition of motor actions. *Cognitive Brain Research, 3*(2), 131–141.

Robins, C. J., Schmidt, H., & Linehan, M. M. (2004). Dialectical behavior therapy: Synthesizing radical acceptance with skillful means. In S. C. Hayes, V.

M. Follette, & M. M. Linehan (Eds.), *Mindfulness and acceptance: Expanding the cognitive-behavioral tradition* (pp. 30–43). New York: Guilford Press.

Robinson, K. J., Mayer, S., Allen, A. B., Terry, M., Chilton, A., & Leary, M. R. (2016). Resisting self-compassion: Why are some people opposed to being kind to themselves? *Self and Identity, 15*(5), 505–524.

Rockliff, H., Gilbert, P., McEwan, K., Lightman, S., & Glover, D. (2008). A pilot exploration of heart rate variability and salivary cortisol responses to compassion-focused imagery. *Clinical Neuropsychiatry, 5*, 132–139.

Rodgers, R. F., Donovan, E., Cousineau, T., Yates, K., McGowan, K., Cook, E., et al. (2018). BodiMojo: Efficacy of a mobile-based intervention in improving body image and self-compassion among adolescents. *Journal of Youth and Adolescence, 47*(7), 1363–1372.

Roemer, L., Orsillo, S. M., & Salters-Pedneault, K. (2008). Efficacy of an acceptance-based behavior therapy for generalized anxiety disorder: Evaluation in a randomized controlled trial. *Journal of Consulting and Clinical Psychology, 76*(6), 1083–1089.

Rogers, C. (1951). A research program in client-centered therapy. *Research Publications of the Association for Research in Nervous and Mental Disease, 31*, 106–113.

Rogers, C. (1962). The interpersonal relationship: The core of guidance. *Harvard Educational Review, 32*(4), 416–429.

Rogers, C. (1980). *A way of being.* Boston: Houghton Mifflin.

Rogers, C. (1995). *On becoming a person: A therapist's view of psychotherapy.* Boston: Houghton Mifflin. (Original work published 1961)

Rose, C., Webel, A., Sullivan, K. M., Cuca, Y. P., Wantland, D., Johnson, M. O., et al. (2014). Self-compassion and risk behavior among people living with HIV/AIDS. *Research in Nursing and Health, 37*(2), 98–106.

Rosenberg, M. (2015). *Non-violent communication: A language of life* (3rd ed.). Encinitas, CA: PuddleDancer Press.

Rothe, K. (2012). Anti-Semitism in Germany today and the intergenerational transmission of guilt and shame. *Psychoanalysis, Culture and Society, 17*(1), 16–34.

Rowe, A. C., Shepstone, L., Carnelley, K. B., Cavanagh, K., & Millings, A. (2016). Attachment security and self-compassion priming increase the likelihood that first-time engagers in mindfulness meditation will continue with mindfulness training. *Mindfulness, 7*(3), 642–650.

Rozin, P., & Royzman, E. B. (2001). Negativity bias, negativity dominance, and contagion. *Personality and Social Psychology Review, 5*(4), 296–320.

Rubia, K. (2009). The neurobiology of meditation and its clinical effectiveness in psychiatric disorders. *Biological Psychology, 82*(1), 1–11.

Ruijgrok-Lupton, P., Crane, R., & Dorjee, D. (2017). Impact of mindfulness-based teacher training on MBSR participant well-being outcomes and course satisfaction. *Mindfulness, 9*(1), 117–128.

Rumi, J. (1999). The guest house. In J. Rumi, *The essential Rumi* (C. Barks, Trans.) (p. 109). New York: Penguin Arkana.

Saarela, M. V., Hlushchuk, Y., Williams, A. C., Schürmann, M., Kalso, E., & Hari, R. (2007). The compassionate brain: Humans detect intensity of pain from another's face. *Cerebral Cortex, 17*(1), 230–237.

Safran, J. D. (1998). *Widening the scope of cognitive therapy: The therapeutic relationship, emotion, and the process of change.* Northvale, NJ: Jason Aronson.

Salmivalli, C., Kaukiainen, A., Kaistaniemi, L., & Lagerspetz, K. M. J. (1999). Self-evaluated self-esteem, peer-evaluated self-esteem, and defensive egotism as predictors of adolescents' participation in bullying situations. *Personality and Social Psychology Bulletin, 25,* 1268–1278.

Salzberg, S. (1995). *Lovingkindness: The revolutionary art of happiness.* Boston: Shambhala.

Salzberg, S. (2011a). Mindfulness and loving-kindness. *Contemporary Buddhism, 12*(1), 177–182.

Salzberg, S. (2011b). *Real happiness: The power of meditation.* New York: Workman.

Santerre-Baillargeon, M., Rosen, N. O., Steben, M., Pâquet, M., Macabena Perez, R., & Bergeron, S. (2018). Does self-compassion benefit couples coping with vulvodynia?: Associations with psychological, sexual, and relationship adjustment. *Clinical Journal of Pain, 34*(7), 629–637.

Santorelli, S., Meleo-Meyer, F., & Koerbel, L. (2017). *Mindfulness-based stress reduction (MBSR): Authorized curriculum guide.* Worcester: University of Massachusetts Medical School, Center for Mindfulness in Medicine, Health Care and Society.

Sartre, J.-P. (1989). *No exit and three other plays* (S. Gilbert, Trans.). New York: Vintage Books.

Sbarra, D. A., Smith, H. L., & Mehl, M. R. (2012). When leaving your ex, love yourself: Observational ratings of self-compassion predict the course of emotional recovery following marital separation. *Psychological Science, 23,* 261–269.

Scarlet, J., Altmeyer, N., Knier, S., & Harpin, R. E. (2017). The effects of Compassion Cultivation Training (CCT) on health-care workers. *Clinical Psychologist, 21*(2), 116–124.

Schanche, E., Stiles, T. C., McCullough, L., Svartberg, M., & Nielsen, G. (2011). The relationship between activating affects, inhibitory affects, and self-compassion in patients with Cluster C personality disorders. *Psychotherapy, 48*(3), 293–303.

Scheff, T., & Mateo, S. (2016). The S-word is taboo: Shame is invisible in modern societies. *Journal of General Practice, 4,* 217.

Schellekens, M. P., Karremans, J. C., van der Drift, M. A., Molema, J., van den Hurk, D. G., Prins, J. B., et al. (2016). Are mindfulness and self-compassion related to psychological distress and communication in couples facing lung cancer?: A dyadic approach. *Mindfulness, 8*(2), 325–336.

Scherer, K. R. (2005). What are emotions?: And how can they be measured? *Social Science Information, 44*(4), 695–729.

Schoenefeld, S. J., & Webb, J. B. (2013). Self-compassion and intuitive eating in college women: Examining the contributions of distress tolerance and body image acceptance and action. *Eating Behaviors, 14*(4), 493–496.

Schuling, R. (2018, October). *Mindfulness-based compassionate living.* Paper presented at the Compassion in Connection conference, Rhinebeck, NY.

Schuling, R., Huijbers, M., Jansen, H., Metzemaekers, R., Van Den Brink, E., Koster, F., et al. (2018). The co-creation and feasibility of a compassion training as a follow-up to mindfulness-based cognitive therapy in patients with recurrent depression. *Mindfulness, 9*(2), 412–422.

Schuling, R., Huijbers, M. J., van Ravesteijn, H., Donders, R., Kuyken, W., & Speckens, A. E. (2016). A parallel-group, randomized controlled trial into the effectiveness of mindfulness-based compassionate living (MBCL) compared to treatment-as-usual in recurrent depression: Trial design and protocol. *Contemporary Clinical Trials, 50*, 77–83.

Schwartz, R. C. (1995). *Internal family systems therapy*. New York: Guilford Press.

Schwartz, R. C. (2013). Moving from acceptance toward transformation with internal family systems therapy (IFS). *Journal of Clinical Psychology, 69*(8), 805–816.

Schwartz, R. C., & Falconer, R. (2017). *Many minds, one self*. Oak Park, IL: Center for Self Leadership.

Scoglio, A. A., Rudat, D. A., Garvert, D., Jarmolowski, M., Jackson, C., & Herman, J. L. (2018). Self-compassion and responses to trauma: The role of emotion regulation. *Journal of Interpersonal Violence, 33*(13), 2016–2036.

Seara-Cardoso, A., & Viding, E. (2015). Functional neuroscience of psychopathic personality in adults. *Journal of Personality, 83*(6), 723–737.

Segal, Z. V., Williams, J. M. G., & Teasdale, J. D. (2013). *Mindfulness-based cognitive therapy for depression* (2nd ed.). New York: Guilford Press.

Seligman, M. E. (2002). Positive psychology, positive prevention, and positive therapy. In C. R. Snyder & S. J. Lopez (Eds.), *Handbook of positive psychology* (pp. 3–12). New York: Oxford University Press.

Senge, P., Kleiner, A., Roberts, C., Ross, R., Roth, G., & Smith, B. (1999). *The dance of change*. New York: Crown Business.

Shahar, B., Szsepsenwol, O., Zilcha-Mano, S., Haim, N., Zamir, O., Levi-Yeshuvi, S., et al. (2015). A wait-list randomized controlled trial of loving-kindness meditation programme for self-criticism. *Clinical Psychology and Psychotherapy, 22*(4), 346–356.

Shapira, L., & Mongrain, L. (2010). The benefits of self-compassion and optimism exercises for individuals vulnerable to depression. *Journal of Positive Psychology, 5*(5), 377–389.

Shapiro, S. L., Astin, J. A., Bishop, S. R., & Cordova, M. (2005). Mindfulness-based stress reduction for health care professionals: Results from a randomized trial. *International Journal of Stress Management, 12*, 164–176.

Shapiro, S. L., Brown, K. W., & Biegel, G. M. (2007). Teaching self-care to caregivers: Effects of mindfulness-based stress reduction on the mental health of therapists in training. *Training and Education in Professional Psychology, 1*(2), 105–115.

Shapiro, S. L., & Carlson, L. E. (2009). *The art and science of mindfulness: Integrating mindfulness into psychology and the helping professions*. Washington, DC: American Psychological Association.

Sharples, B. (2003). *Meditation: Calming the mind*. Melbourne, Australia: Lothian Books.

Shonin, E., & Van Gordon, W. (2016). Thupten Jinpa on compassion and mindfulness. *Mindfulness, 7*, 279–283.

Siegel, D. J. (2012). *The developing mind: How relationships and the brain interact to shape who we are* (2nd ed.). New York: Guilford Press.

Siegel, D. J. (2006). An interpersonal neurobiology approach to psychotherapy. *Psychiatric Annals, 36*(4).

Siegel, D. J. (2010). *The mindful therapist.* New York: Norton.

Siegel, R., & Germer, C. (2012). Wisdom and compassion: Two wings of a bird. In C. Germer & R. Siegel (Eds.), *Wisdom and compassion in psychotherapy* (pp. 7–34). New York: Guilford Press.

Singer, T., & Klimecki, O. M. (2014). Empathy and compassion. *Current Biology, 24*(18), R875–R878.

Singer, T., & Lamm, C. (2009). The social neuroscience of empathy. *Annals of the New York Academy of Sciences, 1156*(1), 81–96.

Singh, A. A., Hays, D. G., & Watson, L. S. (2011). Strength in the face of adversity: Resilience strategies of transgender individuals. *Journal of Counseling and Development, 89*(1), 20–27.

Singh, N. N., Wahler, R. G., Adkins, A. D., Myers, R. E., & The Mindfulness Research Group. (2003). Soles of the feet: A mindfulness-based self-control intervention for aggression by an individual with mild mental retardation and mental illness. *Research in Developmental Disabilities, 24,* 158–169.

Sirois, F. M. (2014). Procrastination and stress: Exploring the role of self-compassion. *Self and Identity, 13*(2), 128–145.

Sirois, F., Bogels, S., & Emerson, L. (2018). Self-compassion improves parental well-being in response to challenging parenting events. *Journal of Psychology.* [Epub ahead of print]

Sirois, F. M., & Hirsch, J. K. (2019). Self-compassion and adherence in five medical samples: The role of stress. *Mindfulness, 10*(1), 46–54.

Sirois, F. M., Kitner, R., & Hirsch, J. K. (2015). Self-compassion, affect, and health-promoting behaviors. *Health Psychology, 34*(6), 661–669.

Sirois, F. M., Molnar, D. S., & Hirsch, J. K. (2015). Self-compassion, stress, and coping in the context of chronic illness. *Self and Identity, 14*(3), 334–347.

Slepian, M. L., Kirby, J. N., & Kalokerinos, E. K. (2019). Shame, guilt, and secrets on the mind. *Emotion.* [Epub ahead of print]

Smeets, E., Neff, K., Alberts, H., & Peters, M. (2014). Meeting suffering with kindness: Effects of a brief self-compassion intervention for female college students. *Journal of Clinical Psychology, 70*(9), 794–807.

Sommers-Spijkerman, M. P. J., Trompetter, H. R., Schreurs, K. M. G., & Bohlmeijer, E. T. (2018). Compassion-focused therapy as guided self-help for enhancing public mental health: A randomized controlled trial. *Journal of Consulting and Clinical Psychology, 86*(2), 101.

Speer, M., Bhanji, J., & Delgado, M. (2014). Savoring the past: Positive memories evoke value representations in the striatum. *Neuron, 84*(4), 847–856.

Spence, N. D., Wells, S., Graham, K., & George, J. (2016). Racial discrimination, cultural resilience, and stress. *Canadian Journal of Psychiatry, 61*(5), 298–307.

Stafford, W. (2013). The way it is. In W. Stafford, *Ask me: 100 essential poems of William Stafford.* Minneapolis, MN: Greywolf Press.

Stebnicki, M. A. (2007). Empathy fatigue: Healing the mind, body, and spirit of professional counselors. *American Journal of Psychiatric Rehabilitation, 10*(4), 317–338.

Stutts, L. A., Leary, M. R., Zeveney, A. S., & Hufnagle, A. S. (2018). A longitudinal analysis of the relationship between self-compassion and the psychological effects of perceived stress. *Self and Identity, 17*(6), 609–626.

Sullivan, H. S. (1964). The illusion of personal individuality. In H. S. Sullivan, *The fusion of psychiatry and social science* (pp. 198–228). New York: Norton. (Original work published 1950)

Svendsen, J. L., Osnes, B., Binder, P. E., Dundas, I., Visted, E., Nordby, H., et al. (2016). Trait self-compassion reflects emotional flexibility through an association with high vagally mediated heart rate variability. *Mindfulness, 7*(5), 1103–1113.

Swann, W. B. (1996). *Self-traps: The elusive quest for higher self-esteem.* New York: Freeman.

Sweezy, M., & Ziskind, E. (Eds.). (2013). *IFS: Internal family systems therapy: New dimensions.* New York: Routledge.

Talbot, N. L. (1996). Women sexually abused as children: The centrality of shame issues and treatment implications. *Psychotherapy: Theory, Research, Practice, Training, 33*(1), 11–18.

Tanaka, M., Wekerle, C., Schmuck, M. L., Paglia-Boak, A., & MAP Research Team. (2011). The linkages among childhood maltreatment, adolescent mental health, and self-compassion in child welfare adolescents. *Child Abuse and Neglect, 35,* 887–898.

Tandler, N., & Petersen, L. E. (2018). Are self-compassionate partners less jealous?: Exploring the mediation effects of anger rumination and willingness to forgive on the association between self-compassion and romantic jealousy. *Current Psychology.* [Epub ahead of print]

Tangney, J. P., & Dearing, R. L. (2002). *Shame and guilt.* New York: Guilford Press.

Taylor, B. L., Strauss, C., Cavanagh, K., & Jones, F. (2014). The effectiveness of self-help mindfulness-based cognitive therapy in a student sample: A randomised controlled trial. *Behaviour Research and Therapy, 63,* 63–69.

Taylor, V. A., Daneault, V., Grant, J., Scavone, G., Breton, E., Roffe-Vidal, S., et al. (2013). Impact of meditation training on the default mode network during a restful state. *Social Cognitive and Affective Neuroscience, 8*(1), 4–14.

Terry, M. L., & Leary, M. R. (2011). Self-compassion, self-regulation, and health. *Self and Identity, 10,* 352–362.

Terry, M. L., Leary, M. R., & Mehta, S. (2013). Self-compassion as a buffer against homesickness, depression, and dissatisfaction in the transition to college. *Self and Identity, 12*(3), 278–290.

Terry, M. L., Leary, M. R., Mehta, S., & Henderson, K. (2013). Self-compassionate reactions to health threats. *Personality and Social Psychology Bulletin, 39*(7), 911–926.

Thompson, B. L., & Waltz, J. (2008). Self-compassion and PTSD symptom severity. *Journal of Traumatic Stress, 21*(6), 556–558.

Tirch, D., Schoendorff, B., & Silberstein, L. R. (2014). *The ACT practitioner's guide to the science of compassion: Tools for fostering psychological flexibility.* Oakland, CA: New Harbinger.

Toole, A. M., & Craighead, L. W. (2016). Brief self-compassion meditation training for body image distress in young adult women. *Body Image, 19,* 104–112.

Treleaven, D. (2018). *Trauma-sensitive mindfulness.* New York: Norton.

Trockel, M., Hamidi, M., Murphy, M. L., de Vries, P. P., & Bohman, B. (2017). *2016 Physician Wellness Survey: Full report*. Stanford, CA: Stanford Medicine, Well MD Center.

Trommer, R. W. (2013). One morning. Retrieved June 10, 2017, from *https://ahundredfallingveils.com/2013/06/11/one-morning*.

Tutu, D., & Tutu, M. (2015). *The book of forgiving*. San Francisco: Harper One.

Twenge, J. M., & Campbell, W. K. (2009). *The narcissism epidemic: Living in the age of entitlement*. New York: Free Press.

Twenge, J. M., Konrath, S., Foster, J. D., Campbell, W. K., & Bushman, B. J. (2008). Egos inflating over time: A cross-temporal meta-analysis of the Narcissistic Personality Inventory. *Journal of Personality, 76*, 875–902.

Umphrey, L. R., & Sherblom, J. C. (2014). The relationship of hope to self-compassion, relational social skill, communication apprehension, and life satisfaction. *International Journal of Wellbeing, 4*(2), 1–18.

Valk, S. L., Bernhardt, B. C., Trautwein, F.-M., Böckler, A., Kanske, P., Guizard, N., et al. (2017). Structural plasticity of the social brain: Differential change after socio-affective and cognitive mental training. *Science Advances, 3*(10), e1700489.

Van Dam, N. T., Sheppard, S. C., Forsyth, J. P., & Earleywine, M. (2011). Self-compassion is a better predictor than mindfulness of symptom severity and quality of life in mixed anxiety and depression. *Journal of Anxiety Disorders, 25*, 123–130.

van den Brink, E., & Koster, F. (2015). *Mindfulness-based compassionate living*. New York: Routledge.

Van Doren, M. (1961). *The happy critic and other essays*. New York: Hill & Wang.

Vazeou-Nieuwenhuis, A., & Schumann, K. (2018). Self-compassionate and apologetic?: How and why having compassion toward the self relates to a willingness to apologize. *Personality and Individual Differences, 124*, 71–76.

Vettese, L. C., Dyer, C. E., Li, W. L., & Wekerle, C. (2011). Does self-compassion mitigate the association between childhood maltreatment and later emotion regulation difficulties?: A preliminary investigation. *International Journal of Mental Health and Addiction, 9*(5), 480.

Viskovich, S., & Pakenham, K. I. (2018). Pilot evaluation of a Web-based acceptance and commitment therapy program to promote mental health skills in university students. *Journal of Clinical Psychology, 74*(12), 2047–2069.

Walcott, D. (1986). Love after love. In D. Walcott, *Collected poems: 1948–1984* (p. 328). New York: Farrar, Straus & Giroux.

Wallmark, E., Safarzadeh, K., Daukantaite, D., & Maddux, R. E. (2012). Promoting altruism through meditation: An 8-week randomized controlled pilot study. *Mindfulness, 4*(3), 223–234.

Wang, S. (2005). A conceptual framework for integrating research related to the physiology of compassion and the wisdom of Buddhist teachings. In P. Gilbert (Ed.), *Compassion: Conceptualisations, research and use in psychotherapy* (pp. 75–120). New York: Routledge.

Wang, X., Chen, Z., Poon, K. T., Teng, F., & Jin, S. (2017). Self-compassion decreases acceptance of own immoral behaviors. *Personality and Individual Differences, 106*, 329–333.

Waring, S. V., & Kelly, A. C. (2019). Trait self-compassion predicts different responses to failure depending on the interpersonal context. *Personality and Individual Differences, 143*, 47–54.

Wasylkiw, L., MacKinnon, A. L., & MacLellan, A. M. (2012). Exploring the link between self-compassion and body image in university women. *Body Image, 9*(2), 236–245.

Wayment, H. A., West, T. N., & Craddock, E. B. (2016). Compassionate values as a resource during the transition to college: Quiet ego, compassionate goals, and self-compassion. *Journal of the First-Year Experience and Students in Transition, 28*(2), 93–114.

Webb, J. B., Fiery, M. F., & Jafari, N. (2016). "You better not leave me shaming!": Conditional indirect effect analyses of anti-fat attitudes, body shame, and fat talk as a function of self-compassion in college women. *Body Image, 18*, 5–13.

Webb, J. B., & Forman, M. J. (2013). Evaluating the indirect effect of self-compassion on binge eating severity through cognitive–affective self-regulatory pathways. *Eating Behaviors, 14*(2), 224–228.

Wei, M., Liao, K., Ku, T., & Shaffer, P. A. (2011). Attachment, self-compassion, empathy, and subjective well-being among college students and community adults. *Journal of Personality, 79*, 191–221.

Weibel, D. T. (2008). A loving-kindness intervention: Boosting compassion for self and others. *Dissertation Abstracts International, 68*(12), 8418B.

Weingarten, K. (2004). Witnessing the effects of political violence in families: Mechanisms of intergenerational transmission and clinical interventions. *Journal of Marital and Family Therapy, 30*(1), 45–59.

Welp, L. R., & Brown, C. M. (2014). Self-compassion, empathy, and helping intentions. *Journal of Positive Psychology, 9*(1), 54–65.

Welwood, J. P. (2019). Unconditional. Retrieved March 11, 2019, from *http://jenniferwelwood.com/poetry*. (Original work published 1998)

Werner, K. H., Jazaieri, H., Goldin, P. R., Ziv, M., Heimberg, R. G., & Gross, J. J. (2012). Self-compassion and social anxiety disorder. *Anxiety, Stress and Coping, 25*(5), 543–558.

Westphal, M., Leahy, R. L., Pala, A. N., & Wupperman, P. (2016). Self-compassion and emotional invalidation mediate the effects of parental indifference on psychopathology. *Psychiatry Research, 242*, 186–191.

Wetterneck, C. T., Lee, E. B., Smith, A. H., & Hart, J. M. (2013). Courage, self-compassion, and values in obsessive–compulsive disorder. *Journal of Contextual Behavioral Science, 2*(3), 68–73.

Whitesman, S., & Mash, R. (2016). Examining the effects of a mindfulness-based professional training module on mindfulness, perceived stress, self-compassion and self-determination. *African Journal of Health Professions Education, 7*(2), 220–223.

Whittle, S., Liu, K., Bastin, C., Harrison, B. J., & Davey, C. G. (2016). Neurodevelopmental correlates of proneness to guilt and shame in adolescence and early adulthood. *Developmental Cognitive Neuroscience, 19*, 51–57.

Whyte, D. (1992). *The poetry of self-compassion* [Audio CD]. Langley, WA: Many Rivers Press.

Whyte, D. (2012). *River flow: New and selected poems*. Langley, WA: Many Rivers Press.

Whyte, D. (2015). *Consolations: The solace, nourishment and underlying meaning of everyday words.* Langley, WA: Many Rivers Press.

Wild, B., Erb, M., & Bartels, M. (2001). Are emotions contagious?: Evoked emotions while viewing emotionally expressive faces: Quality, quantity, time course and gender differences. *Psychiatry Research, 102*(2), 109–124.

Williams, J., & Lynn, S. (2010). Acceptance: An historical and conceptual review. *Imagination, Cognition, and Personality, 30*(1), 5–56.

Williams, J. G., Stark, S. K., & Foster, E. E. (2008). Start today or the very last day?: The relationships among self-compassion, motivation, and procrastination. *American Journal of Psychological Research, 4,* 37–44.

Williams, L. (2014). Compassion. On L. Williams, *Down where the spirit meets the bone* [Audio CD]. Nashville, TN: Highway 20 Records/Thirty Tigers.

Williams, M. (1997). *The ways we touch: Poems.* Champaign: University of Illinois Press.

Williams, M. (2014). *The velveteen rabbit.* New York: Doubleday Books for Young Readers. (Original work published 1922)

Williamson, M. (1996). *A return to love: Reflections on the principles of "A course in miracles."* San Francisco: Harper One.

Wilson, A. C., Mackintosh, K., Power, K., & Chan, S. W. (2018). Effectiveness of self-compassion related therapies: A systematic review and meta-analysis. *Mindfulness.* [Epub ahead of print]

Wong, C. C. Y., & Yeung, N. C. (2017). Self-compassion and posttraumatic growth: Cognitive processes as mediators. *Mindfulness, 8*(4), 1078–1087.

Wood, A. M., Froh, J. J., & Geraghty, A. W. (2010). Gratitude and well-being: A review and theoretical integration. *Clinical Psychology Review, 30*(7), 890–905.

Wood, J. V., Perunovic, W. Q., & Lee, J. W. (2009). Positive self-statements: Power for some, peril for others. *Psychological Science, 20*(7), 860–866.

Woodruff, S. C., Glass, C. R., Arnkoff, D. B., Crowley, K. J., Hindman, R. K., & Hirschhorn, E. W. (2014). Comparing self-compassion, mindfulness, and psychological inflexibility as predictors of psychological health. *Mindfulness, 5*(4), 410–421.

Woods, H., & Proeve, M. (2014). Relationships of mindfulness, self-compassion, and meditation experience with shame-proneness. *Journal of Cognitive Psychotherapy, 28*(1), 20–33.

Wren, A. A., Somers, T. J., Wright, M. A., Goetz, M. C., Leary, M. R., Fras, A. M., et al. (2012). Self-compassion in patients with persistent musculoskeletal pain: Relationship of self-compassion to adjustment to persistent pain. *Journal of Pain and Symptom Management, 43*(4), 759–770.

Xavier, A., Gouveia, J. P., & Cunha, M. (2016). Non-suicidal self-injury in adolescence: The role of shame, self-criticism and rear of self-compassion. *Child and Youth Care Forum, 45*(4), 571–586.

Yadavaia, J. E., Hayes, S. C., & Vilardaga, R. (2014). Using acceptance and commitment therapy to increase self-compassion: A randomized controlled trial. *Journal of Contextual Behavioral Science, 3*(4), 248–257.

Yang, X., & Mak, W. W. (2016). The differential moderating roles of self-compassion and mindfulness in self-stigma and well-being among people living with mental illness or HIV. *Mindfulness, 8*(3), 595–602.

Yang, Y., Zhang, M., & Kou, Y. (2016). Self-compassion and life satisfaction: The mediating role of hope. *Personality and Individual Differences, 98,* 91–95.

Yarnell, L. M., & Neff, K. D. (2013). Self-compassion, interpersonal conflict resolutions, and well-being. *Self and Identity, 12*(2), 146–159.

Yarnell, L. M., Neff, K. D., Davidson, O. A., & Mullarkey, M. (2018). Gender differences in self-compassion: Examining the role of gender role orientation. *Mindfulness.* [Epub ahead of print]

Yarnell, L. M., Stafford, R. E., Neff, K. D., Reilly, E. D., Knox, M. C., & Mullarkey, M. (2015). Meta-analysis of gender differences in self-compassion. *Self and Identity, 14*(5), 499–520.

Yerkes, R. M., & Dodson, J. D. (1908). The relation of strength of stimulus to rapidity of habit-formation. *Journal of Comparative Neurology and Psychology, 18,* 459–482.

Young, J. E., Klosko, J. S., & Weishaar, M. E. (2003). *Schema therapy: A practitioner's guide.* New York: Guilford Press.

Young, S. (2017). Break through pain. Retrieved June 6, 2017, from *http://shinzen. org/Articles/artPain.htm.*

Zeller, M., Yuval, K., Nitzan-Assayag, Y., & Bernstein, A. (2015). Self-compassion in recovery following potentially traumatic stress: Longitudinal study of at-risk youth. *Journal of Abnormal Child Psychology, 43*(4), 645–653.

Zessin, U., Dickhauser, O., & Garbade, S. (2015). The relationship between self-compassion and well-being: A meta-analysis. *Applied Psychology: Health and Well-Being, 7*(3), 340–364.

Zhang, H., Carr, E. R., Garcia-Williams, A. G., Siegelman, A. E., Berke, D., Niles-Carnes, L. V., et al. (2018). Shame and depressive symptoms: Self-compassion and contingent self-worth as mediators? *Journal of Clinical Psychology in Medical Settings, 25*(4), 408–419.

Zhang, J. W., & Chen, S. (2016). Self-compassion promotes personal improvement from regret experiences via acceptance. *Personality and Social Psychology Bulletin, 42*(2), 244–258.

Zhang, J. W., Chen, S., Tomova, T. K., Bilgin, B., Chai, W. J., Ramis, T., et al. (2019). A compassionate self is a true self?: Self-compassion promotes subjective authenticity. *Personality and Social Psychology Bulletin.* [Epub ahead of print]

Index

Note. *t* following a page number indicates a table.

List of Audio Files

Track Number	Title	Run Time	Voice
1	Self-Compassion Break	5:20	Kristin Neff
2	Self-Compassion Break	12:21	Christopher Germer
3	Affectionate Breathing	21:28	Kristin Neff
4	Affectionate Breathing	18:24	Christopher Germer
5	Loving-Kindness for a Loved One	17:08	Kristin Neff
6	Loving-Kindness for a Loved One	14:47	Christopher Germer
7	Finding Loving-Kindness Phrases	23:02	Christopher Germer
8	Loving-Kindness for Ourselves	20:40	Christopher Germer
9	Compassionate Body Scan	23:55	Kristin Neff
10	Compassionate Body Scan	43:36	Christopher Germer
11	Giving and Receiving Compassion	20:48	Kristin Neff
12	Giving and Receiving Compassion	21:20	Christopher Germer
13	Working with Difficult Emotions	16:01	Kristin Neff
14	Working with Difficult Emotions	16:09	Christopher Germer
15	Compassionate Friend	18:09	Kristin Neff
16	Compassionate Friend	15:05	Christopher Germer
17	Compassion with Equanimity	14:38	Christopher Germer

The tracks are available to download or stream from The Guilford Press website at *www.guilford.com/germer4-materials*.

TERMS OF USE FOR DOWNLOADABLE AUDIO FILES